Vascular and Interventional Radiology

A Core Review

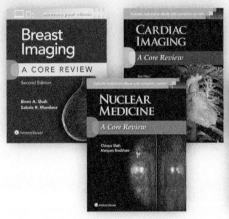
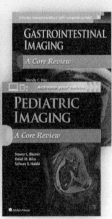
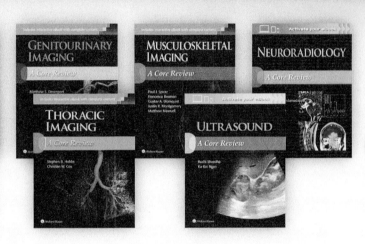
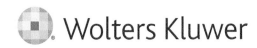

Vascular and Interventional Radiology

A Core Review

EDITORS

Brian Strife, MD

Assistant Professor
VCU Medical Center
Richmond, VA

Jeff Elbich, MD

Assistant Professor
VCU Medical Center
Richmond, VA

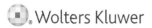 Wolters Kluwer

Philadelphia · Baltimore · New York · London
Buenos Aires · Hong Kong · Sydney · Tokyo

Acquisitions Editor: Sharon Zinner
Development Editor: Sean McGuire
Editorial Coordinator: Lindsay Ries
Marketing Manager: Dan Dressler
Production Project Manager: David Saltzberg
Design Coordinator: Stephen Druding
Manufacturing Coordinator: Beth Welsh
Prepress Vendor: TNQ Technologies

9 8 7 6 5 4

Printed in the United States of America

Library of Congress Cataloging-in-Publication Data

Names: Strife, Brian, editor. | Elbich, Jeff, editor.
Title: Vascular and interventional radiology : a core review / editors, Brian Strife, Jeff Elbich.
Other titles: Vascular and interventional radiology (Strife) | Core review series
Description: Philadelphia : Wolters Kluwer, [2020] | Series: Core review | Includes bibliographical references and index.
Identifiers: LCCN 2019004588 | ISBN 9781496384393 (paperback)
Subjects: | MESH: Radiography, Interventional-methods | Cardiovascular System-diagnostic imaging | Examination Question
Classification: LCC RC78 | NLM WN 18.2 | DDC 616.07/57-dc23
  LC record available at https://lccn.loc.gov/2019004588

shop.lww.com

SERIES FOREWORD

Vascular and Interventional Radiology: A Core Review covers the expanding field of vascular and interventional radiology in a manner that will serve as a useful guide for residents to test their knowledge and review of the material in a question style format that is similar to the core examination.

I believe Drs. Brian Strife and Jeff Elbich have succeeded in producing a book that exemplifies the philosophy and goals of the *Core Review Series*. They have done a magnificent job in covering essential facts and concepts of vascular and interventional radiology including radiology physics. The multiple-choice questions have been divided logically into chapters so as to make it easy for learners to work on particular topics as needed. Each question has a corresponding answer with an explanation of not only why a particular option is correct but also why the other options are incorrect. There are also references provided for each question for those who want to delve more deeply into a specific subject.

The intent of the *Core Review Series* is to provide the resident, fellow, or practicing physician a review of the important conceptual, factual, and practical aspects of a subject by providing approximately 300 multiple-choice questions, in a format similar to the core examination. The *Core Review Series* is not intended to be exhaustive but to provide material likely to be tested on the core examination and that would be required in clinical practice.

As Series Editor of the *Core Review Series*, it has been rewarding to not only be an author of one of the books in this series, but to be able to work with many talented individuals in the profession of radiology across the country who contributed to the series. This series represents countless hours of hard work and dedication by so many that it could not have come together without their participation. It has been very gratifying to see the growing popularity and positive feedback the authors of the *Core Review Series* have received from many reviews. The *Vascular and Interventional Radiology: A Core Review* is the last book in the *Core Review Series*. Exciting work is already underway to updating the earlier books in the *Core Review Series* with the addition of more questions.

Dr. Strife and Dr. Elbich are to be commended on doing an outstanding job. I believe *Vascular and Interventional Radiology: A Core Review* will serve as an excellent resource for residents during their board preparation and a valuable reference for fellows and practicing radiologists.

Biren A. Shah, MD, FACR
Section Chief, Breast Imaging
Site Director of Education
Detroit Medical Center
Clinical Associate Professor of Radiology
Wayne State University School of Medicine
Detroit, Michigan

PREFACE

Passing the Core and Certifying examinations requires comprehensive knowledge of Diagnostic and Interventional Radiology. The purpose of this book is to provide an in-depth case-based review of highly relevant topics in Vascular and Interventional Radiology that practitioners face every day, whether in the private or academic setting. Ten chapters cover the full gamut of pathology from common conditions such as abdominal aortic aneurysms to more rare entities such as vascular malformations. In addition, pre- and postprocedural management is addressed, which is becoming more important than ever in this clinical specialty.

All of the cases are based on actual patients cared for at the Virginia Commonwealth University Medical Center, which is a testament to their relevance in practice, but also to the breadth of knowledge that one must attain to practice safely and skillfully. Vascular and Interventional Radiology, being a technique-based field, enjoys significant variation among practitioners in the application of those techniques, whether among a group's members, different institutions, or different countries. We tried to base the answers and explanations on good science, quality research, or the agreed upon best practice to ensure the information provided is accurate and universal.

Jeff Elbich
Brian Strife

ACKNOWLEDGMENTS

To my adoring wife Randi and our future interventionalists Ben, Henley, and Cam.

Jeff Elbich

I would like to thank my wife Jen and daughter Stella for supporting me throughout this project. Teaching medical students, residents, and fellows about Vascular and Interventional Radiology is my passion. I am indebted to this field and its creators for having the best job anyone could ask for. Specifically, I would like to thank Dr. Barry Stein, Dr. Dan Leung, Dr. Jaime Tisnado, Dr. Malcolm Sydnor, Dr. Dan Komorowski, Dr. Will Fox, and Dr. Shep Morano for exposing me to the field, taking me under their collective wing, and cultivating my interests. Finally, I would like to thank VCU, where I have called home since beginning my medical training more than 16 years ago, for providing a wonderful center to practice and serve our community.

Brian Strife

CONTENTS

1 Fundamentals of Interventional Radiology

QUESTIONS

1. During an endovascular procedure, the access sheath is upsized to 10 Fr. What is the approximate diameter of the hole that the sheath will create in the vessel wall?

   A. 1 mm
   B. 4 mm
   C. 10 mm
   D. 12 mm

2. A noncompliant 8 mm angioplasty balloon is inflated to the nominal pressure, 6 atm. Subsequently, the balloon is deflated and reinflated to 12 atm. How has the hoop stress (T) of the balloon changed when comparing the first to the second inflation?

   A. T increases by 2-fold
   B. T decreases by 2-fold
   C. T increases by 8-fold
   D. T decreases by 4-fold

3. A patient is transferred emergently to the interventional radiology (IR) suite for hemorrhagic shock from extensive pelvic fractures. After the embolization, the patient remains hypotensive and the treating physician would like to increase the rate at which fluid is infused into the patient via the access sheath. Assuming the same pressure and fluid type are administered, by doubling the internal diameter of the access sheath, what change in flow will occur?

   A. Increase 2-fold
   B. Decrease 2-fold
   C. Increase 16-fold
   D. Decrease 16-fold

4. During a lower extremity arterial intervention, the patient is systemically heparinized with 8000 units intravenously. The case concludes 60 minutes later, and the physician is preparing to pull the access sheath and achieve hemostasis with manual pressure. To reverse the remaining active heparin, what dose of protamine sulfate should be administered?

   A. 1 mg
   B. 4 mg
   C. 40 mg
   D. 800 mg

5   For the vessel selected by the catheter, what is an appropriate rate of power injection to study this arterial distribution?

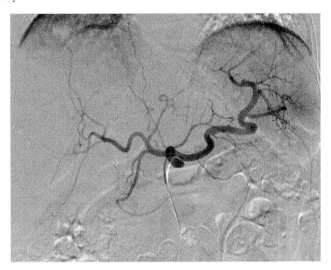

A. 0.5 mL/s
B. 1 mL/s
C. 5 mL/s
D. 15 mL/s

6   Which vessel is identified by the arrow?

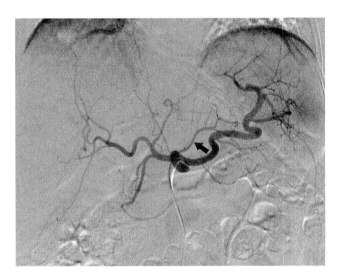

A. Left hepatic artery
B. Left gastric artery
C. Right gastric artery
D. Left inferior phrenic artery

7   As part of a declot procedure to open a thrombosed upper arm arteriovenous graft, the operator needs to anticoagulate the patient with intravenous heparin. What is an appropriate initial dose of heparin to administer? The patient weighs 65 kg.

A. 100 units
B. 500 units
C. 1000 units
D. 5000 units

A. Type 1
B. Type 2
C. Type 3
D. Type 4

22   Which part of this chest tube drainage system will help determine the presence of an air leak?

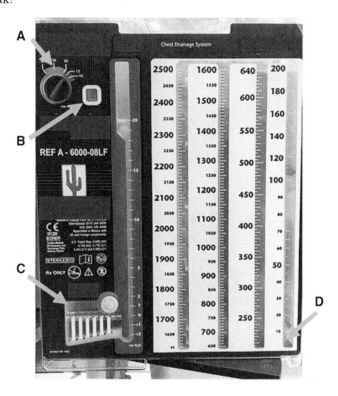

A. A
B. B
C. C
D. D

23   Which of the following is considered a contraindication for vertebroplasty/kyphoplasty?

A. Duration of pain < 1 week
B. Retropulsed bone fragment resulting in myelopathy
C. Treating two vertebral levels in the same setting
D. 50% vertebral body height loss

24   What is the indication for the procedure demonstrated on these images?

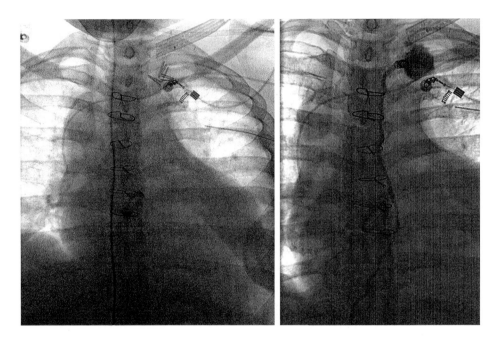

    A. Superior vena cava obstruction
    B. Massive hemoptysis
    C. High-output chylothorax
    D. Laceration to the internal thoracic artery

25   What modality is most often used to access the cisterna chyli for potential thoracic duct embolization?

    A. Fluoroscopy
    B. Ultrasound
    C. Magnetic resonance imaging (MRI)
    D. Computed tomography (CT)

26   A patient with normal body habitus requires left groin arterial access for a right lower extremity arterial intervention. What would be the best approach in this patient?

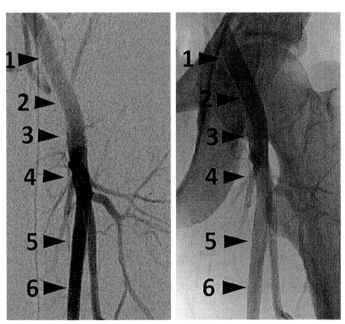

A. Skin entry 1; arteriotomy 2
B. Skin entry 6; arteriotomy 5
C. Skin entry 5; arteriotomy 4
D. Skin entry 3; arteriotomy 2

27 Which artery represents the right colic artery?

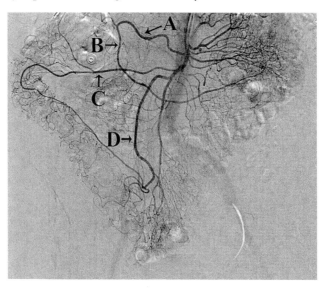

A. A
B. B
C. C
D. D

28 What is the course of the microcatheter in this angiogram demonstrating active extravasation (catheter tip marked with arrows)?

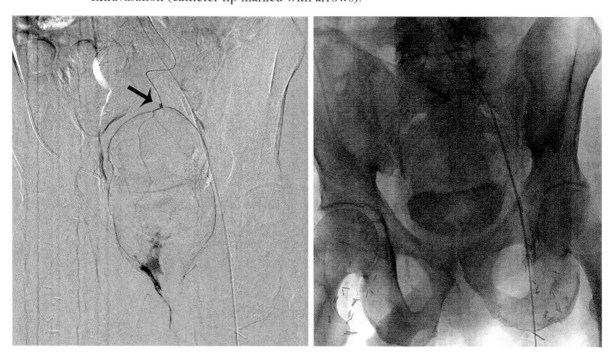

A. Inferior mesenteric artery → superior hemorrhoidal artery
B. Left internal iliac artery → cystic artery
C. Aortic bifurcation → median sacral artery
D. Left internal iliac artery → uterine artery

29   Where is the catheter positioned to create this image?

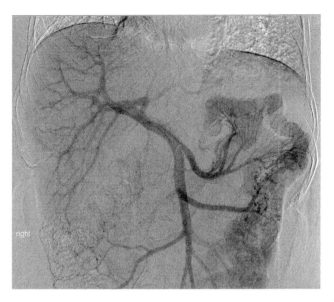

A. Superior mesenteric artery (SMA)
B. Superior mesenteric vein
C. Main portal vein
D. Inferior vena cava

30   After wire and catheter manipulation into a right hepatic artery branch, angiography shows spasm (arrow) at the catheter tip. Which of the following is the most appropriate next step?

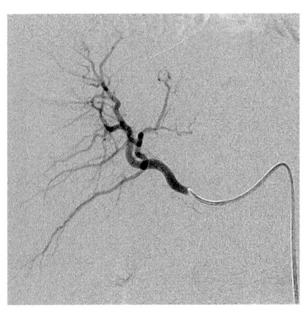
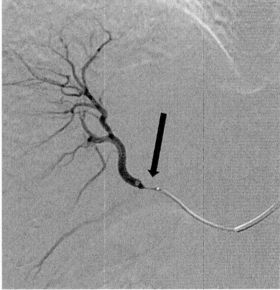

A. Fentanyl 50 mcg intra-arterial
B. Nitroglycerin 50 mcg intra-arterial
C. Nitrous oxide 50 mg inhaled
D. Vasopressin 0.2 units/min intravenous

31 During a transjugular intrahepatic portosystemic shunt (TIPS) procedure, the operator makes a needle throw from the right hepatic vein toward the right portal vein. Blood is then easily aspirated confirming intraluminal needle tip position. Based on these sequential digital subtraction angiography (DSA) images obtained by injecting the needle with contrast, which of the following "next steps" is correct?

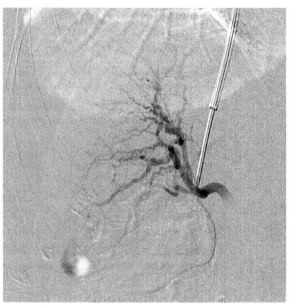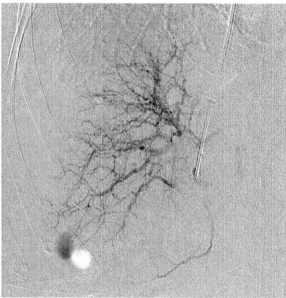

A. Right portal vein access is too central; make a more peripheral throw
B. Advance wire and then dilate the parenchymal tract for subsequent stent placement
C. Incorrect vessel accessed; reposition needle or make a new throw

32 Which of the following is considered a temporary embolic agent?

A. Amplatzer vascular plug
B. Gelatin foam slurry
C. Polyvinyl alcohol particles
D. N-butyl cyanoacrylate glue

33 Which of the following is true regarding pulmonary artery catheter angiography?

A. Power injection for right pulmonary artery is 5 cc/s for 10 cc total
B. Right common femoral artery access is preferred
C. Inject and image on inspiratory hold
D. Right bundle branch block is a contraindication

34 Which of the following conditions is most likely to benefit from systemic beta blocker therapy?

A. Infantile hemangioma
B. Venous malformation
C. Lymphatic malformation
D. Arteriovenous malformation (AVM)

ANSWERS AND EXPLANATIONS

1 **Answer B.**   Understanding device sizes is important basic knowledge for the interventional radiologist. Many devices have the diameter reported in "French" (Fr); 1 Fr = 0.33 mm, 3 Fr = 1 mm. In addition, sheaths are described by their inner diameter (ID), ie, what size device they can accept. The outer diameter (OD) of a sheath, which defines the size of the hole created, is roughly 1.5 to 2 Fr larger than the reported ID. In this example, a standard 10 Fr sheath produces a hole that is about 12 Fr; 12 Fr × 1 mm/3 Fr = 4 mm. Unlike sheaths, the reported diameter of a catheter is the OD.

Reference: Kaufman JA. Invasive vascular diagnosis. In: Mauro MA, Murphy KP, Thomson KR, et al. *Image-Guided Interventions*. Saunders; 2008:39-61.

2 **Answer A.**   The dilating force or hoop stress (T) of a balloon is directly proportional to the diameter (D) multiplied by the pressure (P). In this example, the balloon is first inflated to the nominal pressure, which is the pressure whereby the balloon reaches its stated diameter. Noncompliant balloons by definition do not dilate significantly beyond their stated diameter, even at pressures much greater than nominal. On the second inflation, the pressure doubles; however, you can assume that the balloon diameter stays the same. T = P × D; this is the law of Laplace.

Reference: Sarin S, Turba U, Angle F, et al. Balloon catheters. In: Mauro MA, Murphy KP, Thomson KR, et al. *Image-Guided Interventions*. Saunders; 2008:75-84.

3 **Answer C.**   This question relates to the properties that govern simple flow in a tube. This is Poiseuille's law. Of all the variables in the equation, the radius (r) has the greatest impact on the flow. Doubling the internal diameter of the sheath will obviously double its radius. If 1 is the initial diameter, $1^4 = 1$; when doubled, $2^4 = 16$.

$$Q = \frac{\Delta P \, \pi \, r^4}{8 \, \eta \, l}$$

Q, flow; *P*, pressure; *r*, radius; *η*, viscosity; *l*, tubing length.

Reference: Bakal C. Diagnostic catheters and guidewires. In: Mauro MA, Murphy KP, Thomson KR, et al. *Image-Guided Interventions*. Saunders; 2008:65-73.

4 **Answer C.**   Intravenous heparin is commonly used in endovascular procedures for periprocedural anticoagulation. Heparin binds and activates the enzyme antithrombin III, causing a conformational change and subsequent binding and inactivation of thrombin and factor Xa. The plasma half-life is between 60 and 90 minutes, sometimes longer, depending on the initial dose. Heparin is reversed by the drug protamine sulfate. For use in heparin reversal, 1 mg of protamine sulfate will inactivate approximately 100 units of active heparin. In the current case, after 1 hour, there is approximately 4000 to 5000 units of active heparin remaining in the patient. A 40 mg dose of protamine sulfate would be appropriate for reversal. Notably, protamine sulfate should be administered slowly to avoid hypotension and anaphylactoid-like reactions.

Reference: Cook BW. Anticoagulation management. *Semin Intervent Radiol*. 2010;27(4):360-367.

5 **Answer C.**   The vessel selected by the catheter is the celiac artery, which is a medium-sized vessel typically around 6 to 8 mm in diameter. From a size standpoint, it is analogous to a common femoral artery. When describing angiographic power injections, it is commonly stated "x for y," where x is the rate of injection in mL/s and y is total volume of the injection. "Five for fifteen" is an injection of 5 mL/s for a total volume of 15 mL. Naturally, the injection duration is 3 seconds.

Common injection rates that one should be familiar with include

Thoracic aorta 20 mL/s

Abdominal aorta 15 mL/s

Abdominal aortic bifurcation/iliac arteries 5 to 10 mL/s

Femoropopliteal arteries 4 to 6 mL/s

Celiac/SMA 4 to 6 mL/s

Main pulmonary artery 20 mL/s

Selective right or left pulmonary artery 10 mL/s

Inferior vena cava 10 to 20 mL/s

These injections are reasonable reference rates that should be adjusted based on the individual patient and goal of the angiographic study. Most injections using a power injector will be carried out for a duration of 2 to 3 seconds. It can be useful to carry out the injection for several additional seconds when trying to opacify a large vascular bed, to detect a small or peripheral bleed, or to study the venous out-flow of an organ. For instance, one can inject the celiac or splenic artery with 5 for 25, and obtain fairly good images of the portal venous system after the arterial and parenchymal phases have been imaged.

Reference: Farsad K, Keller FS, Kandarpa K. Vascular access and catheter-directed angiography. In: Kandarpa K, Machan L, Durham J. *Handbook of Interventional Radiologic Procedures*. Lippincott Williams & Wilkins; 2016:1-26.

6 **Answer B.**   The angiogram depicts classic celiac artery anatomy with three terminal branches: the left gastric artery (coursing leftward and cephalad), splenic artery (coursing leftward), and common hepatic artery (coursing rightward). Many variants of the celiac artery, SMA, and their respective branches exist and are of considerable significance to interventional radiologists and surgeons. A few common hepatic arterial variants are shown below.

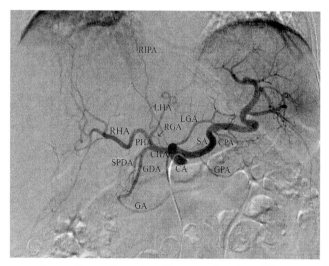

Figure 6-1   Image from celiac angiography with conventional arterial anatomy. CA, celiac artery; CHA, common hepatic artery; CPA, caudal pancreatic artery; GPA, greater pancreatic artery; GA, gastroepiploic artery; GDA, gastroduodenal artery; LGA, left gastric artery; LHA, left hepatic artery; PHA, proper hepatic artery; SPDA, superior pancreaticoduodenal artery; RGA, right gastric artery; RHA, right hepatic artery; RIPA, right inferior phrenic artery; SA, splenic artery.

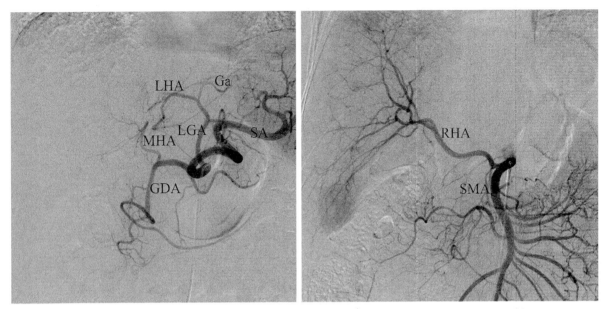

Figure 6-2   Images from celiac (left) and superior mesenteric artery (SMA) (right) angiography. There is variant anatomy with a replaced left hepatic artery off the left gastric artery and a replaced right hepatic artery off the proximal SMA. Note the presence of a middle hepatic artery (MHA) that perfuses segment 4 only of the left hepatic lobe. Ga, gastric branches.

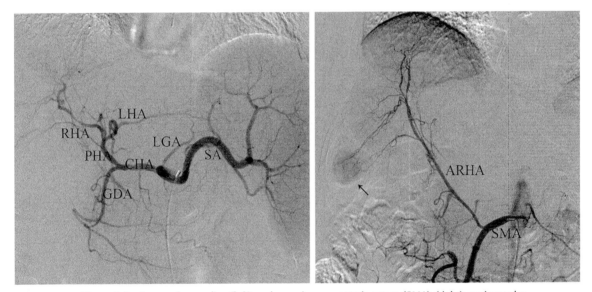

Figure 6-3   Images from celiac (left) and superior mesenteric artery (SMA) (right) angiography. There is variant anatomy with an accessory right hepatic artery (ARHA) off the proximal SMA. Note that it perfuses a hypervascular tumor (arrow) at the caudal tip of the right lobe that would have been missed if the variant went unrecognized. The accessory right or left hepatic artery often perfuses different segments of the lobe than its "normal" arterial companion.

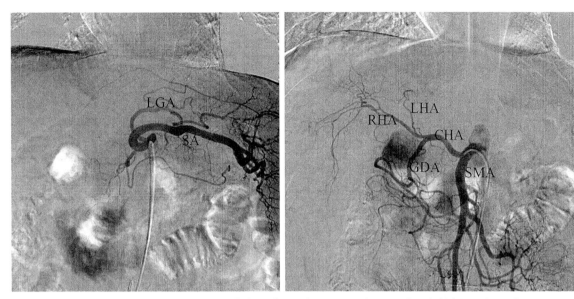

Figure 6-4 Images from celiac (left) and superior mesenteric artery (SMA) (right) angiography. There is variant anatomy with a completely replaced common hepatic artery off the proximal SMA.

References: Covey AM, Brody LA, Maluccio MA, Getrajdman GI, Brown KT. Variant hepatic arterial anatomy revisited: digital subtraction angiography performed in 600 patients. *Radiology*. 2002;224(2):542-547.

Uflacker R. *Atlas of Vascular Anatomy: An Angiographic Approach*. Lippincott Williams & Wilkins; 2007:457-654.

Wang Y, Cheng C, Wang L, Li R, Chen JH, Gong SG. Anatomical variations in the origins of the celiac axis and the superior mesenteric artery: MDCT angiographic findings and their probable embryological mechanisms. *Eur Radiol*. 2014;24(8):1777-1784.

White RD, Weir-mccall JR, Sullivan CM, et al. The celiac axis revisited: anatomic variants, pathologic features, and implications for modern endovascular management. *Radiographics*. 2015;35(3):879-898.

7 **Answer D.** For procedural anticoagulation in an adult patient, the initial dose of intravenous heparin can be given empirically or weight based. A reasonable empiric dose is 5000 units with additional 1000 units given after each additional hour for longer procedures. Weight-based dosing is typically 50 to 100 units/kg. Notably, there are no firm evidence-based guidelines for anticoagulation dosing or use during endovascular procedures, hence the range of options.

Reference: Cook BW. Anticoagulation management. *Semin Intervent Radiol*. 2010;27(4):360-367.

8 **Answer B.** An ACT is ideally established in the patient immediately before administering anticoagulation such as heparin. This level serves as the baseline or pre-anticoagulation measurement. If unavailable, one can assume the baseline ACT to be <150 seconds. During the procedure, an ACT of 1.5 to 2.5 times baseline is the goal for therapeutic anticoagulation. If no baseline is available, an ACT >200 seconds is often used to define therapeutic anticoagulation.

Reference: Cook BW. Anticoagulation management. *Semin Intervent Radiol*. 2010;27(4):360-367.

9 **Answer B.** The most commonly used wire calibers for interventional procedures are 0.038″, 0.035″, 0.018″, and 0.014″. Knowing which needles will accommodate the different sized wires helps with procedural planning and efficiency. Typical needles used for access are 21 gauge, which will accept a 0.018″ to 0.021″ wire, and 18 gauge, which will accept a 0.035″ to 0.038″ wire.

Reference: Bakal C. Diagnostic catheters and guidewires. In: Mauro MA, Murphy KP, Thomson KR, et al. *Image-Guided Interventions*. Saunders; 2008:65-73.

10   **Answer B.**   A meta-analysis from 2012 demonstrated that for patients undergoing large-volume paracentesis (>5 L), albumin repletion improved survival (odds ratio for death of 0.64). The mechanism of injury during large-volume paracentesis is not well understood, with several theories describing the complex interplay of third spacing, altered abdominal pressure and cardiac blood return as well as decreased peripheral vascular resistance. Given the meta-analysis data, the AASLD (American Association for the Study of Liver Diseases) recommends an infusion of albumin of 6 to 8 g/L of ascites removed for large-volume paracentesis (choice B).

Reference: Bernardi M, Carceni P, Navickis RJ, Wilkes MM. Albumin infusion in patients undergoing large-volume paracentesis: a meta-analysis of randomized trials. *Hepatology.* 2012;55:1172-1181.

AASLD Practice Guidelines: Management of Adult Patients With Ascites due to Cirrhosis: Update 2012.

11   **Answer A.**   Leaving a drain in a chronic, recurring sterile fluid collection carries a significant risk of infection, especially when the life expectancy of the patient is greater than 3 months. Studies have shown good catheter patency for tunneled drains in both cirrhotic ascites and hepatic hydrothorax; however, adoption of the practice has been thwarted by a realistic fear of infectious complications. Medical management, serial large-volume paracentesis/thoracentesis, portosystemic shunt creation, and peritoneovenous shunt (Denver shunt) creation are more favored options in this patient population. Patients with advanced cancer can develop malignant ascites, and when this occurs, the life expectancy is typically short (<3 mo). Placing an external drainage catheter (often tunneled) in these patients has been found to be relatively safe and acceptable for palliation.

References: Kathpalia P, Bhatia A, Robertazzi S, et al. Indwelling peritoneal catheters in patients with cirrhosis and refractory ascites. *Intern Med J.* 2015;45(10):1026-1031.

Orman ES, Lok AS. Outcomes of patients with chest tube insertion for hepatic hydrothorax. *Hepatol Int.* 2009;3(4):582-586.

Reinglas J, Amjadi K, Petrcich B, Momoli F, Shaw-stiffel T. The palliative management of refractory cirrhotic ascites using the PleurX (©) Catheter. *Can J Gastroenterol Hepatol.* 2016;2016:4680543.

12   **Answer C.**   The image depicts standing or stationary waves, an occasionally seen angiographic phenomenon in which the arterial wall has a beaded appearance similar to a crinkle-cut French fry. The exact mechanism is unknown, and it is generally considered a benign artifact with no clinical significance. Although fibromuscular dysplasia (discussed elsewhere in this book) can have a similar appearance, standing waves can involve long segments of arteries with a more symmetric and uniform beading pattern. Standing waves are also more often found in the arteries of the extremities.

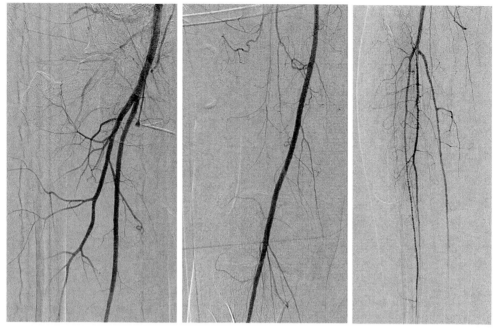

Figure 12-1   Companion case of lower extremity angiogram demonstrating standing waves involving multiple different arteries of the same limb.

References: Lehrer H. The physiology of angiographic arterial waves. *Radiology*. 1967;89(1):11-19.

Sharma AM, Gornik HL. Standing arterial waves is NOT fibromuscular dysplasia. *Circ Cardiovasc Interv*. 2012;5(1):e9-e11.

13   **Answer D.**   Of all the contrast agents listed, carbon dioxide gas has the lowest viscosity by far. It is approximately 400× less viscous than water-soluble contrast mediums (choices A through C). Lipiodol, the first iodinated contrast agent, is several times more viscous than water-soluble contrast. The ultralow viscosity of CO_2 gas translates to rapid diffusion, which can elucidate subtle findings such as small hemorrhages, endoleaks, or collateral vessels. It can also be used with a wedged catheter to retrograde opacify vascular structures across a capillary or sinusoidal bed (see Figure 31-1, wedged portography during TIPS planning).

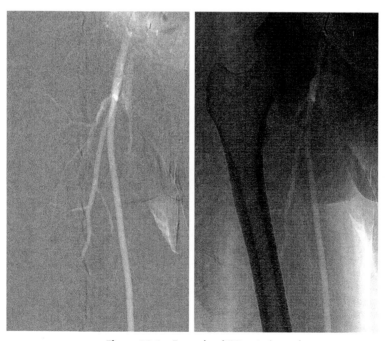

Figure 13-1   Example of CO_2 arteriography.

References: Cho KJ. Carbon dioxide angiography: scientific principles and practice. *Vasc Specialist Int*. 2015;31(3):67-80.

Nadolski GJ, Stavropoulos SW. Contrast alternatives for iodinated contrast allergy and renal dysfunction: options and limitations. *J Vasc Surg*. 2013;57(2):593-598.

14   Answer C.   This case is worth showing, as it is not seen everyday. The images demonstrate angiography of the right internal iliac artery distribution. The vessel of interest is actually the uterine artery, which is extending far cephalad and off the field of view. Normally, the uterine artery arises from the internal iliac artery anterior division, courses medially, and has a characteristic appearance with an initial descending segment, transverse segment, and finally an ascending segment terminating in the periuterine arterial plexus in the midpelvis (see Figure 14-1). In a gravid or postpartum uterus, the organ is enlarged and the arteries cover a much larger territory as seen in this case. The case example angiogram was performed in a woman with uncontrolled postpartum hemorrhage. This can be treated with catheter-directed particle or gelfoam embolization, often avoiding the morbidity of a hysterectomy.

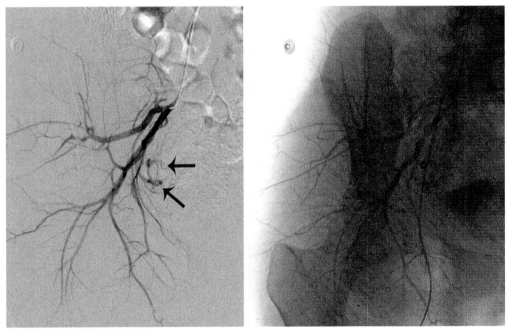

Figure 14-1   Angiography from the right internal iliac artery in a nulligravid woman demonstrating the uterine artery (arrows).

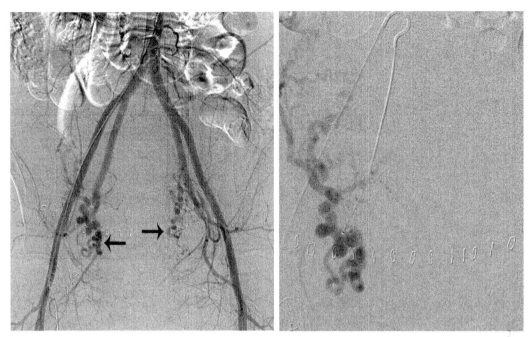

Figure 14-2 Companion case of postpartum hemorrhage in a 34-year-old female. digital subtraction angiography (DSA) image from pelvic angiogram (left) demonstrates massive enlargement of the uterine arteries (arrows). The right uterine artery is selected with a microcatheter (right), and angiography highlights the abnormal course and caliber of the vessel. Bilateral uterine artery embolization is subsequently performed with cessation of bleeding.

References: Kirby JM, Kachura JR, Rajan DK, et al. Arterial embolization for primary postpartum hemorrhage. *J Vasc Interv Radiol*. 2009;20(8):1036-1045.

Newsome J, Martin JG, Bercu Z, Shah J, Shekhani H, Peters G. Postpartum hemorrhage. *Tech Vasc Interv Radiol*. 2017;20(4):266-273.

15   **Answer A.**   Presented are sequential DSA images of the inferior mesenteric artery and its branches. In the arterial phase, there is a "ghost" of something in the region of the left colon. Over the next 2 images, the ghost separates into a white oval and a more cranial dark oval. This is an example of registration artifact that can occur with DSA technique. The unsubtracted image confirms that the finding is due to retained barium in the colon (see Figure 15-1) and not active bleeding with extravasated contrast. DSA technique begins with a preinjection mask image, which is produced by subtracting out all preexisting densities (such as bone, bowel, retained contrast) resulting in an initial homogeneous light gray image. From this point forward, only changes in attenuation will be shown as they occur over time. With arteriography, crystal clear images of the injected vessels can be produced without the background noise of nonvascular structures. In real life, however, some degree of artifact is unavoidable (from bowel motility, beating heart) even if the patient does a good job of holding their breath. More than just academic knowledge, registration artifact can result in some truly confusing images and false positives, especially when looking for subtle bleeds in the gastrointestinal (GI) tract. To avoid this error, the unsubtracted images should be reviewed to appreciate preexisting densities.

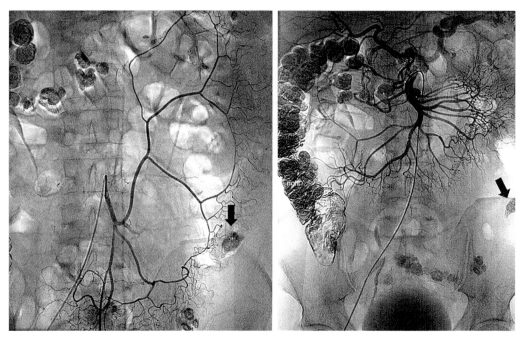

Figure 15-1 Unsubtracted images from inferior mesenteric artery (IMA) (left) and superior mesenteric artery (SMA) (right) angiography show the retained barium (arrows) in the left colon producing the registration artifact seen in the case example.

Reference: Pooley RA, Mckinney JM, Miller DA. The AAPM/RSNA physics tutorial for residents: digital fluoroscopy. *Radiographics*. 2001;21(2):521-534.

16   **Answer C.**   The images show an embolic protection device. The device is essentially a working wire with a fine mesh metal filter basket at its terminus. The operator can perform interventions over the wire and then remove the wire and filter at the conclusion of the intervention. The filter is designed to catch debris, whether clot or atheroma, that can embolize during arterial interventions. The most common locations to use such a device are the carotid and lower extremity arteries, as embolized plaque or clot in these territories can cause significant end organ damage.

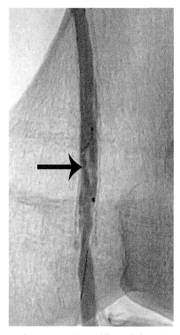

Figure 16-1 Magnified image demonstrating a filling defect (arrow) within the filter of the embolic protection device following balloon angioplasty of the superficial femoral artery. The embolized plaque was subsequently removed by withdrawing the filter into a larger catheter.

Reference: Metzger DC. Embolic protection in carotid artery stenting: new options. *Tech Vasc Interv Radiol.* 2011;14(2):86-94.

17   Answer B.   The best strategy for this patient will allow safe and timely exchange of the damaged nephrostomy catheter. The two safety components to the procedure are avoiding a reaction to iodinated contrast agents and ensuring accurate positioning of the new tube. In general, when a patient reports an anaphylactoid reaction to iodinated contrast, we avoid using it entirely unless there is truly no alternative. Premedication with steroids and histamine blockers can reduce the severity of contrast reactions but will not prevent a life-threatening anaphylactoid reaction. Interestingly, both vascular and nonvascular (GI, urinary collecting system) contrast administration can result in an adverse reaction. Alternative agents should be entertained, with gadolinium and air/gas being the obvious choices. Gadolinium attenuates X-rays, giving a similar appearance to traditional iodinated agents during fluoroscopic procedures. A nephrostomy catheter exchange can easily be performed with this agent. Gentle injection of CO_2 gas or room air could also be used as a negative contrast agent.

Reference: Davis PL. Anaphylactoid reactions to the nonvascular administration of water-soluble iodinated contrast media. *AJR Am J Roentgenol.* 2015;204(6):1140-1145.

18   Answer B.   Intravenous sedation in the IR suite most often consists of giving an opiate for pain relief as well as a benzodiazepine for anxiolysis. If the goal is moderate sedation, the dosing should be such that the patient will protect their airway without intervention, will maintain adequate ventilation, and will respond purposefully to physical and verbal stimuli. Fentanyl, a short-acting opiate, is typically given in intravenous bolus doses of 25 to 100 mcg. Midazolam, a short-acting benzodiazepine, is typically given in intravenous bolus doses of 0.5 to 2 mg. Both have a fairly rapid onset of action and work well for procedures lasting 30 to 60 minutes. Although these are good starting doses to know, each patient's medication needs will be different depending on multiple factors including underlying comorbidities, chronic pain medication use, and procedure type among others.

Reference: Johnson S. Sedation and analgesia in the performance of interventional procedures. *Semin Intervent Radiol.* 2010;27(4):368-373.

19   Answer A.   High-quality angiographic evaluation of the vasculature relies on comprehensive knowledge of anatomy and how different fluoroscopic projections will depict the anatomy. Evaluation of the aortic arch and its branch vessels is best accomplished with certain projections. Practically, these projections are termed for the position of the image intensifier/detector, but classic radiologic nomenclature uses the position of the patient in relation to the radiation source. The best projection for evaluation of the thoracic aortic arch is a steep LAO (patient is RPO to the source). On the RAO and AP comparison images below, note the difficulty in distinguishing the great vessel origins. While not a great projection for the great vessel origins, RAO splays out the brachiocephalic bifurcation nicely. A few additional projections to know include (1) using the contralateral oblique to evaluate the common iliac artery bifurcation and (2) using the ipsilateral oblique to evaluate the common femoral artery bifurcation.

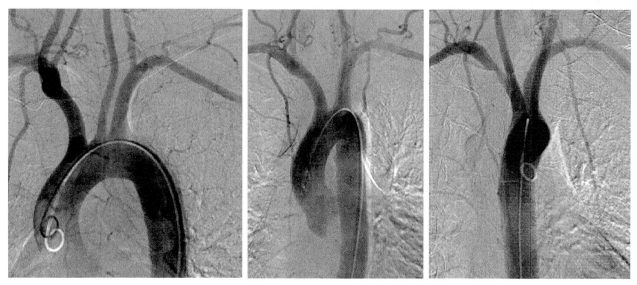

Figure 19-1   Thoracic aortography in the left anterior oblique (LAO) (left), anteroposterior (AP) (middle), and right anterior oblique (RAO) (right) projections.

Reference: Heng R, Soon KH, Ang SG, et al. Vascular anatomy of the thorax, including the heart. In: Mauro MA, Murphy KP, Thomson KR, et al. *Image-Guided Interventions.* Saunders; 2008:351-364.

20   **Answer D.**   The typical left aortic arch with 3 great vessel origins occurs 70% to 80% of the time. The first artery is the brachiocephalic trunk, followed by the left common carotid artery, and finally the left subclavian artery. There are several variations in the populace. The most common variation is a common trunk of the brachiocephalic and left common carotid artery (see Figure 20-1), occurring 21% to 27% of the time.

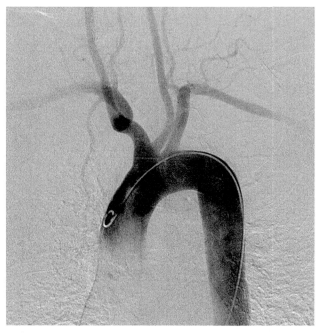

Figure 20-1   Left anterior oblique (LAO) thoracic aortography with a common trunk of the brachiocephalic and left common carotid artery.

In the case example, there are 2 arch variations present. First, there is a common origin of the right common carotid and left common carotid artery. There is also an aberrant right subclavian artery arising distal to the left subclavian artery (see Figure 20-2, single white arrowhead). The aberrant right subclavian artery is present in 0.5% to 2% of the population and is an important variant to recognize, as it is associated with congenital vascular anomalies including patent ductus arteriosus, aortic coarctation, ventricular septal defect, and carotid/vertebral anomalies. Because of its typically retroesophageal course, it can cause esophageal compression, and when symptomatic, the condition is known as "dysphagia lusoria." Also worth knowing is that the vessel origin can become aneurysmal, termed a Kommerell diverticulum (see Figure 20-3).

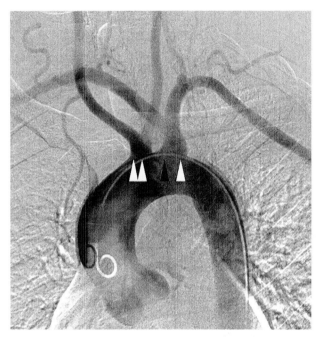

Figure 20-2   Left anterior oblique (LAO) thoracic aortography with common trunk of the right and left common carotid arteries (double white arrowhead), followed by the left subclavian artery in normal position (black arrowhead), and finally the aberrant right subclavian artery (single white arrowhead).

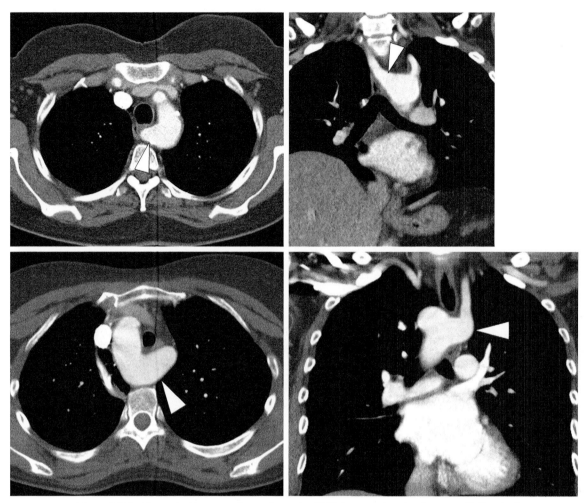

Figure 20-3   Computed tomography angiography (CTA) images showing Kommerell diverticulum (arrowheads) at the origin of an aberrant subclavian artery. On the top, the patient has a left arch with an aberrant right subclavian artery. On the bottom, the patient has a right arch with an aberrant left subclavian artery. Although asymptomatic in most patients, a Kommerell diverticulum has been associated with dissection and rupture.

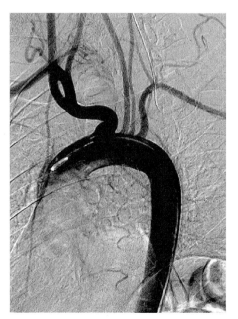

Figure 20-4   Left anterior oblique (LAO) thoracic aortography depicting another variation worth knowing: the "4-vessel arch" where the left vertebral artery arises directly from the arch proximal to the left subclavian artery.

References: Hanneman K, Newman B, Chan F. Congenital variants and anomalies of the aortic arch. *Radiographics*. 2017;37(1):32-51.

Heng R, Soon KH, Ang SG, et al. Vascular anatomy of the thorax, including the heart. In: Mauro MA, Murphy KP, Thomson KR, et al. *Image-Guided Interventions*. Saunders; 2008:351-364.

21　Answer C. Even with standard branch anatomy, not all aortic arches are equal. Increasing age and longstanding hypertension can produce elongation or unfolding of the arch, often with increased steepness. These changes in arch geometry directly affect the operator's ability to perform selective catheterizations and interventions, particularly from a groin approach. There are a few different methods that classify the arch as type 1, 2, or 3, with type 3 providing the greatest degree of difficulty. The type can be defined by measuring the distance (D) between the brachiocephalic artery origin to the cephalad margin of the arch. The left common carotid artery or the brachiocephalic trunk diameter is used as a reference unit distance. When D < 1 reference vessel diameter, it is a type 1. When D is between 1 and 2 reference vessel diameters, it is a type 2. When D is >2 reference vessel diameters, it is a type 3.

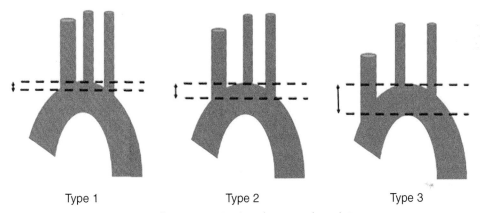

Type 1　　　　Type 2　　　　Type 3

Figure 21-1　Aortic arch types 1 through 3.

References: Madhwal S, Rajagopal V, Bhatt DL, Bajzer CT, Whitlow P, Kapadia SR. Predictors of difficult carotid stenting as determined by aortic arch angiography. *J Invasive Cardiol*. 2008;20(5):200-204.

Uflacker R. *Thoracic aorta and arteries of the trunk*. In: *Atlas of Vascular Anatomy: An Angiographic Approach*. Lippincott Williams & Wilkins; 2007:133-193.

22　Answer C. The chest tube output (from the patient) drains into the collection chamber labeled D. As fluid fills the chamber, it falls dependently allowing output quantification. The collection chamber also communicates with the water seal section labeled C. The connection between C and D exists at the cephalad aspect of the device; therefore fluid will fall dependently, but gas can transfer into and through the water seal. If there is a continued flow of gas into the system (air leak), it will suction through the blue water chamber creating bubbles. Examining the water seal during exhalation or a cough helps detect an ongoing air leak. When present, it indicates an ongoing source of air, such as a leak in the tubing or from inside the patient, such as due to a pneumothorax or bronchopleural fistula.

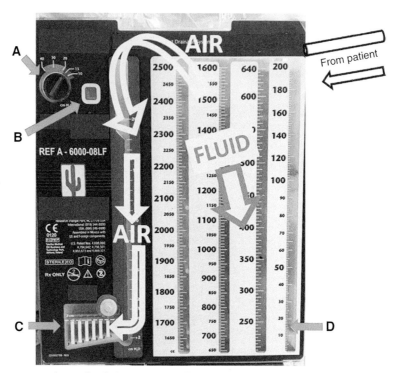

Figure 22-1 Chest tube drainage system. The output tube connects to the upper right. Fluid fills the collection chambers (D). Air leak (if present) escapes through communications at the top and can be detected in the water seal section (C). Letter A delineates the suction strength in centimeters of H$_2$O. Letter B points to an indicator as to whether suction is on or off.

Reference: Cerfolio RJ, Bryant AS, Singh S, Bass CS, Bartolucci AA. The management of chest tubes in patients with a pneumothorax and an air leak after pulmonary resection. *Chest.* 2005;128(2):816-820.

23   **Answer B.** Vertebral augmentation includes both vertebroplasty and kyphoplasty procedures. Vertebroplasty is percutaneous injection of cement (polymethyl methacrylate) into the vertebral body. Kyphoplasty includes adjunctive balloon inflation within the vertebral body with the intention of creating a cavity for additional cement injection, and possibly restoring vertebral body height. Both techniques are effective. The typical indication is a symptomatic compression fracture(s) from underlying osteoporosis or neoplasm. As discussed elsewhere, preprocedure imaging evaluation is critical (whether MRI, nuclear scan, or CT) to evaluate the proposed level of treatment as well as other conditions, which may be causing the patient's pain. The goal of the procedure is pain relief, which will quickly improve the patient's functional status and avoid the morbidity associated with prolonged immobility and chronic pain medication usage. Therefore, treating with <1 week of pain is acceptable and arguably preferable. Regarding technique, access into the vertebral body is often a trans- or parapedicular and treating more than one level at a time is not unusual. Some have suggested a limit on the number of levels treated in a single setting as marrow displacement during the procedure can result in fat emboli syndrome. If there is bony retropulsion from the fracture, the addition of cement to the vertebral body may further displace the fragment posteriorly and worsen the spinal canal compromise. If the retropulsion is so severe that it is causing myelopathy, vertebral augmentation should be avoided (choice B correct).

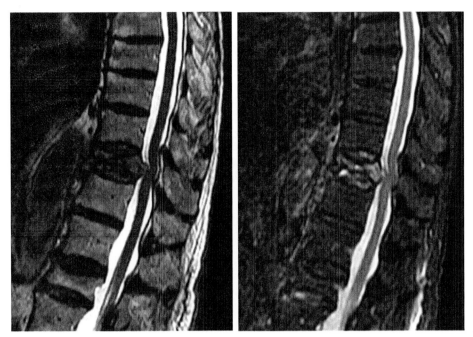

Figure 23-1   Sagittal T2 (left) and STIR (short-TI inversion recovery) (right) magnetic resonance (MR) images in a patient with an acute compression fracture of T10. There is significant height loss, high signal intensity within the vertebral body, and bony retropulsion causing canal compromise. There is corresponding high signal in the spinal cord. The patient was symptomatic with lower extremity weakness. Vertebral augmentation was not offered to the patient.

References: Baerlocher MO, Saad WE, Dariushnia S, et al. Quality improvement guidelines for percutaneous vertebroplasty. *J Vasc Interv Radiol*. 2014;25(2):165-170.

Nussbaum DA, Gailloud P, Murphy K. A review of complications associated with vertebroplasty and kyphoplasty as reported to the Food and Drug Administration medical device related website. *J Vasc Interv Radiol*. 2004;15(11):1185-1192.

24   Answer C.   The image on the left demonstrates recent surgery in the left hemithorax with clips overlying the left clavicle, a left chest tube, and a left neck drain. The image on the right demonstrates a new contrast-filled tubular structure extending from the abdomen just right of midline, which ascends in the thorax just left of midline. At the most superior extent, there is a coil pack and an adjacent pool of extravasated contrast. While the caliber and location of this structure could be confused for an internal mammary artery, the path does not quite fit as it crosses midline and has no visible branches. The images are from a lymphangiogram with thoracic duct embolization using coils and an nBCA glue:lipiodol mixture. The thoracic duct normally arises from the cisterna chyli at the thoracolumbar junction, just right of midline, ascends in the thorax just left of midline, and empties into left internal jugular vein as it joins the subclavian vein. The most common setting for this procedure is traumatic or iatrogenic thoracic duct injury with resultant chylothorax. Initial conservative management for chyle leak includes low-fat diet or total parenteral nutrition, octreotide infusion, and tube drainage of the leak. If the leak is of high output or refractory to conservative measures, traditionally surgical ligation of the thoracic duct was performed. More recently, percutaneous transcatheter embolization of the thoracic duct (and other chyle leaks) has gained popularity because of its reasonable clinical success, low morbidity, and minimal recovery time.

References: Itkin M, Chen EH. Thoracic duct embolization. *Semin Intervent Radiol*. 2011;28(2):261-266.

Itkin M, Kucharczuk JC, Kwak A, Trerotola SO, Kaiser LR. Nonoperative thoracic duct embolization for traumatic thoracic duct leak: experience in 109 patients. *J Thorac Cardiovasc Surg*. 2010;139(3):584-589.

25   **Answer A.**   Although the cisterna chyli can often be seen with transabdominal ultrasound, CT, and MRI, fluoroscopy is used most commonly for image-guided needle access. The procedure begins with lymphangiography. Traditionally, this was performed with a dorsal foot cut down onto delicate pedal lymphatics. Contemporary practice largely uses ultrasound-guided percutaneous access to the inguinal lymph nodes, with direct injection of lipiodol into the node. The lipiodol is infused slowly with gradual opacification of the iliolumbar lymphatics, which coalesce into the cisterna chyli near the thoracolumbar junction (see Figure 25-1). In adults, we typically inject 5 cc of lipiodol per side, followed by a 5 cc saline flush. Once a dominant lumbar lymphatic channel, or better yet the cisterna chyli, becomes opacified, a 21- or 22-gauge needle is then advanced from a right of mid-line subxiphoid approach into the target (see Figure 25-2). After careful wire manipulation, a microcatheter is advanced into the thoracic duct and direct ductography is performed with either additional lipiodol or water-soluble contrast. Subsequent embolization is then performed if indicated. In some cases, the operator may not be able to catheterize the thoracic duct. Lipiodol lymphangiography alone may seal the leak in many of these cases. If not, thoracic duct needle disruption can be performed. Other techniques for thoracic duct access include a transvenous retrograde catheterization of the duct as it empties into the venous system and direct ultrasound-guided access into the duct in the lower cervical region.

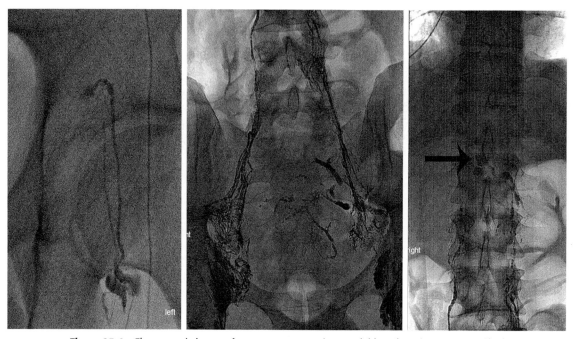

Figure 25-1   Fluoroscopic images from percutaneous intranodal lymphangiogram. Magnified image in the left groin (left) shows a 25 g needle infusing lipiodol into a lymph node with drainage into small lymphatic channels. After 5 cc of lipiodol is administered to each groin, there is excellent opacification of the iliolumbar lymphatics (middle) with the ducts coalescing into the cisterna chyli (arrow) near the thoracolumbar junction.

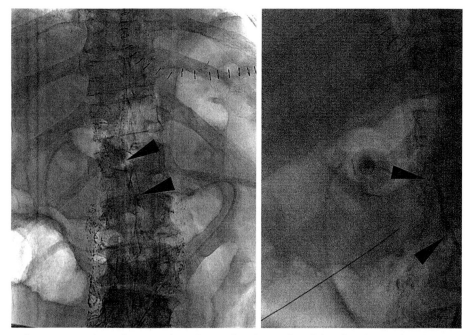

Figure 25-2 Companion case of a patient undergoing study with lymphangiogram for refractory chylothorax. A combination of anteroposterior (AP) (left) and steep oblique (right) fluoroscopy is used to guide a 22 g needle transabdominally into the cisterna chyli (arrowheads). A wire is then finessed cephalad, over which a catheter can be passed to perform additional ductography and intervention.

References: Binkert CA, Yucel EK, Davison BD, Sugarbaker DJ, Baum RA. Percutaneous treatment of high-output chylothorax with embolization or needle disruption technique. *J Vasc Interv Radiol.* 2005;16(9):1257-1262.

Guevara CJ, Rialon KL, Ramaswamy RS, Kim SK, Darcy MD. US-guided, direct puncture retrograde thoracic duct access, lymphangiography, and embolization: feasibility and efficacy. *J Vasc Interv Radiol.* 2016;27(12):1890-1896.

Itkin M, Kucharczuk JC, Kwak A, Trerotola SO, Kaiser LR. Nonoperative thoracic duct embolization for traumatic thoracic duct leak: experience in 109 patients. *J Thorac Cardiovasc Surg.* 2010;139(3):584-589.

Nadolski GJ, Itkin M. Feasibility of ultrasound-guided intranodal lymphangiogram for thoracic duct embolization. *J Vasc Interv Radiol.* 2012;23(5):613-616.

26   **Answer D.**   Arrowhead 1 points to the left external iliac artery. Arrowhead 2 points to the common femoral artery directly over the middle third of the left femoral head. Arrowhead 3 points to the common femoral artery at the inferior margin of the femoral head. Arrowhead 4 points to the common femoral bifurcation. Arrowheads 5 and 6 point to the proximal superficial femoral artery. For lower extremity arterial interventions, the access is commonly obtained in retrograde fashion on the contralateral side. The operator works up and over the aortic bifurcation, allowing himself or herself to be positioned alongside the lower extremities of the patient. Ideally, the arteriotomy is located directly over the midportion or middle third of the femoral head, in a healthy segment of artery. The femoral head serves as a backstop for manual compression if needed. Access more proximal can result in retroperitoneal hemorrhage with inadvertent puncture through the back wall of the artery. Manual compression may also be less successful in this proximal segment, as the artery dives deep into the pelvis. Access more distal can result in injury or access to branches such as the profunda femoris and superficial femoral arteries. For this patient, the skin puncture should occur at arrowhead 3 with needle entry into the artery at arrowhead 2. With obese patients, the skin puncture may begin closer to arrowhead 4 to accommodate for a longer subcutaneous tract to the artery.

Reference: Farsad K, Keller FS, Kandarpa K. Vascular access and catheter-directed angiography. In: Kandarpa K, Machan L, Durham J. *Handbook of Interventional Radiologic Procedures.* Lippincott Williams & Wilkins; 2016:1-26.

27 **Answer C.** In the case example, the diagnostic catheter has selected the SMA, with the catheter tip just beyond the pancreaticoduodenal branches. As with all arteriograms, it is helpful to picture the underlying organ anatomy (see Figure 27-1) to help identify the various branches. Artery branch A is the middle colic artery, which classically extends for a few centimeters and then branches in a "T" configuration giving rise to right and left (artery branch B) branches that extend out along the transverse colon. The right and left branches anastomose with the right colic and left colic arteries, respectively, forming the marginal artery of the colon. The artery marked C is the right colic artery and D is the ileocolic artery. The smaller artery branches coming off the SMA left of midline are termed jejunal and ileal branches.

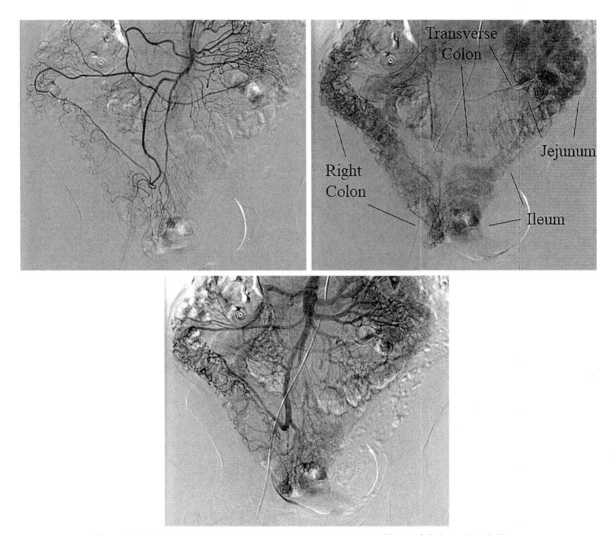

Figure 27-1 Superior mesenteric artery (SMA) angiography with arterial phase (top left), parenchymal phase (top right), and venous phase (bottom).

Reference: Uflacker R. *Atlas of Vascular Anatomy: An Angiographic Approach.* Lippincott Williams & Wilkins; 2007:457-654.

28 **Answer A.** The subtracted and native images from this arteriogram demonstrate an artery bifurcation at the tip of the catheter with right and left branches draping down over a pelvic structure with active extravasation and contrast pouring out to the bottom field of view. The native image confirms the bleeding organ is not the bladder (note the Foley catheter). The only arterial branch pattern that makes sense in this scenario is the superior hemorrhoidal artery (superior rectal), which is the terminal branch of the inferior mesenteric artery. The extravasation occurs into the rectal lumen and is spilling out the anus. The cystic and uterine arteries are paired with each side supplying approximately half of the respective organ, and not crossing midline. The median sacral artery is a reasonable choice for a midline artery but largely supplies the sacrum and coccyx.

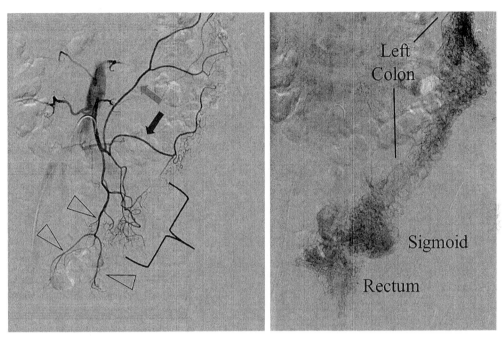

Figure 28-1   Digital subtraction angiography (DSA) from selective inferior mesenteric artery (IMA) catheterization demonstrating the main arterial branches. Light gray arrow, left colic artery ascending branch; dark gray arrow, left colic artery descending branch; bracket, sigmoid branches; open arrowheads, superior hemorrhoidal artery.

Reference: Uflacker R. *Atlas of Vascular Anatomy: An Angiographic Approach*. Lippincott Williams & Wilkins; 2007:457-654.

29   Answer A.   This is a DSA image of the portal venous system. Figure 29-1 delineates the anatomy present. To opacify the draining branches to the superior mesenteric vein and subsequently the main portal vein, a delayed image from a SMA injection was obtained. A prolonged SMA injection will fill the artery bed, perfuse the jejunum through the transverse colon, and ultimately fill the venous bed. Although direct (transhepatic, transsplenic, or transjugular intrahepatic) and indirect (wedged hepatic vein) portal venography can also be performed, it is not possible to opacify the entire venous bed against the direction of flow.

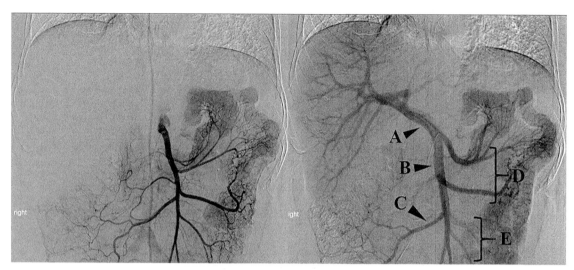

Figure 29-1   Left image shows a diagnostic catheter in the superior mesenteric artery (SMA) with arteriogram. A prolonged injection is performed to obtain the image on the right depicting the venous drainage of the SMA distribution. A, main portal vein; B, superior mesenteric vein; C, right colic vein; D, jejunal veins; E, ileal veins.

Reference: Uflacker R. *Atlas of Vascular Anatomy: An Angiographic Approach*. Lippincott Williams & Wilkins; 2007:457-654.

30   **Answer B.**   With catheter- or wire-induced vasospasm, the operator can inject nitroglycerin directly through the catheter for acute treatment. The onset of action is nearly immediate. Typical bolus doses range between 50 and 300 μg. It is uncommon to see any significant drop in blood pressure, although caution should be taken in patients actively taking phosphodiesterase 5 inhibitors such as sildenafil or tadalafil, as concomitant administration is considered contraindicated for 24 to 48 hours depending on the drug. Intra-arterial nitroglycerin can also be given preemptively, just before vessel interrogation or intervention. The plasma half-life is 1 to 4 minutes. Time is also a reasonable alternative, as spasm often subsides once the inciting or aggravating agent has been removed. Another common vasodilator used in practice is intra-arterial verapamil (calcium channel blocker, 2.5-5 mg bolus dose). The onset of action is a few minutes, with duration of action lasting up to 20 minutes. Papaverine and tolazoline are additional alternatives if available. Nitrous oxide, a vascular smooth muscle–relaxing agent, mainly affects the pulmonary vasculature when inhaled.

Vasopressin causes vasoconstriction and is used intravenously for the treatment of shock. Its current role in IR is mainly in the treatment of GI bleeding. With a catheter positioned in the culprit mesenteric artery, an infusion is begun at 0.2 units/min. After 20 minutes, repeat angiography is performed. If the bleeding has stopped, the infusion is continued for 12 to 24 hours, followed by a gradual dose reduction over 6 to 12 hours. If bleeding persists, the dose can be increased up to 0.4 units/min. This technique has largely been replaced by superselective embolization, but in cases of diffuse mucosal bleeding or inability to perform superselective catheterization, it remains a useful treatment strategy.

References: Cherian MP, Mehta P, Kalyanpur TM, Hedgire SS, Narsinghpura KS. Arterial interventions in gastrointestinal bleeding. *Semin Intervent Radiol*. 2009;26(3):184-196.

Oppenheimer J, Ray CE, Kondo KL. Miscellaneous pharmaceutical agents in interventional radiology. *Semin Intervent Radiol*. 2010;27(4):422-430.

31   **Answer C.**   There are multiple branching tubular structures in the liver, and sometimes distinguishing them from one another can be difficult. In the case example, the operator has accessed the right hepatic artery rather than the right portal vein. Typically, hepatic arteries are smaller in caliber and more tortuous as they branch peripherally. Named branches such as the cystic artery can often be identified (see Figure 31-1). Real time angiography demonstrates pulsatile forward flow, rather than a continuous slow flow. Conversely, the portal vessels tend to be straighter and larger, and other clues such as the presence of a periumbilical vein or varix may be seen (see Figure 31-1).

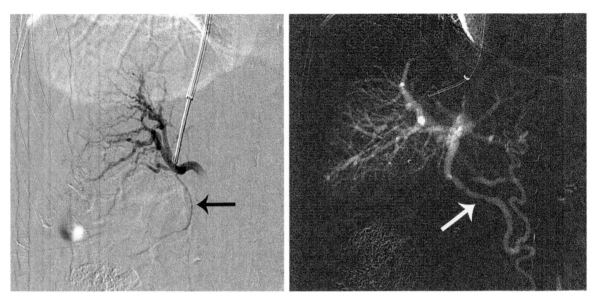

Figure 31-1   Left image from the case example demonstrates the operator has accessed the right hepatic artery. In addition to the overall appearance, the cystic artery is seen (black arrow) confirming arterial entry. Right image is a wedged CO_2 portogram obtained in the same patient depicting the portal venous system. Note the large periumbilical vein (white arrow), which came off the left portal vein.

In addition to the arteries and portal veins of the liver, the operator may access the hepatic veins or the biliary tree. The former is easy to identify, as contrast will flow centrally toward the right atrium in large straight veins and empty into the inferior vena cava. Cholangiography can initially look similar to hepatic arterial or portal venous angiograms; however, with time and additional injection of contrast, slow hepatofugal flow will progress toward the hilum and will not immediately wash out. Dependent biliary branches will fill first, with nondependent (left lobe) branches often filling later on. In the absence of obstruction, the contrast will eventually drain into the bowel.

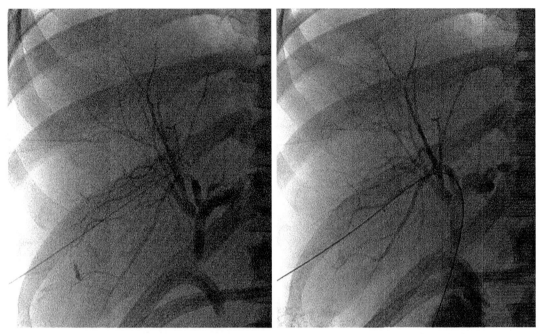

Figure 31-2 Percutaneous biliary access with cholangiogram demonstrating the typical appearance of the nondilated biliary tree. Note the branches are straight, similar to portal veins, but smaller in caliber with limited peripheral arborization. Contrast drains into the bowel. Also in this example is a common variant with the right posterior duct draining into the left main duct.

Reference: Ripamonti R, Ferral H, Alonzo M, Patel NH. Transjugular intrahepatic portosystemic shunt-related complications and practical solutions. *Semin Intervent Radiol.* 2006;23(2):165-176.

32 Answer B. Autologous clot was the first agent used for transcatheter embolization but was limited in application because of clot lysis over time. In contemporary practice, gelatin is the most common temporary agent used and comes in several forms (powder, foam block, beads). The duration of occlusion is typically days to weeks, and its most common application is embolization of traumatic hemorrhage. Numerous permanent embolic agents exist, and their application is wide ranging and dependent on the pathology being treated, location of embolization, risk of nontarget embolization, operator experience, and patient coagulation among others. A combination of agents can be used, most commonly in situations where both proximal and distal vascular occlusion is desired (think portal vein embolization with particles and coils) or to augment control over an embolic agent (think coils and glue in AVM embolization).

Embolic agents of IR

- Temporary
  - Autologous clot
    - Percutaneous biopsy tract
  - Gelatin
    - Traumatic hemorrhage
    - Percutaneous biopsy tract
  - Thrombin
    - Percutaneous injection of pseudoaneurysm
- Permanent
  - Metallic coils (pushable, detachable), vascular plugs (covered or uncovered)
    - Traumatic vessel injury, GI bleeding, aneurysm and pseudoaneurysm occlusion, arteriovenous fistula closure, pulmonary AVM embolization, small and large vessel occlusion, portal vein embolization
  - Particles

- Benign and malignant tumor embolization, bronchial and GI hemorrhage, portal vein embolization, partial splenic embolization
  - o Liquid (nBCA glue, Onyx)
    - Vascular malformations, thoracic duct embolization, portal vein embolization, small vessel hemorrhage, eg, GI/bronchial/inferior epigastric, partial splenic embolization, aneurysm endoleak embolization

References: Ray CE, Bauer JR. Embolization agents. In: Mauro MA, Murphy KP, Thomson KR, et al. *Image-Guided Interventions*. Saunders; 2008:131-139.

Vaidya S, Tozer KR, Chen J. An overview of embolic agents. *Semin Intervent Radiol.* 2008;25(3):204-215.

33 **Answer C.** Although catheter angiography has largely been replaced by computed tomography angiography (CTA) for the diagnosis of acute pulmonary embolism, it remains an important diagnostic and therapeutic technique that carries some unique risks and challenges. Venous access via the internal jugular or common femoral veins is preferred. To perform the catheterization, we use an angled pigtail catheter or flow-directed balloon catheter to quickly negotiate into the right ventricular (RV) outflow tract, thereby minimizing contact and irritation with the right atrium and ventricle. Before catheterization, a baseline electrocardiogram should be obtained to evaluate for an underlying heart block. The catheter or sheath when placed through right atrium, right ventricle, and outflow tract can induce a right bundle branch block. If the patient has an underlying left bundle branch block, complete heart block can ensue. If known, patients with a left bundle branch block undergoing a pulmonary artery catheterization should have immediate access to pacing equipment. In additional to right bundle branch block, traversing the right-sided heart often results in arrhythmias, and sustained ventricular tachycardia can occur necessitating treatment.

Once the catheter is maneuvered into the main pulmonary artery, the intravascular pressure is measured. Normal main pulmonary artery pressure (PAP) is roughly 25/10 mmHg with a mean around 15 mmHg. Pulmonary hypertension is defined as resting mean PAP >25 mmHg. To study the pulmonary artery distribution, power injection of the catheter is appropriate. Over the years, there has been some controversy regarding power injection in the setting of elevated pressures (RV end diastolic pressure >20 mmHg or systolic PAP >80 mmHg), as fatal complications have occurred. Modern experience with low-osmolar nonionic contrast agents indicates that power injection is safe; however, operators may choose to tailor their injection parameters depending on the clinical scenario and observed hemodynamics. The volume of blood in the pulmonary vasculature is massive requiring large-volume power injections to adequately study the distribution. Appropriate injections for the main pulmonary artery are 15 to 30 mL/s; right or left pulmonary artery 10 to 20 mL/s. If the patient is able, imaging should be performed on full inspiration to expand the lung, which will spread out and optimize visualization of the vessels and underlying pathology.

References: Mills SR, Jackson DC, Older RA, Heaston DK, Moore AV. The incidence, etiologies, and avoidance of complications of pulmonary angiography in a large series. *Radiology.* 1980;136(2):295-299.

Nicod P, Peterson K, Levine M, et al. Pulmonary angiography in severe chronic pulmonary hypertension. *Ann Intern Med.* 1987;107(4):565-568.

Nilsson T, Carlsson A, Mâre K. Pulmonary angiography: a safe procedure with modern contrast media and technique. *Eur Radiol.* 1998;8(1):86-89.

Smith TP, Lee VS, Hudson ER, et al. Prospective evaluation of pulmonary artery pressures during pulmonary angiography performed with low-osmolar nonionic contrast media. *J Vasc Interv Radiol.* 1996;7(2):207-212.

34   **Answer A.**   Hemangiomas are the most common vascular tumors and may present fully grown at birth (congenital type) or may appear after birth (infantile type). They can be superficial or deep and solitary or multifocal. The overwhelming majority (about 90%) will involute on their own over time and leave the patient with normal to mildly blemished skin. When hemangiomas cause complications, therapy is indicated. Therapies include resection and reconstruction, topical or locally directed treatments, and systemic treatments. For years, systemic treatment was dominated by corticosteroids; however, in the past decade, beta blocker therapy with propranolol has emerged as a promising treatment with significant regression occurring in the majority of patients treated.

On ultrasound, hemangiomas are usually well circumscribed with heterogeneous echogenicity and intense low-resistance perilesional and internal vascularity. On MRI, they are often well defined, iso- to hyperintense on T1/hyperintense on T2 relative to muscle, with high flow vascularity characterized by flow voids, early homogenous enhancement, and lack of early venous drainage.

Radiologists should be familiar with the modern classification of vascular anomalies, as described by the International Society for the Study of Vascular Anomalies (ISSVA), which can be accessed for free online. This classification scheme breaks down anomalies into two major groups, vascular tumors and vascular malformations, and provides a universal descriptive terminology that accurately reflects current understanding of vascular anomalies. A few entities are worth showing in greater detail (see Figures 34-1 to 34-4).

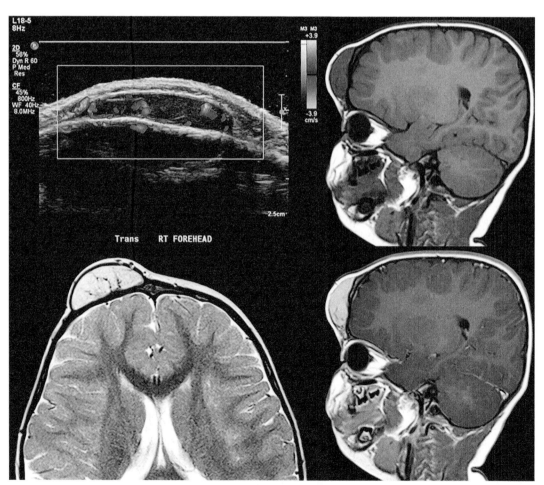

Figure 34-1   Infantile hemangioma. A 2-year-old with growing forehead mass. Ultrasound shows a circumscribed heterogeneously hypoechoic mass with internal vascularity. Magnetic resonance imaging (MRI) performed 6 months later shows enlargement of the mass which is T2 hyperintense with internal flow voids (bottom left), T1 isointense (top right), and diffusely enhancing with gadolinium (bottom right).

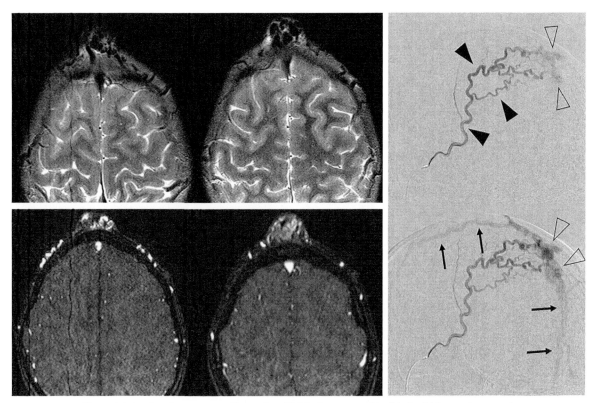

Figure 34-2 Arteriovenous malformation (AVM). A 13-year-old with throbbing scalp mass that demonstrates a palpable thrill on physical examination. Axial T2 MR images (top) show a superficial mass comprised entirely of flow voids. Axial time-of-flight (TOF) MR images (bottom) highlight the enlarged feeding arteries and draining veins in the surrounding soft tissue of the scalp. Digital subtraction angiography (DSA) images obtained after selecting out the superficial temporal artery demonstrate hypertrophied arterial feeders (solid arrowheads), the palpable mass (open arrowheads), and early filling of enlarged draining veins (arrows). AVMs are characterized by an abnormal connection(s) between an artery and vein without an intervening capillary bed.

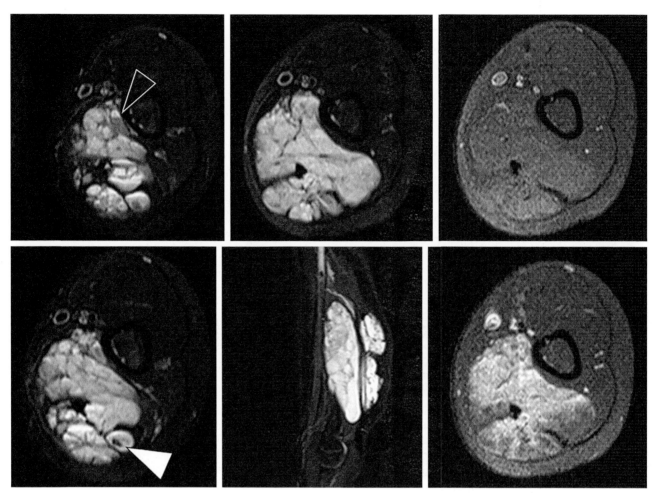

Figure 34-3 Venous malformation (VM). A 10-year-old with enlarging mass in the left upper arm. T2 FS MRI images show a high signal intensity mass with cystic spaces and thin septations centered in the posterior muscle compartment. There is a low signal intensity filling defect (white arrowhead) consistent with a phlebolith as well as a fluid-fluid level (open arrowhead). T1 FS pre (top right) and post (bottom right) contrast images show near homogenous enhancement of the mass. VMs typically display progressive intralesional enhancement over time.

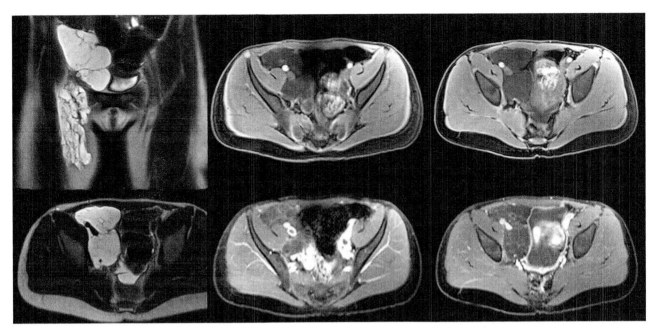

Figure 34-4   Lymphatic malformation (LM). A 7-year-old with a right groin mass evaluated with MRI. Coronal and axial T2 (left images) show high signal intensity mass with large cystic spaces and thin internal septations extending from the mid-thigh, crossing the inguinal ligament, and extending cephalad with intrapelvic component. Axial T1 FS GRE pre (top) and post (bottom) contrast images show peripheral enhancement and thin enhancing septations.

References: Jarrett DY, Ali M, Chaudry G. Imaging of vascular anomalies. *Dermatol Clin.* 2013;31(2):251-266.

Tekes A, Koshy J, Kalayci TO, et al. S.E. Mitchell Vascular Anomalies Flow Chart (SEMVAFC): a visual pathway combining clinical and imaging findings for classification of soft-tissue vascular anomalies. *Clin Radiol.* 2014;69(5):443-457.

2 Arterial Interventions

1. An 85-year-old male undergoes endovascular aortic repair (EVAR) for a 6 cm abdominal aortic aneurysm. The 6-month follow-up computed tomography angiography (CTA) with arterial (left) and delayed (right) phase images shows what complication?

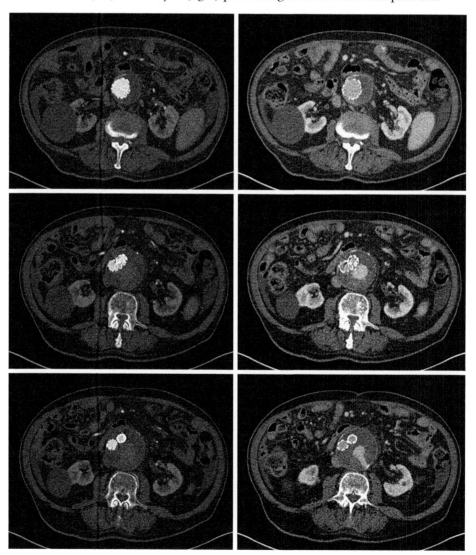

A. Vasculitis
B. Vasospasm
C. Thromboangiitis obliterans
D. Atheroemboli

11 A 78-year-old female presents with abdominal pain. Based on the CTA images below, what is the most likely diagnosis?

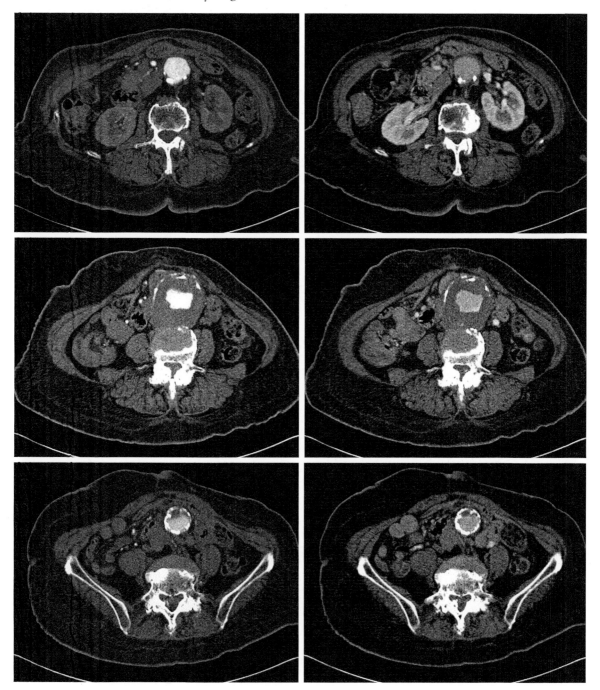

A. Retroperitoneal fibrosis
B. Infectious aortitis with abscess formation
C. Abdominal aortic injury with active extravasation
D. Abdominal aortic aneurysm with features of impending rupture

12   A 45-year-old female presents for embolization of an intrasplenic arterial pseudoaneurysm due to blunt trauma. The interventional radiology (IR) physician obtains the following angiographic images from the initial selective catheterization. Which is the correct interpretation?

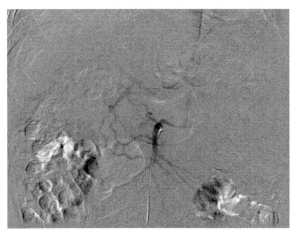 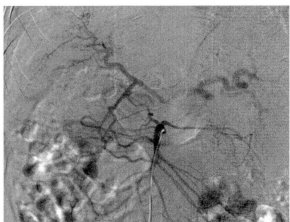

A. Celiac artery stenosis
B. SMA stenosis
C. Common origin of the celiac and SMA
D. Arc of Buhler

13   When evaluating a patient with suspected median arcuate ligament syndrome (MALS), which technique will help discern the etiology of the celiac artery stenosis?

A. Angiogram with Valsalva
B. Angiogram with carbon dioxide
C. Angiogram in lateral view with separate inspiration and expiration injections
D. Angiogram after eating

14   A 60-year-old male presents with bright red blood per rectum. He is hypotensive and placed on pressor support. A CTA is performed to evaluate the source, and active bleeding is identified in the rectum. Surgery and Gastroenterology services decline intervention. The patient is brought to IR for angiography and embolization.

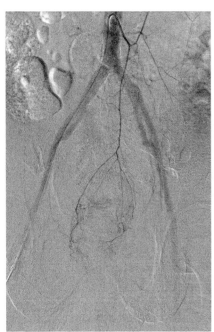 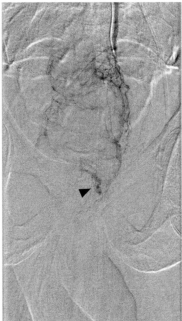 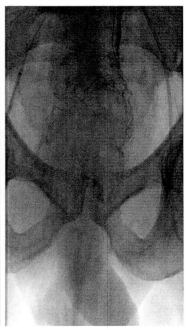

A branch of the superior rectal artery is selected with a microcatheter, and active bleeding (arrowhead) is identified and subsequently treated with Gelfoam slurry embolization. Despite a good technical result, the patient continues to have bright red blood per rectum and hypotension in the angiography suite. What should be done next?

    A. Transfer to the intensive care unit (ICU) as the bleeding will likely stop

    B. Refer to surgery for operative intervention

    C. Perform additional angiography to evaluate for a bleed at a different location in the bowel

    D. Perform additional angiography to evaluate for collateral flow to the rectal bleed

15 What is the most likely clinical presentation for this patient?

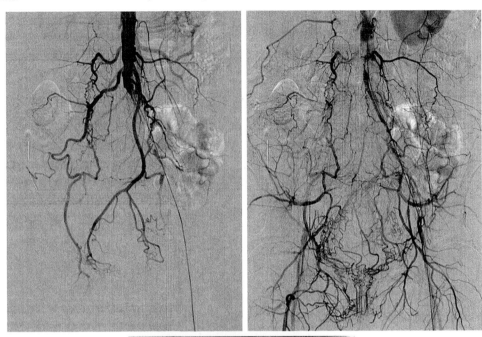

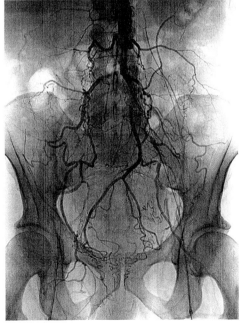

    A. Acute abdominal pain and bloody stools

    B. Chronic bilateral lower extremity swelling and varicose veins

    C. Progressive buttock claudication and impotence

    D. Abrupt-onset cold and painful lower extremities

16   What collateral arterial pathway is delineated by the arrowheads?

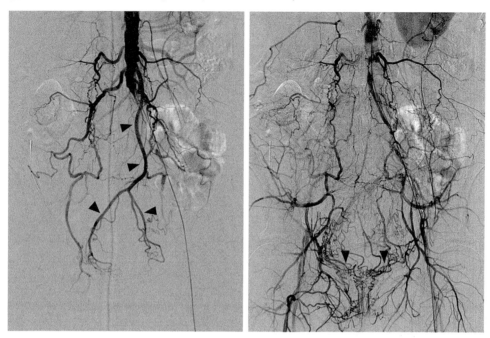

A. Inferior mesenteric artery (IMA) >> superior rectal artery >> middle and inferior rectal arteries >> internal iliac artery

B. Median sacral artery >> iliolumbar artery >> external iliac artery >> internal iliac artery

C. Lumbar artery >> deep circumflex iliac artery >> external iliac artery

D. SMA >> iliocolic artery >> sigmoidal artery >> internal iliac artery

17   After a diagnostic arteriogram, the common femoral arterial access is closed with manual pressure. Three days later, there is swelling in the right groin. Ultrasound (US) images below. Which of the following is a contraindication to percutaneous thrombin injection?

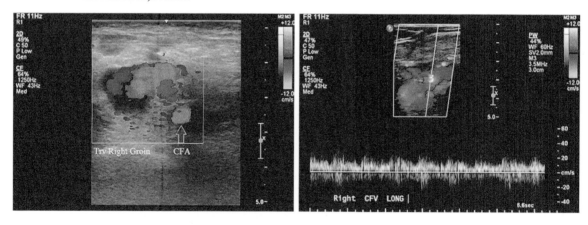

A. Pseudoaneurysm sac diameter <3 cm

B. Pseudoaneurysm with fistula to adjacent deep vein

C. Narrow pseudoaneurysm neck

D. Pseudoaneurysm arising from the common femoral artery

18   Which arrow denotes the recommended needle tip position for ultrasound-guided thrombin injection of a common femoral artery pseudoaneurysm?

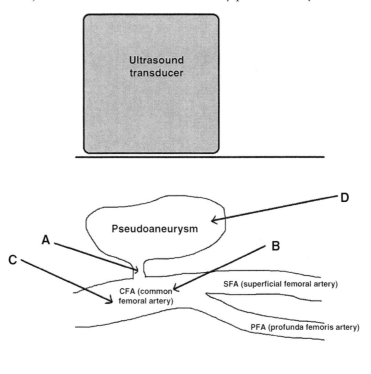

A. A
B. B
C. C
D. D

19   An otherwise healthy 25-year-old male undergoes placement of a stent graft to repair a traumatic pseudoaneurysm of the descending thoracic aorta. Which complication is the patient least at risk of developing?

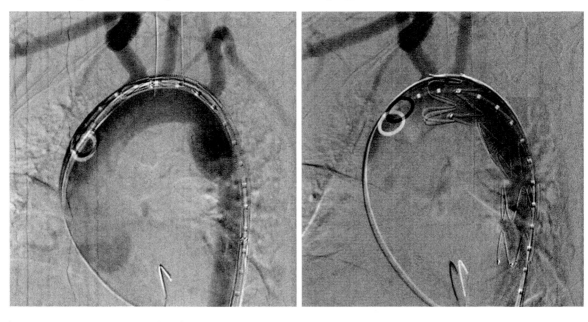

A. Myocardial ischemia
B. Cerebral ischemia
C. Left arm ischemia
D. Spinal cord ischemia

20   To further evaluate a young patient with left calf claudication, a bilateral lower extremity angiogram is performed with DSA images below obtained at the popliteal artery level in the neutral position (left image) and with plantar flexion with resistance (right image). What is the most likely pathology?

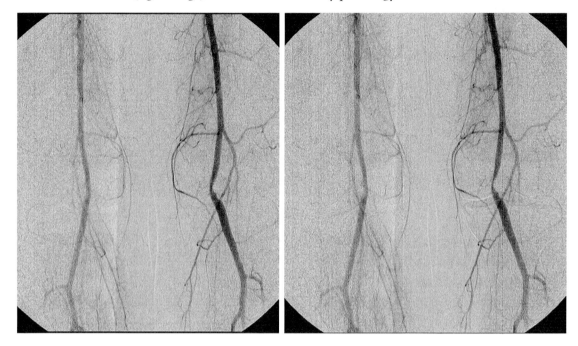

    A. Cystic adventitial disease
    B. Aneurysm with mural thrombus
    C. Arterial entrapment
    D. Atherosclerotic plaque

21   Following ejection from a motor vehicle, a middle-aged female is brought to the emergency room (ER) for blunt trauma evaluation. Chest and pelvic radiographs are quickly obtained, demonstrating multiple rib and complex pelvic fractures. The patient is hypotensive and transported directly to the interventional suite for angiography. Which is the correct interpretation of the pelvic angiogram?

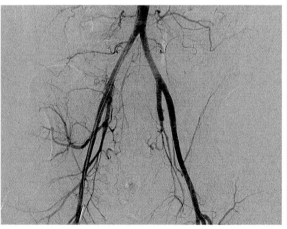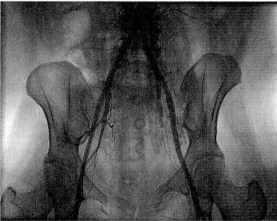

    A. No evidence of vascular injury, study complete
    B. No evidence of vascular injury, additional images needed
    C. Evidence of vascular injury, study complete
    D. Evidence of vascular injury, additional images needed

22   An elderly female with massive hemoptysis from the left lower lobe of the lung presents for bronchial angiography and embolization. Particle embolization from the demonstrated catheter position may result in nontarget embolization to which territory?

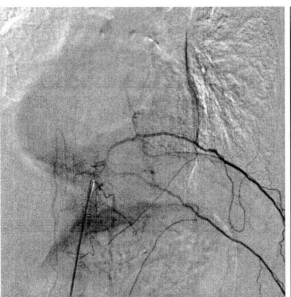 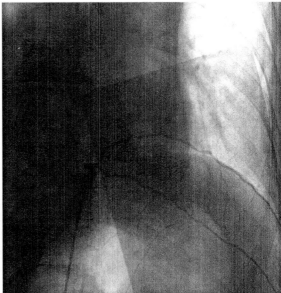

 A. Spinal cord
 B. Esophagus
 C. Stomach
 D. Diaphragm

23   A 37-year-old construction worker presents with numbness, tingling, and discoloration of the third digit in the right hand. Based on the angiographic images, what is the most likely diagnosis?

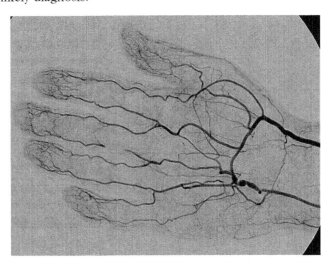

 A. Normal angiogram
 B. Vasculitis
 C. Posttraumatic aneurysm with distal embolus
 D. Raynaud disease

24   A lower extremity angiogram is performed to evaluate a patient with acute limb ischemia. An embolus is identified in the dorsalis pedis artery at the level of the ankle and successfully aspirated with restoration of flow to the foot (not shown). Pre- and postintervention images of the tibial runoff below show what complication from the procedure?

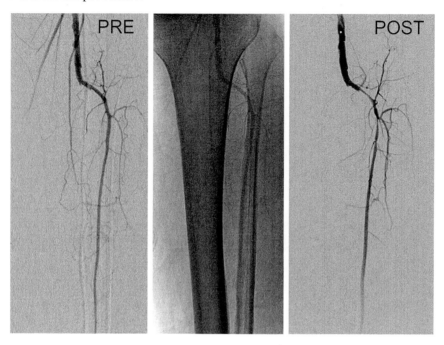

A. Spasm
B. Thrombosis
C. Rupture
D. Atherosclerosis

25   An elderly female undergoes seemingly uneventful renal angiography, angio-
     plasty, and stenting for renovascular hypertension due to left renal artery stenosis.
     Immediately following the procedure, the patient becomes hypotensive and tachy-
     cardic. The case images are quickly reviewed for any clue to the patient's change
     in status while contrast-enhanced computed tomography (CECT) is rapidly per-
     formed. Based on the images presented, what is the most likely diagnosis?

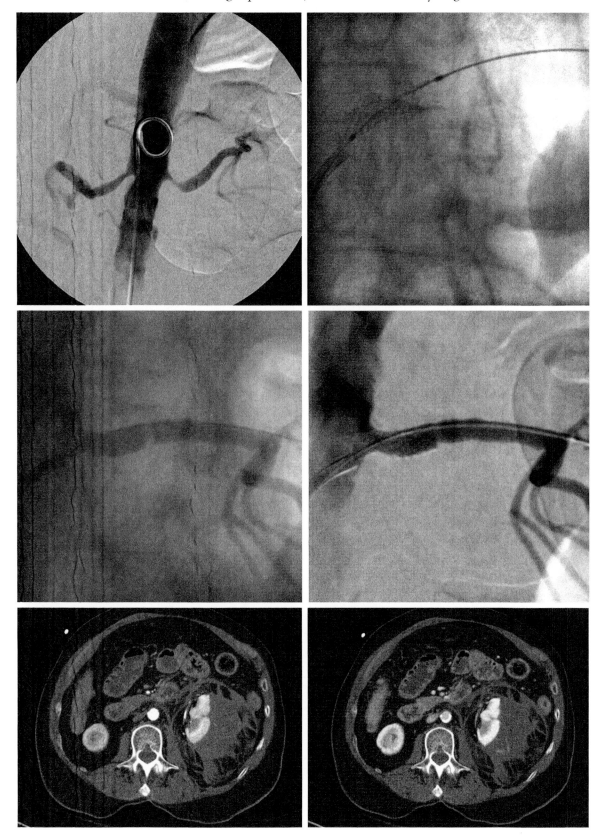

A. Main renal artery rupture
B. Guidewire perforation of the renal capsule
C. Expected post-procedure change following relief of left renal artery stenosis
D. Access site complication
E. Large left renal infarction

26 With respect to fibromuscular dysplasia (FMD), what is the most commonly involved artery?

A. Vertebral artery
B. Renal artery
C. Common femoral artery
D. SMA

27 Following an ultrasound-guided paracentesis in the left lower abdomen, a patient becomes hypotensive and develops a large ecchymosis near the access site. What artery should have been assessed with ultrasound at the time of paracentesis?

A. Left common femoral artery
B. Left inferior epigastric artery
C. Left internal mammary artery
D. Left hypogastric artery

28 A hypotensive patient is taken to IR for embolization of a left abdominal wall expanding hematoma. From a right common femoral artery access, a catheter is positioned in the left external iliac artery, and an angiogram is obtained. What artery is indicated by the black arrowheads?

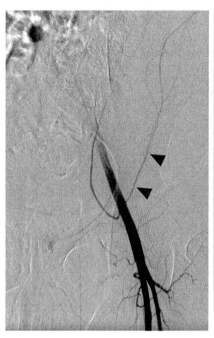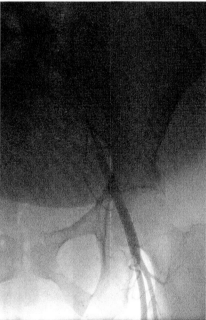

A. Obturator artery
B. Lateral circumflex femoral artery
C. Deep circumflex iliac artery
D. Inferior epigastric artery

29   A 29-year-old female is involved in a motor vehicle accident and sustains significant
      blunt trauma. A multiphase CECT is performed (arterial phase, top images; portal
      venous phase, middle images; delayed phase, bottom images). What is the diagnosis?

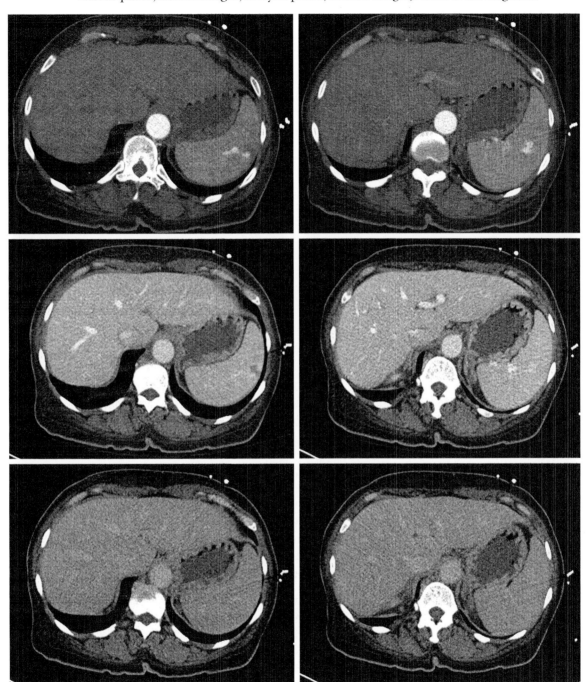

A. Splenic laceration with active bleeding
B. Splenic laceration with pseudoaneurysm formation
C. Splenic hemangioma
D. Normal variation in perfusion

30   Which of the following is an appropriate adjunctive treatment for a hemodynam-
     ically stable adult patient with blunt splenic injury and intrasplenic pseudoaneu-
     rysm formation?

     A. Distal main splenic artery covered stent
     B. Proximal main splenic artery embolization with coils
     C. Proximal main splenic artery embolization with particles
     D. Distal main splenic artery thrombin injection

31   Following a proximal splenic artery embolization for blunt splenic injury with
     intrasplenic pseudoaneurysm formation, a CECT is performed to reevaluate the
     injury. Which is the correct interpretation?

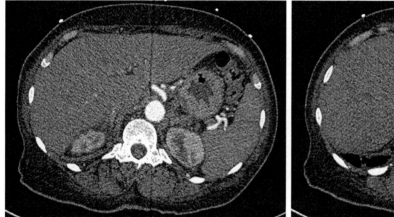
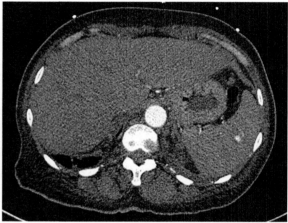

     A. Expected findings after proximal splenic artery embolization
     B. Treatment failure with patent splenic artery branches despite embolization
     C. Treatment failure with persistent filling of intrasplenic pseudoaneurysm

32   A patient presents for radioembolization treatment of the left hepatic lobe.
     Angiography demonstrates an enlarged gastrohepatic trunk with significant tortuos-
     ity (arrowhead).

     A microcatheter is advanced and after several unsuccessful attempts to cross the tor-
     tuous segment, a repeat angiogram is performed with early (middle) and delayed (right)
     phase images.

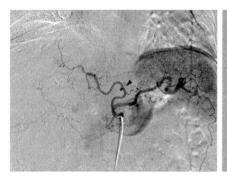
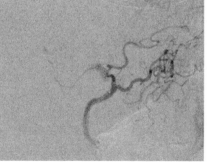
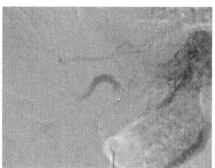

     What is the most likely explanation?

     A. Arterial thrombosis
     B. Arterial rupture
     C. Arterial dissection

33   What is the most likely pathology being demonstrated in this angiogram of the liver?

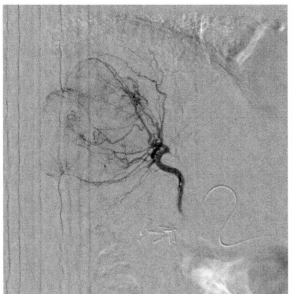 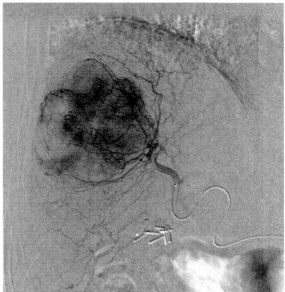

    A. Traumatic injury
    B. Hepatocellular carcinoma
    C. Hemangioma
    D. Cyst

34   In this patient with a painful left arm mass about to undergo surgical resection and reconstruction, what is the most likely purpose of this endovascular procedure?

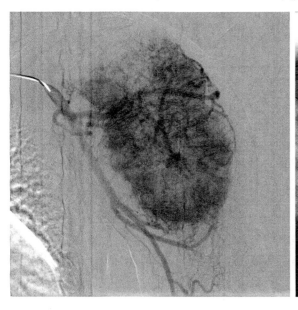 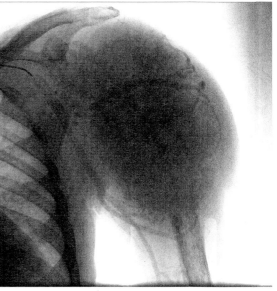

    A. A diagnostic study to establish pathology
    B. A diagnostic study to assist with operative planning
    C. An interventional procedure to reduce intraoperative bleeding
    D. An interventional procedure to reduce postoperative swelling and pain

35   Based on North American Symptomatic Carotid Endarterectomy Trial (NASCET)
     criteria, what percent stenosis is demonstrated on this carotid angiogram?

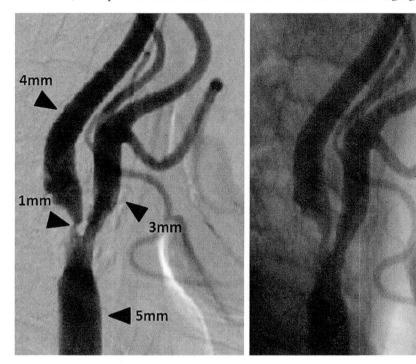

   A. 60%

   B. 75%

   C. 80%

   D. 90%

36   An otherwise healthy 65-year-old male presents with a nonhealing right foot ulcer.
     A CECT of the affected extremity is performed. Based on the images, which of the
     following is the best treatment plan for this lesion?

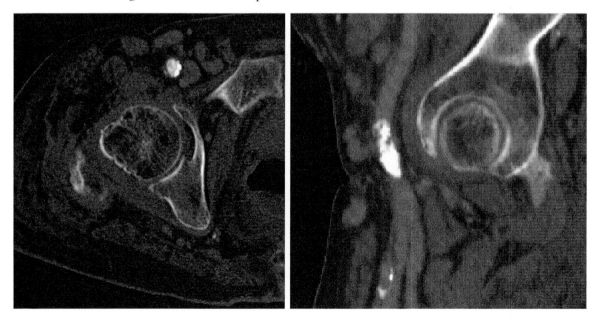

   A. Angioplasty

   B. Bare-metal stent

   C. Covered stent

   D. Surgical consult

37   A 35-year-old male presents for evaluation of an ulcer at the tip of thumb. For diagnostic evaluation, a catheter is placed in the brachial artery and an arteriogram is
obtained. Which of the following best explains the findings?

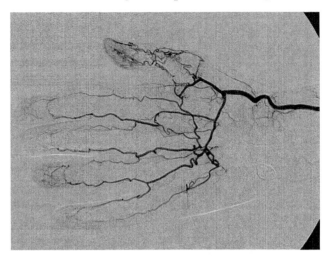

A. Buerger disease
B. Septic emboli
C. Atherosclerosis
D. Primary Raynaud disease

38   A CTA is performed in preparation for EVAR of an infrarenal abdominal aortic aneurysm. Which of the following is true?

A. Accessory renal arteries are a contraindication to EVAR
B. IMA occlusion increases endoleak risk after EVAR
C. Increased aneurysm neck length is a favorable characteristic for EVAR
D. Angulation at the aneurysm neck reduces endoleak risk after EVAR

ANSWERS AND EXPLANATIONS

1 **Answer B.** The arterial phase images show a patent endograft and faint increased attenuation within the excluded aneurysm sac in the mid segment, where the graft becomes bifurcated. A left lumbar artery is visible coursing toward the aneurysm sac between the vertebral body and the psoas muscle. The delayed phase images show dense contrast accumulation within the aneurysm sac at the lumbar level with visible left lumbar artery as the feeding artery. This is a type 2 endoleak by definition (endoleak types defined in the following question). Other arteries often responsible for a type 2 endoleak include the IMA and median sacral artery.

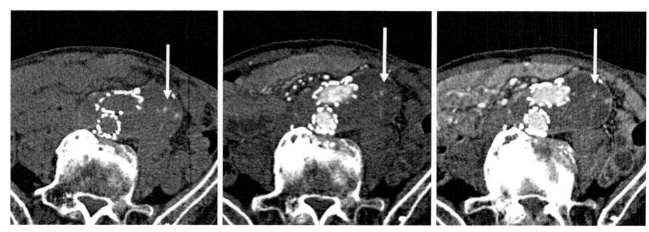

Figure 1-1 Companion case with computed tomography angiography (CTA) following endovascular aortic repair (EVAR) for abdominal aortic aneurysm (AAA) showing high-attenuation foci in the sac (arrows) suspicious for an endoleak. Careful comparison shows these are present before administration of intravenous contrast (left) and unchanged in the arterial (middle) and delayed (right) phases of imaging. These foci represent calcifications in the thrombosed aneurysm sac.

References: Chen J, Stavropoulos SW. Management of endoleaks. *Semin Intervent Radiol.* 2015;32(3):259-264.

O'Mara JE, Bersin RM. Endovascular management of abdominal aortic aneurysms: the year in review. *Curr Treat Options Cardiovasc Med.* 2016;18(8):54.

2 **Answer C.** The most accepted indication for the treatment of a type 2 endoleak is the growth of the aneurysm sac by 5 mm. Additional and perhaps more controversial indications include persistent endoleak on follow-up imaging, large feeding or draining artery, and high flow within the aneurysm sac. Percutaneous embolization techniques are first line in the treatment of type 2 endoleaks, with surgery reserved for refractory endoleaks or cases where embolization is not feasible. Surveillance is not appropriate in this case, as the aneurysm sac has grown by 1 cm in 6 months. A growing aneurysm is at risk for rupture. Placing a second endograft within the original endograft will have no effect on a leak that is not occurring at a seal site.

TABLE 2-1   Endoleak Classification

Endoleak Type	Pathology	Risk	Management
1a 1b	Failure of the stent graft to achieve a circumferential seal. This can occur at the proximal attachment site (1a) or distal attachment sites (1b).	Continued systemic pressurization of the aneurysm sac can lead to rupture.	Immediate fix with balloon remodeling and/or additional fixation with extension cuff, stents, or other devices. Rarely aneurysm sac embolization.
2	Retrograde collateral arterial flow to the aneurysm sac by branch vessels. Most commonly the inferior mesenteric artery or a lumbar artery.	Continued variable pressurization of the aneurysm sac can result in aneurysm sac enlargement and, ultimately, aneurysm rupture.	Elective fix in cases of aneurysm sac growth by 5 mm on follow-up imaging. First-line treatment is embolization of the nidus and/or feeding artery.
3	Leak or separation between stent graft components. Less commonly tear or hole in the stent graft fabric.	Continued systemic pressurization of the aneurysm sac can lead to rupture.	Immediate fix with stent grafts.
4	Graft porosity. Identified immediately after stent graft deployment.	Continued variable pressurization of the aneurysm sac.	Resolves on its own once procedural anticoagulation wears off.
5	Unknown. By definition, an enlarging aneurysm sac without a demonstrable endoleak.	Continued variable pressurization of the aneurysm sac.	Not clear. Conversion to an open repair or second endograft.

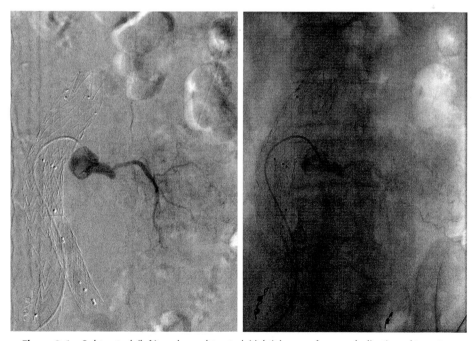

Figure 2-1 Subtracted (left) and unsubtracted (right) images from embolization of type 2 endoleak arising from left lumbar artery as seen in question 1. The operator uses a transseal technique whereby the catheter is advanced from the arterial access in the groin and passed between the wall of the iliac artery and fabric of the iliac limb of the endograft. The catheter courses cephalad in this plane, ultimately reaching the aneurysm sac and endoleak nidus. Note the morphology of contrast accumulation in the sac mirrors the computed tomography (CT) images from question 1, with a large left lumbar artery seen feeding the endoleak. The artery is subsequently embolized with coils, and the nidus is closed with glue.

References: Chen J, Stavropoulos SW. Management of endoleaks. *Semin Intervent Radiol.* 2015;32(3):259-264.

O'Mara JE, Bersin RM. Endovascular management of abdominal aortic aneurysms: the year in review. *Curr Treat Options Cardiovasc Med.* 2016;18(8):54.

3   **Answer B.**   The images show single-level arterial occlusive disease in the left lower extremity. Specifically, there is a long-segment occlusion, chronic in appearance, involving approximately 20 cm of the SFA with reconstitution distally. There is compensatory hypertrophy of the profunda femoris artery with prominent thigh collaterals that have formed because of the chronicity of the arterial obstruction. There is no flow-limiting inflow (iliac) or tibial artery disease. This patient likely presents with intermittent claudication, with reduced ankle-brachial index (ABI) to the range 0.70 to 0.75 (normal ABI 0.9-1.1).

Many clinicians use Rutherford's categorization of chronic peripheral arterial disease in their patient assessment.

Category 0: Asymptomatic

Category 1: Mild claudication

Category 2: Moderate claudication

Category 3: Severe claudication

Category 4: Rest pain

Category 5: Minor tissue loss/ulcer

Category 6: Major tissue loss/gangrene

Regarding the other answer choices: Severe aortoiliac arterial occlusive disease often produces Leriche syndrome, which presents as diminished or absent common femoral artery pulses, buttock claudication, and impotence. An abrupt onset of pain in a pulseless leg is consistent with acute limb-threatening ischemia (ALI). This can be due to in situ disease with thrombosis or distant embolus occluding otherwise normal arteries in the leg. This is not the case in this question, as the images presented show a chronic arterial occlusion with hypertrophied collaterals. Critical limb ischemia (CLI) is the combination of severely reduced ABI (typically < 0.3-0.4) with concomitant rest pain, tissue loss, and/or gangrene. These patients often have severe multilevel arterial occlusive disease, and there is a high associated rate of limb amputation (30% per year) and mortality (25% per year).

Reference: Bailey MA, Griffin KJ, Scott DJ. Clinical assessment of patients with peripheral arterial disease. *Semin Intervent Radiol.* 2014;31(4):292-299.

4   **Answer C.**   Primary patency is the time from the original intervention performed to restore vessel patency (SFA recanalization with stenting) until the time that a second intervention is required to treat thrombosis or stenosis. Primary-assisted patency is the time from the original intervention performed to restore vessel patency plus additional time gained from a second intervention to keep the vessel patent, such as balloon angioplasty or atherectomy. Secondary patency is the time from the original intervention performed to restore vessel patency plus additional time gained from an intervention to restore patency once the vessel thromboses or occludes, such as catheter-directed fibrinolysis or thrombectomy. Secondary patency concludes when further intervention to restore patency to the vessel is abandoned.

SFA recanalization
with stenting

In-stent stenosis treated
with angioplasty

Stent thrombosis treated
with tPA lysis

Stent thrombosis, vessel abandoned
and femoral-popliteal bypass is performed

⬇   ⬇   ⬇   ⬇

Time 0   9 months   15 months   21 months

——— Primary patency ———

——— Primary-assisted patency ——————

———Secondary patency ——————————————————

Figure 4-1 Graphic representation of primary, primary-assisted, and secondary patency. SFA, superficial femoral artery; tPA, tissue plasminogen activator.

Reference: Stoner MC, Calligaro KD, Chaer RA, et al. Reporting standards of the society for vascular surgery for endovascular treatment of chronic lower extremity peripheral artery disease. *J Vasc Surg*. 2016;64(1):e1-e21.

5 **Answer C.** This patient is presenting with acute limb-threatening ischemia or ALI. This differs from CLI in that there is often not an insidious course of intermittent claudication or known peripheral arterial disease. The etiology is often embolic, from cardiac or aortic pathology, or even paradoxically from the venous system through a right-to-left cardiac shunt. Extensive in situ thrombosis (thrombus formation at the site of preexisting atherosclerotic disease) can also produce ALI. The presentation is abrupt, with a classic progression that is clinically assessed. We use the Rutherford assessment to classify the patient presentation and help with treatment decisions. As noted below, when the sensory and motor function are absent in the affected extremity, irreversible tissue ischemia is present, and operative assessment is warranted.

TABLE 5-1 Rutherford Assessment for Acute Limb-Threatening Ischemia

Class	Limb Prognosis	Sensory Examination	Motor Examination	Arterial Doppler	Venous Doppler
I viable	Salvageable with urgent intervention	Normal	Normal	Present	Present
IIa	Salvageable with urgent intervention	Diminished	Normal	Absent	Present
IIb	Salvageable with immediate intervention	Diminished	Diminished	Absent	Present
III	Irreversible tissue damage	Absent	Absent	Absent	Absent

Adapted from Rutherford RB, Baker JD, Ernst C, et al. Recommended standards for reports dealing with lower extremity ischemia: revised version. *J Vasc Surg*. 1997;26(3):517-538.

For patients with Class I, IIa, or IIb presentation, the choice between endovascular and surgical revascularization is dependent on a number of factors including local expertise, resource availability, and type of reconstruction needed among others.

References: Bailey MA, Griffin KJ, Scott DJ. Clinical assessment of patients with peripheral arterial disease. *Semin Intervent Radiol*. 2014;31(4):292-299.

Rutherford RB, Baker JD, Ernst C, et al. Recommended standards for reports dealing with lower extremity ischemia: revised version. *J Vasc Surg*. 1997;26(3):517-538.

6   **Answer C.**   This is an iatrogenic injury related to the celiac artery catheterization performed 1 week prior. Mesenteric arterial pseudoaneurysms warrant urgent treatment at any size, as there is no way to compress the injury if there is rupture, the surgical treatment is challenging, and the risk of rupture is unpredictable. Pseudoaneurysms are by definition contained ruptures of the parent vessel, with fewer than 3 layers of vessel wall remaining intact. Choice A is inappropriate in a patient with an unexplained dropping hemoglobin level, and there is virtually no risk to the patient if the celiac artery undergoes thrombosis. The SMA is patent and will provide collateral circulation to all 3 celiac artery branches via the pancreaticoduodenal arcade. Similarly, open major surgery with ligation and arterial bypass is unnecessary with an intact SMA, particularly in a 79-year-old. The celiac artery can be sacrificed with an embolization procedure that occludes the artery proximal and distal to the neck of the pseudoaneurysm, also known as isolation technique. A stent graft would also be appropriate if an adequate seal could be achieved to exclude the pseudoaneurysm and prevent further filling.

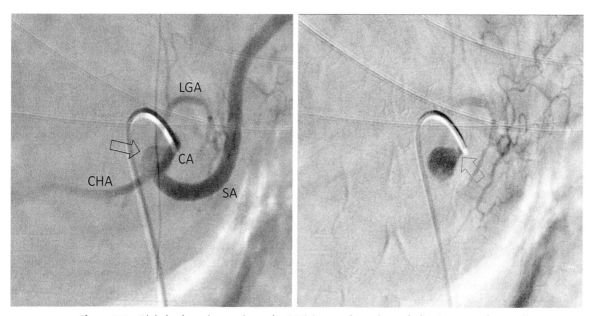

Figure 6-1   Digital subtraction angiography DSA) images from the embolization procedure. Celiac angiogram shows the saccular pseudoaneurysm (black arrow) arising from the mid segment of the artery. Note the narrow neck (red arrow) on the more delayed phase image on the right. CA, celiac artery; CHA, common hepatic artery; LGA, left gastric artery; SA, splenic artery.

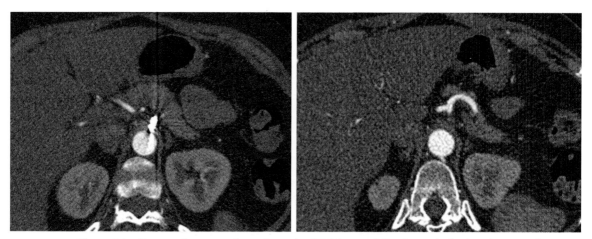

Figure 6-2   Computed tomography angiography (CTA) images following embolization show metallic artifact from the coil pack within the celiac artery (left) and patent common hepatic and splenic arteries (right), which are filling via collateral circulation off the superior mesenteric artery. There is no evidence of end-organ ischemia on the remaining images.

Reference: Hemp JH, Sabri SS. Endovascular management of visceral arterial aneurysms. *Tech Vasc Interv Radiol*. 2015;18(1):14-23.

7 **Answer B.** The duplex ultrasound result indicates a flow-limiting stenosis in the proximal segment of the bypass graft (peak systolic velocity, PSV >300 cm/s), with markedly reduced flow beyond the stenosis (graft flow velocity, GFV <45 cm/s). Pursuing surveillance imaging in 6 months (choice A) is too long to wait and may change the intervention from a simple balloon angioplasty of a focal stenosis to a multiday admission to lyse open a thrombosed bypass. Surgical revision at this time is not necessary, as the bypass is still patent and the duplex ultrasound shows a stenosis that certainly warrants attempted endovascular treatment.

TABLE 7-1 Arterial Duplex Ultrasound Surveillance of Lower Extremity Bypass Graft With Guidance-Based Peak Systolic Velocity (PSV) and Graft Flow Velocity (GFV)

Risk of Bypass Thrombosis	PSV	PSV Ratio	GFV (Avg Over Consecutive Nonstenotic Segments)	Management
High	>300 cm/s	>3.5	<45 cm/s	Immediate intervention
Intermediate	>300 cm/s	>3.5	>45 cm/s	Elective intervention
Low	<300 cm/s	<2.0	>45 cm/s	Continued observation

Adapted from Dhanoa D, Baerlocher MO, Benko AJ, et al. Position statement on noninvasive imaging of peripheral arterial disease by the society of interventional radiology and the Canadian Interventional Radiology Association. *J Vasc Interv Radiol*. 2016;27(7):947-951.

Reference: Dhanoa D, Baerlocher MO, Benko AJ, et al. Position statement on noninvasive imaging of peripheral arterial disease by the society of interventional radiology and the Canadian Interventional Radiology Association. *J Vasc Interv Radiol*. 2016;27(7):947-951.

8 **Answer A.** The DSA images from selective right and left subclavian arteriography demonstrate symmetric long-segment stenoses of the subclavian, axillary, and visualized brachial artery segments. This appearance is most consistent with a large cell vasculitis. Although there is overlap between TA and GCA, there are some distinguishing features that help narrow down the diagnosis. TA is likely to affect patients under the age of 50 years, whereas GCA often presents after the age of 50 years. TA also has a strong female predominance. The vessels affected can be helpful as well: TA primarily involves the main branches of the aorta whereas GCA often involves the extracranial external carotid arterial branches.

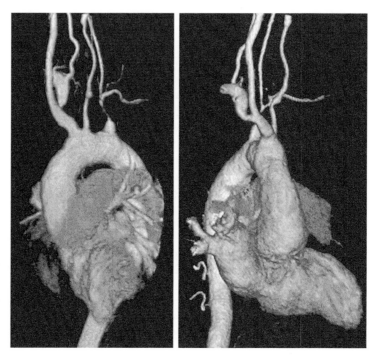

Figure 8-1 Three-dimensional volume rendered magnetic resonance angiography (MRA) images in another patient with known Takayasu arteritis (TA). Left anterior oblique (LAO) (left) image demonstrating severe stenosis of the proximal left subclavian artery. Right anterior oblique (RAO) (right) image demonstrating aneurysm formation of the proximal right subclavian artery.

Reference: Serra R, Butrico L, Fugetto F, et al. Updates in pathophysiology, diagnosis and management of takayasu arteritis. *Ann Vasc Surg.* 2016;35:210-225.

9   **Answer A.**   TA is a complex disease process with management including medical, endovascular, and/or surgical treatments. The course of the disease is often phasic with an early or prepulseless phase, a vascular inflammatory phase, and a late quiescent phase. A sequential triphasic pattern is not common, and phases may coexist. Although treatment regimens may vary, a generally agreed upon concept is to avoid any surgical or endovascular treatments during the active inflammatory phase of the disease. Inflammatory activity can be assessed by measuring the ESR. When active inflammation is absent or reduced, invasive treatments can be performed.

Reference: Serra R, Butrico L, Fugetto F, et al. Updates in pathophysiology, diagnosis and management of takayasu arteritis. *Ann Vasc Surg.* 2016;35:210-225.

10   **Answer D.**   This is a classic presentation of blue toe syndrome, for which there are many causes. Embolism is the most common etiology, often from focal shaggy atherosclerotic plaques or underlying aneurysms that thrombose and embolize clot fragments down into the small arteries of toes and feet. As in this case, the pedal pulses can remain palpable as the larger arteries of the leg are unaffected by the emboli. In the first image, there is smooth narrowing of the proximal and mid SFA from early atherosclerotic plaque formation; however, in the distal segment, there is a focal ledge-like filling defect from a bulky eccentric atherosclerotic plaque.

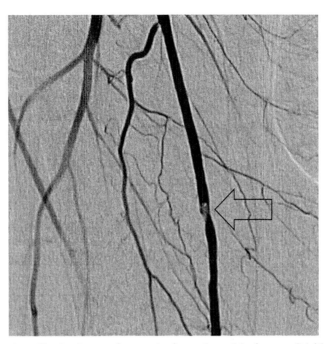

Figure 10-1   Magnification image of eccentric plaque (arrow) in the superficial femoral artery (SFA) responsible for distal emboli.

Vasculitides can manifest as stenoses, occlusions, and/or aneurysms often affecting more than 1 artery or segment. Vasospasm or vasoconstriction can occur from traumatic injury, shock, medications such as ergots, or exposure to extreme cold. Focal or diffuse smooth narrowing and sometimes occlusion can occur. Thromboangiitis obliterans or Buerger disease typically affects younger patients with a history of heavy smoking and involves the small- to medium-sized arteries and veins of the upper and lower extremities. In the lower extremities, the tibial arteries are often affected with multifocal occlusions and formation of collateral arteries with a characteristic "corkscrew" appearance.

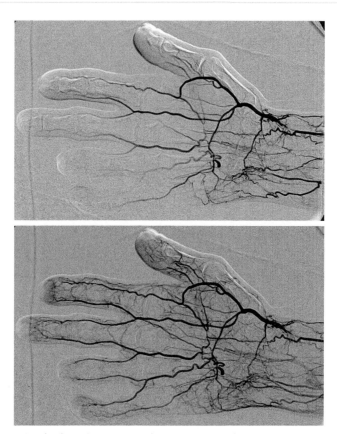

Figure 10-2 Digital subtraction angiography (DSA) images from upper extremity angiography in a young male with suspected Buerger disease demonstrate occlusion of the distal radial and ulnar arteries, corkscrew collateral formation, and occlusion of the proper digital arteries of the thumb.

Reference: Matchett WJ, Mcfarland DR, Eidt JF, Moursi MM. Blue toe syndrome: treatment with intra-arterial stents and review of therapies. *J Vasc Interv Radiol.* 2000;11(5):585-592.

11   **Answer D.**   The CTA images demonstrate iodinated contrast filling an irregular infrarenal abdominal aortic lumen. Note the atherosclerotic calcifications displaced both anteriorly and posteriorly in comparison to the aortic lumen, indicating the true aortic diameter is significantly greater than that depicted by the contrast-filled lumen. This appearance is consistent with an abdominal aortic aneurysm with mural thrombus formation. Additionally, on the bottom left image the posterior wall of the aorta is concave and inseparable from the adjacent lumbar vertebral body; a CT sign known as the "draped aorta sign" and associated with contained and/or impending rupture of the aneurysm. This high-risk feature should be identified and reported to the referring physician. Two phases of contrast-enhanced imaging are presented, with no periaortic accumulation or change in appearance of the aortic luminal contrast to indicate active extravasation. While retroperitoneal fibrosis often involves the distal abdominal aorta and bifurcation, displaced aortic wall calcifications should not be present. The fibrosis can cause luminal narrowing of the aorta and inferior vena cava and also involve adjacent structures such as the ureters causing medial deviation and obstruction with upstream hydroureteronephrosis. Infectious aortitis is fairly uncommon with the most common offending agents being tuberculosis, syphilis, salmonella, *Escherichia coli*, and streptococcus. The CT appearance includes aortic wall thickening, periaortic fluid and/or soft tissue, pseudoaneurysm formation (often saccular), and rarely gas formation.

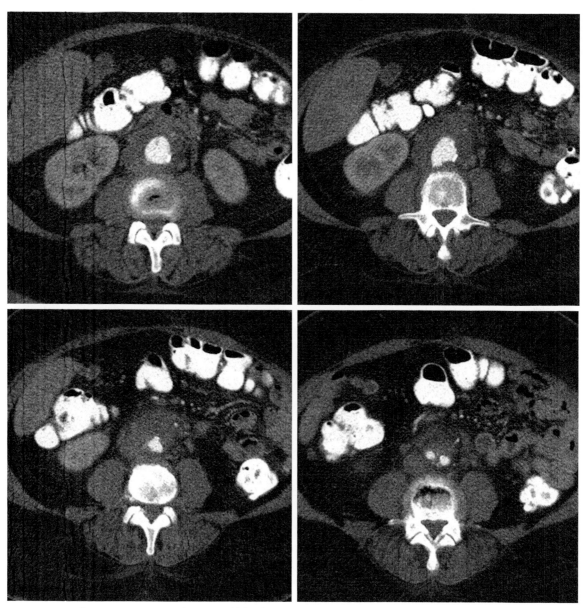

Figure 11-1 Companion case of infectious aortitis in 68-year-old female that presented with fevers and back pain. There is ill-defined periaortic low attenuation and stranding. Also note the saccular outpouching of the aortic lumen in the top right image.

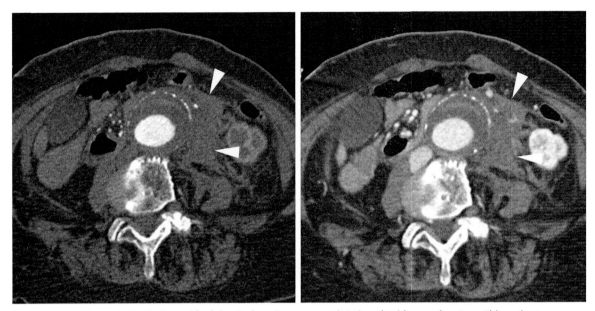

Figure 11-2 Patient with abdominal aortic aneurysm (AAA) and evidence of rupture. This patient has an AAA with well-seen calcified wall that is surrounded by blood (arrowheads) in the retroperitoneum. Although there is no active bleeding on this 2-phase contrast-enhanced computed tomography (CECT), this is a vascular emergency.

Reference: Halliday KE, Al-Kutoubi A. Draped aorta: CT sign of contained leak of aortic aneurysms. *Radiology*. 1996;199(1):41-43.

12   Answer A. On the images provided, the catheter has selected the SMA, evidenced by iodinated contrast first filling the SMA. On the subsequent image, the branches of the celiac artery are now filling with contrast. This appearance is classic for underlying celiac artery stenosis with hypertrophy of the pancreaticoduodenal arcade, which retrograde fills the gastroduodenal artery (GDA) and provides inflow to all 3 celiac artery branches. With a common origin, both the celiac and SMA branches will fill simultaneously. The Arc of Buhler is a rare persistent embryonic connection between the celiac and SMA. A visible connecting vessel is seen when this variant is present.

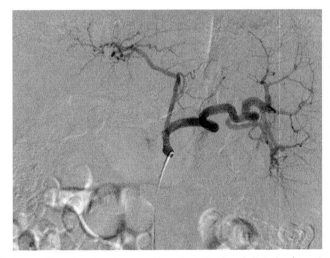

Figure 12-1 The celiac artery is subsequently catheterized and digital subtraction angiography (DSA) demonstrates the splenic artery and left gastric artery filling from the injection. There is no opacification of the common hepatic artery due to retrograde flow of nonopacified blood coming from the gastroduodenal artery (GDA). Note the variant anatomy with replaced left hepatic artery off the left gastric artery.

Reference: White RD, Weir-Mccall JR, Sullivan CM, et al. The celiac axis revisited: anatomic variants, pathologic features, and implications for modern endovascular management. *Radiographics.* 2015;35(3):879-898.

13   **Answer C.**   An intrinsic stenosis of the celiac artery from atherosclerosis should be unaffected on angiography by any provocative maneuver. Median arcuate ligament compression, an extrinsic mass effect on the superior aspect of the celiac artery, can be better demonstrated with inspiration and expiration angiograms in the lateral projection. On inspiration, the diaphragm moves down, displacing the intra-abdominal organs caudally, lessening the effect of the median arcuate ligament on the celiac artery. In expiration, the diaphragm and intra-abdominal organs move cephalad, pulling up on the celiac artery, worsening the effect (and stenosis) of the median arcuate ligament on the celiac artery.

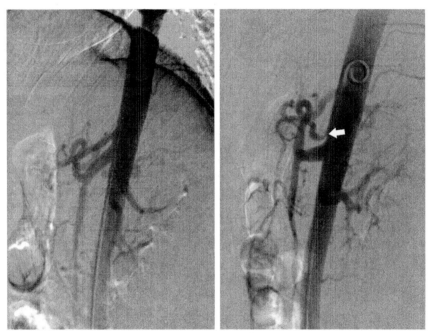

Figure 13-1   Digital subtraction angiography (DSA) images from abdominal aortography in the lateral projection. Inspiration image (left) shows widely patent celiac and superior mesenteric arteries. Expiration image (right) shows moderate focal narrowing (arrow) just beyond the origin of the celiac artery due to median arcuate ligament compression. This patient was a healthy 37-year-old female being evaluated as a donor for living donor liver transplantation.

Reference: Tracci MC. Median arcuate ligament compression of the mesenteric vasculature. *Tech Vasc Interv Radiol.* 2015;18(1):43-50.

14   **Answer D.**   The angiogram shows selective catheterization of the IMA with subsequent microcatheterization of the superior rectal artery and demonstration of the bleed. Following embolization, the patient continues with overt bleeding from below and hypotension. Following successful embolization at other sites of GI bleeding such as the stomach, small bowel, or colon, patients often continue to have blood and/or melena from below, as they pass residual blood in the bowels. This is an expected finding and not associated with a continued drop in hemoglobin or clinical deterioration (hypotension). In this case, however, as the bleed originated from the rectum, continued blood from below with hypotension is concerning for persistent bleeding despite embolization and warrants further investigation. The rectum receives its blood from the IMA via the superior rectal artery as well as the middle and inferior rectal arteries, which are branches from the anterior division of the internal iliac arteries. Subsequent selection of the left internal iliac artery and anterior division truck demonstrates collateral flow with continued bleeding into the lumen of the rectum (see Figure 14-1). The middle rectal artery is treated with Gelfoam slurry, resulting in immediate cessation of the bleeding and stabilization of the patient.

While the majority of GI bleeding is intermittent, the actively bleeding patient with hypotension should be resuscitated and undergo treatment, whether endoscopic, endovascular, or surgical. As the patient was already in the IR suite, transfer back to the ICU or referral to surgery is not appropriate (choices A and B). Multifocal bleeding in the bowel is extremely uncommon, and both the CTA and catheter angiogram confirmed the clinical diagnosis of lower GI bleeding. There is no reason to pursue investigatory angiography in a different segment of bowel (choice C).

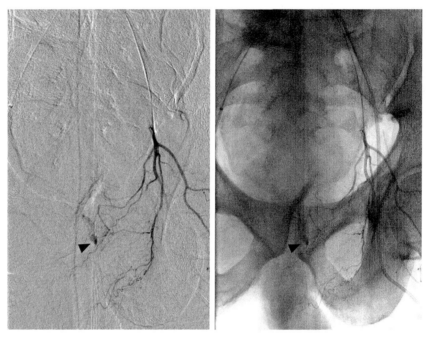

Figure 14-1 Angiography from the anterior division of the left internal iliac artery demonstrates persistent rectal bleeding (arrowheads) from collateral flow through the middle rectal artery.

Reference: Lee JH, Lee KH, Chung WS, Hur J, Won JY, Lee DY. Transcatheter embolization of the middle sacral artery: collateral feeder in recurrent rectal bleeding. *AJR Am J Roentgenol.* 2004;182(4):1055-1057.

15 **Answer C.** The angiographic images depict occlusion of the distal infrarenal abdominal aorta and bilateral common and external iliac arteries. Note the faint reconstitution of the bilateral common femoral arteries and proximal segments of the profunda femoris artery and SFA on the later phase image. We can confidently state the condition is chronic because of the extensive large and tortuous collaterals that have formed, which circumvent the arterial obstruction and allow for a viable pelvis and lower extremities. Also note the irregular wall of the aorta due to underlying atherosclerotic disease. This is the angiographic picture of Leriche syndrome, which is characterized clinically by diminished common femoral artery pulses, buttock claudication, and impotence. Choices A and D can be excluded based on acuity. Choice B is almost certainly related to venous pathology, which is clearly not depicted here.

Reference: Ahmed S, Raman SP, Fishman EK. CT angiography and 3D imaging in aortoiliac occlusive disease: collateral pathways in Leriche syndrome. *Abdom Radiol (NY).* 2017;42(9):2346-2357.

16 **Answer A.**   Collateral arterial pathways in aortoiliac occlusive disease are important to recognize and can present diagnostic and therapeutic challenges. A collateral pathway forms to bypass the level of arterial obstruction and provide blood flow to those tissues normally perfused by the involved artery. In the case of aortoiliac occlusive disease or Leriche syndrome, blood flow is compromised to the pelvis and bilateral lower extremities. The DSA image on the left shows the classic appearance of the superior rectal (hemorrhoidal) artery as it descends into the pelvis and gives off right and left lateral branches that appear to drape around the rectum. The DSA image on the right shows tremendous collateral formation in the pelvis near the termination of the superior rectal artery, with filling of internal iliac artery branches (middle and inferior rectal arteries). This pathway brings flow to the pelvis via the internal iliac artery branches and can bring flow to the lower extremities via the external iliac arteries (if patent, via retrograde internal iliac artery flow) or via other collaterals (obturator arteries >> upper thigh).

Important collateral pathways to be familiar with include the following:

1) Subclavian artery >> internal thoracic artery >> superior epigastric artery >> inferior epigastric artery >> external iliac artery (aka pathway of Winslow)

2) SMA >> IMA >> superior rectal artery >> middle and inferior rectal arteries >> internal iliac artery >> external iliac artery

3) Lumbar, intercostal and subcostal arteries >> deep circumflex iliac artery >> external iliac artery

4) Lumbar, intercostal and subcostal arteries >> lateral sacral and iliolumbar arteries >> internal iliac artery >> external iliac artery

Reference: Ahmed S, Raman SP, Fishman EK. CT angiography and 3D imaging in aortoiliac occlusive disease: collateral pathways in Leriche syndrome. *Abdom Radiol (NY)*. 2017;42(9):2346-2357.

17 **Answer B.**   Following arterial access in the groin, complications can occur including pseudoaneurysm formation, hematoma formation, arterial thrombosis, arterial dissection, and arteriovenous fistula (AVF) formation among others. When pseudoaneurysms form, patients most commonly present with a pulsatile groin mass after a recent catheterization procedure. Ultrasound is the modality of choice for evaluation, as it can detect and define virtually all access-related complications. When assessing pseudoaneurysms, it is important to identify the parent artery, arterial patency of the affected extremity, pseudoaneurysm size and neck morphology, and presence or absence of arteriovenous fistula. In the case presented, the color Doppler image demonstrates an oval pseudoaneurysm arising from the common femoral artery measuring approximately 2.5 cm with classic to-and-fro flow (yin-yang sign). On the spectral Doppler image, the common femoral vein is sampled with spectral tracing showing an arterialized vein with continuous diastolic flow, classic for an AVF. Additional images (not shown) demonstrate connection of the adjacent deep vein to the pseudoaneurysm.

Once detected, pseudoaneurysms can be observed or treated with ultrasound-guided compression, ultrasound-guided thrombin injection, or surgical repair. Various algorithms for management exist. More complex endovascular interventions can also be used but are beyond the scope of this book. Ultrasound-guided thrombin injection is the most common technique used in current practice. Contraindications to the technique include infection of the overlying skin or tissues, concomitant arteriovenous fistula, inability to visualize the needle, and/or a short wide neck. With an AVF, thrombin can directly enter the systemic venous system leading to venous thromboembolic complications. Pseudoaneurysm size becomes important as many small ones (less than 1 or 2 cm) will spontaneously thrombose without intervention, and operators may choose serial ultrasound over immediate intervention. Notably, thrombin injection of pseudoaneurysms <1 cm increases the risk of parent artery thrombosis. Having a narrow neck and common femoral artery origin are not unfavorable features for thrombin injection.

Reference: Stone PA, Campbell JE, Aburahma AF. Femoral pseudoaneurysms after percutaneous access. *J Vasc Surg*. 2014;60(5):1359-1366.

18 **Answer D.** When performing ultrasound-guided percutaneous thrombin injection for groin access pseudoaneurysms, the preferred technique is to place the needle tip into the pseudoaneurysm sac, away from the neck or communication with the parent artery. The injection is typically performed with a small syringe (1 mL) containing reconstituted thrombin in a concentration of 1000 U/mL. Live color and grayscale ultrasound during slow injection demonstrates the echogenic clot forming at the needle tip and ultimately filling the volume of the pseudoaneurysm sac. At completion, there should be no demonstrable flow in the pseudoaneurysm and the parent artery remains patent. Injection near the neck (choice A) can result in accidental parent artery injection (leading the thrombosis and limb ischemia) or incomplete pseudoaneurysm thrombosis. Injection into the parent artery upstream or downstream (choices C and B) from the neck will not effectively deliver thrombin to the pseudoaneurysm and will virtually guarantee parent artery thrombosis.

Reference: Stone PA, Campbell JE, Aburahma AF. Femoral pseudoaneurysms after percutaneous access. *J Vasc Surg*. 2014;60(5):1359-1366.

19 **Answer A.** The DSA images depict ongoing thoracic endovascular aortic repair or TEVAR, for a traumatic pseudoaneurysm of the descending thoracic aorta. On the predeployment image (left), the constrained endograft has been advanced into position over a stiff wire, and a flush aortogram in a steep left anterior oblique position demonstrates the normal arch anatomy. After stent graft deployment, repeat flush aortogram (right) shows successful exclusion of the pseudoaneurysm; however, there is nonopacification of the left subclavian artery. A carotid to subclavian arterial bypass is not visualized. The risks to the patient in this scenario are actually quite low but include cerebral ischemia via diminished flow to the ipsilateral vertebral artery, left arm ischemia via diminished flow to the subclavian artery, and spinal cord ischemia via diminished flow to the intercostal and spinal arteries. Notably, acute left arm ischemia is rarely seen despite the somewhat unnerving angiographic appearance due to robust collateral pathways in the neck and shoulder region. Chronic arm ischemia or claudication is more likely to occur. The left internal thoracic artery (mammary) also experiences reduced flow, as it is a branch of the subclavian artery; however, in the absence of prior usage as a bypass conduit for coronary artery disease, low flow or occlusion presents no risk to the patient.

Reference: Findeiss LK, Cody ME. Endovascular repair of thoracic aortic aneurysms. *Semin Intervent Radiol*. 2011;28(1):107-117.

20 **Answer C.** DSA images centered about the right and left popliteal arteries demonstrate abnormal medial deviation of both arteries at the level of the knee joint with moderate to severe stenosis on the left, which is worse with plantar flexion against resistance. The history, appearance, and provocative effect are classic for popliteal artery entrapment syndrome (PAES). Popliteal artery entrapment typically occurs secondary to one of several anatomic variants involving the musculotendinous structures of the popliteal fossa. The entrapment can occur bilaterally, and result in stenosis, occlusion, or aneurysmal degeneration of the affected popliteal artery. When symptomatic, treatment is typically surgical reconstruction. Although conventional angiography is an excellent tool for evaluation, dynamic ultrasound, CTA, and magnetic resonance angiography (MRA) have become first-line diagnostic tools in modern practice. Other conditions affecting

the popliteal artery (choices A, B, and D) can present as a stenosis, but the medial deviation and provocative effect are unique to PAES. It is important to remember that a significant limitation of angiography is its inability to visualize extraluminal pathology.

References: Corneloup L, Labanère C, Chevalier L, et al. Presentation, diagnosis, and management of popliteal artery entrapment syndrome: 11 years of experience with 61 legs. *Scand J Med Sci Sports*. 2017;00:1-7.

Liu Y, Sun Y, He X, et al. Imaging diagnosis and surgical treatment of popliteal artery entrapment syndrome: a single-center experience. *Ann Vasc Surg*. 2014;28(2):330-337.

21 **Answer D.** Pelvic angiography and intervention for trauma is one of the most rewarding aspects of IR. Embolization for pelvic bleeding can truly be lifesaving. In this case, the unsubtracted image demonstrates left sacral ala and bilateral superior rami fractures. The subtracted image demonstrates normal appearance of the visualized infrarenal abdominal aorta, bilateral common iliac, bilateral external iliac, and right internal iliac arteries. Although there is no evidence of active bleeding, there is a clear paucity of left hemipelvis arterial branches. Note the normal right superior gluteal artery (largest branch of the internal iliac artery, posterior division) and absent left superior gluteal artery due to proximal injury with occlusion. Although there is no active bleeding from the vessel stump, embolization is warranted, as the stump may be intermittently bleeding and over time can form a pseudoaneurysm.

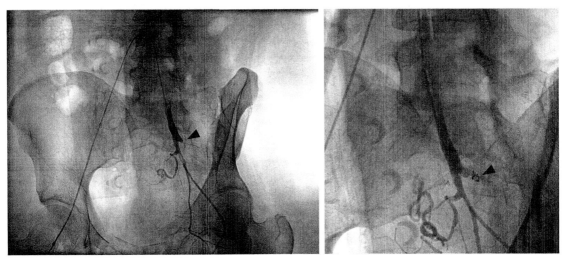

Figure 21-1 Unsubtracted images from left superior gluteal artery stump embolization with coils (arrowheads).

Although there is evidence of vascular injury on the initial angiogram in this case, one should not clear the pelvis with nonselective angiography alone. Bilateral selective internal iliac angiography in multiple obliquities should be performed with quality power injections to completely evaluate the vasculature for injury. Subsequent embolization is carried out with various agents such as Gelfoam slurry, coils, or glue depending on the location and type of injury.

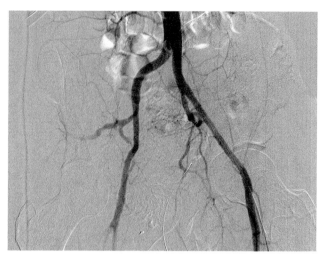

Figure 21-2   Companion case of a patient with blunt trauma, pelvic fractures, and hypotension evaluated with angiography. Nonselective right anterior oblique (RAO) pelvic arteriogram shows no evidence of injury. Selective interrogation of the right internal iliac artery is then performed (see Figure 21-3).

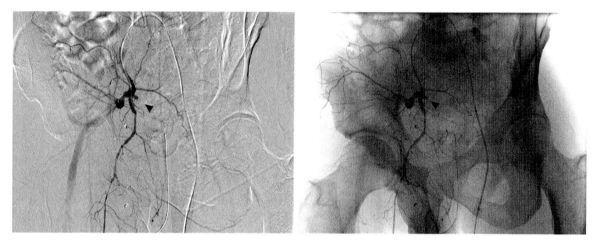

Figure 21-3   Selective left anterior oblique (LAO) angiography from the right internal iliac artery demonstrates an anterior division injury with vessel stump which is not appreciated by the operator (arrowheads). No embolization performed. Approximately 10 days later, the patient experiences a sudden drop in hemoglobin with associated pelvic pain and a computed tomography angiography (CTA) is obtained (see Figure 21-4).

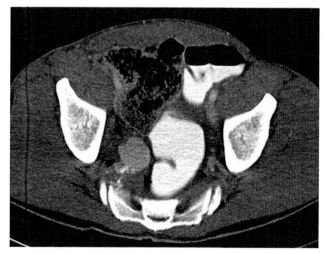

Figure 21-4   Pelvic CTA demonstrates interval development of a large pseudoaneurysm (arrowheads) in the region of the right internal iliac artery with adjacent hematoma. The patient returns to IR and undergoes a lengthy complex embolization to occlude the pseudoaneurysm and an associated arteriovenous fistula arising from the injured anterior division branch artery.

Reference: Scemama U, Dabadie A, Varoquaux A, et al. Pelvic trauma and vascular emergencies. *Diagn Interv Imaging*. 2015;96(7-8):717-729.

22 **Answer A.**   The subtracted and unsubstracted images from a selective arterial catheterization in the thorax demonstrate opacification of 2 left-sided intercostal arteries arising from a common trunk. The diaphragm is visible, localizing the artery to the lower thoracic region. Additionally, there is a medially directed branch that ascends over a short segment, makes a hairpin loop, and descends in the midline over the spinal column. This branch has the classic appearance of the great anterior radiculomedullary artery or artery of Adamkiewicz. This artery ultimately anastomoses with the anterior spinal artery, which provides blood supply to the lower thoracic and lumbar spinal cord. The artery most commonly arises from a left intercostal artery in the lower thoracic region. Particle embolization from the demonstrated catheter position can cause permanent spinal cord ischemia. Operators need to be aware of this uncommonly seen branch to avoid a potentially catastrophic complication.

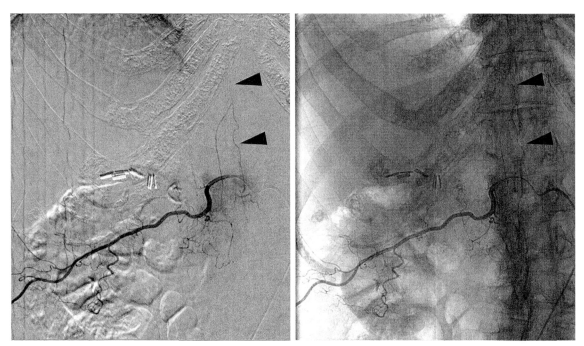

Figure 22-1   Companion case of the anterior spinal artery (arrowheads) with communication to the right L2 lumbar artery.

Reference: Yoon W, Kim JK, Kim YH, Chung TW, Kang HK. Bronchial and nonbronchial systemic artery embolization for life-threatening hemoptysis: a comprehensive review. *Radiographics*. 2002;22(6):1395-1409.

23 **Answer C.**   The image demonstrates fusiform aneurysmal dilatation of the ulnar artery just proximal to the palmar arch. Moving peripherally, there is a short-segment occlusion of the third digit proper digital artery consistent with an embolus. This is hypothenar hammer syndrome, a classic vascular syndrome characterized by repetitive trauma to the hypothenar region of the hand, where the ulnar artery takes a relatively superficial and unprotected course over the hook of the hamate bone. Over time, intimal injury can lead to hyperplasia, fibrosis, and fusiform aneurysmal dilatation. Partial or complete thrombosis can occur with resultant downstream embolization manifested by signs and symptoms of digital ischemia. Obtaining an accurate occupational history is often the most important first step in diagnosing this condition. A similar condition can occur over the thenar aspect

of the palm with injury to the radial artery. Vasculitides can certainly affect the medium and small arteries of the hand but would be expected to demonstrate a more global abnormality involving multiple digits with areas of stenosis, occlusion, collateral formation, and distal embolization. Raynaud disease can present similarly, but the predominant pattern is short-segment stenosis and occlusions that may be fixed or responsive to vasodilator injection. Raynaud disease can be primary or secondary to an underlying condition such as connective tissue disease.

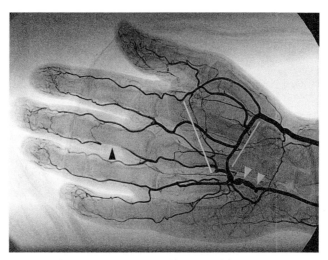

Figure 23-1   Right-hand angiogram with partial bony overlay demonstrating fusiform aneurysm of the distal ulnar artery (blue arrowheads), with associated short-segment embolic occlusion of the proper digital artery (black arrowhead). Superficial (green line) and deep (blue line) palmar arterial arches.

References: Gardiner GA, Tan A. Repetitive blunt trauma and arterial injury in the hand. *Cardiovasc Intervent Radiol*. 2017;40(11):1659-1668.

Wong VW, Katz RD, Higgins JP. Interpretation of upper extremity arteriography: vascular anatomy and pathology [corrected]. *Hand Clin*. 2015;31(1):121-134.

24   **Answer A.**   When considering a lower extremity arterial intervention, the entire arterial course from the aortic bifurcation through the foot is routinely studied before any intervention has taken place. Following an intervention, the runoff is often restudied to ensure no complication occurs from the procedure itself. In this case, the patient has an intervention performed in the dorsalis pedis artery, which is the continuation of the anterior tibial artery into the foot. To perform that intervention, a wire and catheter are advanced from the groin (contra- or ipsilateral approach) down the leg, through the popliteal and anterior tibial arteries to reach the embolus in the dorsalis pedis artery. The images presented pre and post intervention are centered about the knee where the popliteal artery gives off the anterior tibial artery. In this patient, there is only single vessel runoff via the anterior tibial artery, due to chronic occlusion of the tibioperoneal trunk, posterior tibial, and peroneal arteries. On the preintervention image, the anterior tibial artery is widely patent without stenosis. On the postintervention image, there are smooth-walled segments of moderate to severe narrowing with intervening more normal caliber artery. Note the preserved flow in the side branches. This is the appearance of arteriospasm and occurred from wire and catheter irritation of the vessel. If severe and persistent, it can lead to diminished distal flow and ultimately arterial thrombosis. This patient was treated with intra-arterial nitroglycerin and repeat angiogram demonstrated complete resolution (see Figure 24-1). Other complications operators should be familiar with include dissection, thrombosis, rupture, and distal embolism, which are discussed elsewhere in this book.

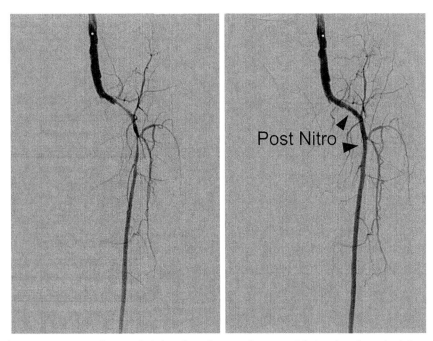

Figure 24-1 Pre and post administration of 200 µg intra-arterial nitroglycerin to the left anterior tibial artery with complete relief of arteriospasm (arrowheads).

References: Razavi MK. Detection and treatment of acute thromboembolic events in the lower extremities. *Tech Vasc Interv Radiol.* 2011;14(2):80-85.

25 **Answer B.** Renal artery intervention for renovascular hypertension can be a relatively simple and straightforward arterial intervention; however, small errors in technique can be disastrous. The images from the intervention show stenting of a moderate proximal left renal artery stenosis. Note the operator has collimated in such a way that the entire length of the guidewire is not visible during the intervention, particularly the distal intrarenal segment. The wire used has a visible transition point from proximal stiff (less dense) to distal floppy (more dense) that is visible in the upper right image. On the final images after the stent has been deployed, the transition point is no longer visible, suspicious for inadvertent advancement of the wire. There is no evidence of main renal artery rupture. Following the procedure, shock occurs and CECT demonstrates a large subcapsular hematoma involving the left kidney with small jet of extravasating contrast and dependent pooling. This is due to guidewire perforation of the renal capsule.

Expected postprocedure changes on imaging include a normal-appearing kidney and occasionally a striated enhancement pattern. If substantial plaque is encountered during the procedure, distal emboli can occur with the development of wedge-shaped peripheral nonenhancing infarctions. Clinically, patients can develop hypotension in the recovery period due to diminished circulating angiotensin II. Access-site complications such as dissection, thrombosis, and pseudoaneurysm formation do not produce shock. A retroperitoneal hematoma from high (above the inguinal ligament) groin access or posterior artery wall needle transgression could present similarly, but the CECT demonstrates subcapsular hematoma, indicating a renal source.

References: Carr TM, Sabri SS, Turba UC, et al. Stenting for atherosclerotic renal artery stenosis. *Tech Vasc Interv Radiol.* 2010;13(2):134-145.

Morris CS, Bonnevie GJ, Najarian KE. Nonsurgical treatment of acute iatrogenic renal artery injuries occurring after renal artery angioplasty and stenting. *AJR Am J Roentgenol.* 2001;177(6):1353-1357.

26   Answer B.   FMD is an uncommon disease of unknown etiology affecting medium-sized arteries in 1 or more vascular territories. The most common site of pathology is the renal arteries, followed by the extracranial carotid arteries. Less common involvement of the vertebral arteries, mesenteric arteries, upper and lower extremity arteries, as well as intracranial carotid arteries has been described. Presentation is dictated by the anatomic site of the disease, with renovascular hypertension as the leading symptom. The majority of the patients are female. On radiologic studies, dissection, stenosis, beading, aneurysm, and occlusion may be identified. There are several different types of FMD based on histology, with medial fibroplasia being most common.

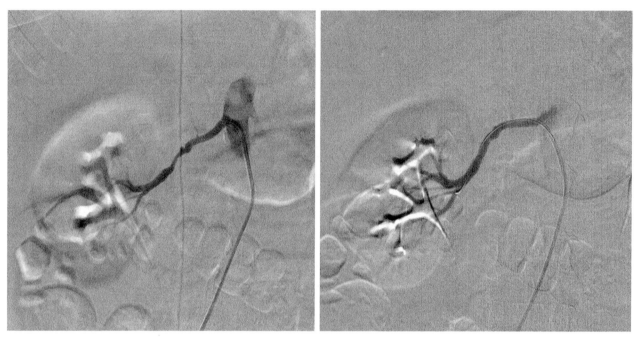

Figure 26-1   A 50-year-old female with refractory hypertension studied with angiography. Preintervention digital subtraction angiography (DSA) image on the left shows beading of the mid segment right renal artery consistent with fibromuscular dysplasia (FMD). Following angioplasty alone (right image), there is no residual stenosis. Unlike atherosclerotic lesions in the renal arteries, FMD tends to respond well to angioplasty alone with stenting reserved for complications and refractory lesions.

References: Sharma AM, Kline B. The United States registry for fibromuscular dysplasia: new findings and breaking myths. *Tech Vasc Interv Radiol*. 2014;17(4):258-263.

Shivapour DM, Erwin P, Kim ESh. Epidemiology of fibromuscular dysplasia: a review of the literature. *Vasc Med*. 2016;21(4):376-381.

27   Answer B.   When performing paracentesis in the lower abdominal region off midline, the inferior epigastric arteries can be accidentally traversed. They arise from the distal external iliac arteries, often traveling caudally at first then immediately looping cranial and coursing medially between the posterior rectus sheath and the rectus abdominis muscle. The arteries eventually give off multiple branches that perforate the muscle and spread out over the abdominal wall. The inferior epigastric artery should be identified on ultrasound when planning for paracentesis. Of note, when compared with blind paracentesis, ultrasound guidance is associated with fewer adverse events including bleeding complications. Choice A would be an unacceptable location for paracentesis, below the inguinal ligament; choice C is the cephalad communicating artery via the superior epigastric artery in the thorax. Traversing the hypogastric artery (aka internal iliac artery) during paracentesis would be an egregious complication.

References: Patel PA, Ernst FR, Gunnarsson CL. Evaluation of hospital complications and costs associated with using ultrasound guidance during abdominal paracentesis procedures. *J Med Econ.* 2012;15(1):1-7.

Sekiguchi H, Suzuki J, Daniels CE. Making paracentesis safer: a proposal for the use of bedside abdominal and vascular ultrasonography to prevent a fatal complication. *Chest.* 2013;143(4):1136-1139.

28 Answer C.   The deep circumflex iliac artery is another important artery in the lower abdominal wall that can be traversed during percutaneous procedures such as paracentesis or abscess drainage, especially with a more lateral approach. The artery comes off the distal external iliac artery, coursing cephalad and lateral. The artery pierces the transversus abdominis muscle and ascends between it and the overlying internal oblique muscle. It can often be identified on CECT. The inferior epigastric artery is present on the images; however, it is the more medial artery arising opposite from the deep circumflex iliac artery. These 2 arteries are the vascular landmark for the inguinal ligament demarcating intrapelvic external iliac artery from infrainguinal common femoral artery. The obturator artery is deep within the pelvis typically arising from the anterior division of the internal iliac artery. The lateral circumflex femoral artery arises in the proximal thigh.

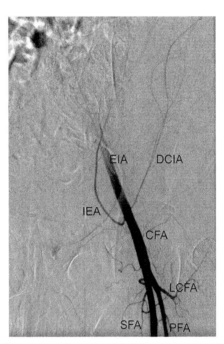

Figure 28-1   Digital subtraction angiography (DSA) from left external iliac artery injection. CFA, common femoral artery; DCIA, deep circumflex iliac artery; EIA, external iliac artery; IEA, inferior epigastric artery; LCFA, lateral circumflex femoral artery; PFA, profunda femoris artery; SFA, superficial femoral artery.

References: Park SW, Ko SY, Yoon SY, et al. Transcatheter arterial embolization for hemoperitoneum: unusual manifestation of iatrogenic injury to abdominal muscular arteries. *Abdom Imaging.* 2011;36(1):74-78.

Satija B, Kumar S, Duggal RK, Kohli S. Deep circumflex iliac artery pseudoaneurysm as a complication of paracentesis. *J Clin Imaging Sci.* 2012;2:10.

29 Answer B.   The arterial phase images show abnormal round and linear contrast enhancement within the splenic parenchyma. On the portal venous and delayed phase images, there is gradual washout without pooling or spreading of the abnormal contrast. These findings are consistent with intrasplenic pseudoaneurysm formation. Note the adjacent linear low-attenuation lacerations best seen on the arterial and portal venous phase images. Active bleeding (choice A) within the spleen is uncommon; however, if present, should show increasing accumulation of extravasated contrast into an expanding intrasplenic hematoma. More commonly, active bleeding from splenic trauma is seen when the laceration extends to the capsule and extravasation into the perisplenic space occurs. As in almost all organ traumas, multiphase imaging helps tremendously with the identification and characterization of injuries, particularly vascular injuries. Choice C, a common but benign splenic vascular lesion, is often a well-circumscribed mass(es) with gradual centripetal or homogenous enhancement.

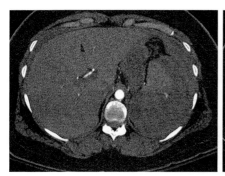 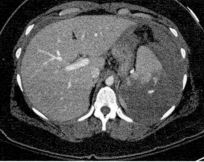 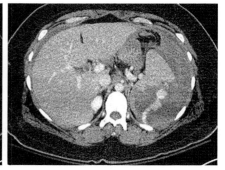

Figure 29-1   Companion case. Three-phase contrast-enhanced computed tomography (CECT) demonstrating high-grade splenic injury with perisplenic hematoma. Note the subcentimeter focus of contrast in the spleen (arterial phase, left image) that enlarges and extends beyond the parenchymal edge on the portal venous and delayed phase images consistent with active bleeding.

References: Boscak A, Shanmuganathan K. Splenic trauma: what is new? *Radiol Clin North Am.* 2012;50(1):105-122.

Melikian R, Goldberg S, Strife BJ, Halvorsen RA. Comparison of MDCT protocols in trauma patients with suspected splenic injury: superior results with protocol that includes arterial and portal venous phase imaging. *Diagn Interv Radiol.* 2016;22(5):395-399.

30   **Answer B.**   Current management of blunt splenic injury in adults consists of operative and nonoperative strategies, with splenic arterial embolization (SAE) frequently used as an adjunctive therapy. The technique uses one of 2 methods: proximal or distal SAE. With proximal SAE, the splenic artery is occluded distal to the dorsal pancreatic artery (often the first downgoing branch) with the use of coils or a vascular plug. Diminished arterial pressure beyond the embolization site promotes hemostasis and healing of splenic injuries, whereas collateral arterial pathways (pancreatic and gastric) reconstitute the distal splenic artery, maintaining viable perfusion to the splenic parenchyma. With distal SAE, a peripheral branch(es) of the splenic artery is occluded, frequently with coils, Gelfoam, or other embolic agents. Collateral arterial pathways do not exist this far peripherally, and the splenic injury is effectively treated through feeding artery thrombosis and focal tissue devascularization (infarct). Occasionally, both methods are used in a single procedure. There is no consensus opinion on the appropriate application of the techniques as both provide a high rate of splenic salvage, often 90% or greater, with a low complication rate. In our practice, we use proximal SAE as long as there is no demonstrable active bleeding on angiography. If there is active bleeding, we perform a distal SAE at that site to achieve immediate hemostasis.

Choice A is appropriate for cases of main splenic artery injury, not intrasplenic pseudoaneurysm formation. Choices C and D would likely result in total or near total infarction of the spleen. Particles are flow-directed embolics and will lodge in the distal artery/arteriole depending on their size, producing end-organ ischemia. Thrombin injected into a high-flow artery like the splenic will cause immediate thrombosis of the entire vascular territory. Remember, the goals of SAE for trauma are control of the injury AND preservation of the spleen.

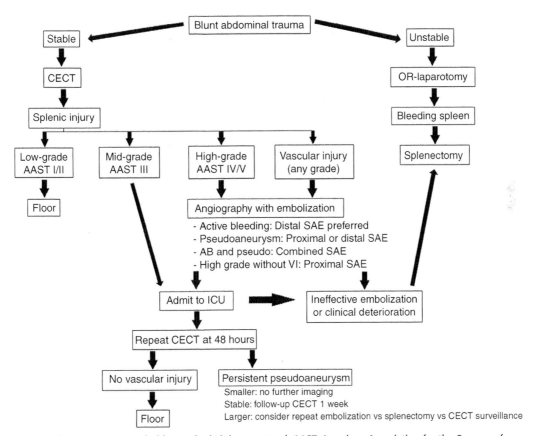

Figure 30-1 Sample blunt splenic injury protocol. AAST, American Association for the Surgery of Trauma; AB, active bleeding; CECT, contrast-enhanced computed tomography; ICU, intensive care unit; OR, operating room; SAE, splenic arterial embolization; VI, vascular injury.

References: Coccolini F, Montori G, Catena F, et al. Splenic trauma: WSES classification and guidelines for adult and pediatric patients. *World J Emerg Surg.* 2017;12:40.

Imbrogno BF, Ray CE. Splenic artery embolization in blunt trauma. *Semin Intervent Radiol.* 2012;29(2):147-149.

Schnüriger B, Inaba K, Konstantinidis A, Lustenberger T, Chan LS, Demetriades D. Outcomes of proximal versus distal splenic artery embolization after trauma: a systematic review and meta-analysis. *J Trauma.* 2011;70(1):252-260.

31   **Answer A.** With proximal embolization, a coil pack or vascular plug is deployed in the proximal to mid splenic artery, ideally just beyond the dorsal pancreatic artery such that pancreatic and short gastric collaterals will reconstitute the distal main splenic artery. It is an expected finding to see contrast opacification in the main splenic artery proximal and distal to the coil pack or plug, as a result of the collateral arterial filling. Additionally, when the procedure is performed in the setting of intrasplenic pseudoaneurysm, it is common to see persistent pseudoaneurysm filling after embolization, particularly on early follow-up examinations. This

warrants no further treatment. Naturally, if there are enlarging pseudoaneurysms or evidence of interval splenic rupture despite proximal embolization, surgical splenectomy should be considered.

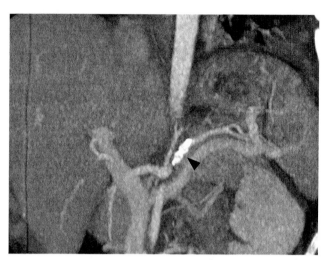

Figure 31-1   Coronal oblique contrast-enhanced computed tomography (CECT) image after proximal splenic artery embolization with a vascular plug. The plug (arrowhead) is clearly seen in the proximal main splenic artery with expected opacification of the artery distal to the plug from collaterals.

Reference: Haan JM, Marmery H, Shanmuganathan K, Mirvis SE, Scalea TM. Experience with splenic main coil embolization and significance of new or persistent pseudoaneurysm: reembolize, operate, or observe. *J Trauma*. 2007;63(3):615-619.

32   **Answer C.**   The images obtained after attempted catheterization of the tortuous artery segment demonstrate a discrete terminus to the normal-looking artery, with an abnormal wire-thin lumen beyond. On the delayed phase image, there is contrast retention in a relatively larger distal artery segment. This appearance is classic for an arterial dissection with dyssynchronous filling of the true (smaller) and false (larger) lumen. The images show no extraluminal contrast to indicate vessel rupture and no filling defect or complete occlusion to suggest thrombosis. With dissection, if the false lumen becomes pressurized and expanded (as in this case), it can compress the true lumen with virtually no downstream passage of contrast (or blood). With a little luck, a wire can be passed through the true lumen beyond the site of pathology and subsequently dilated with balloon angioplasty, restoring normal perfusion and hopefully eliminating flow in the false lumen.

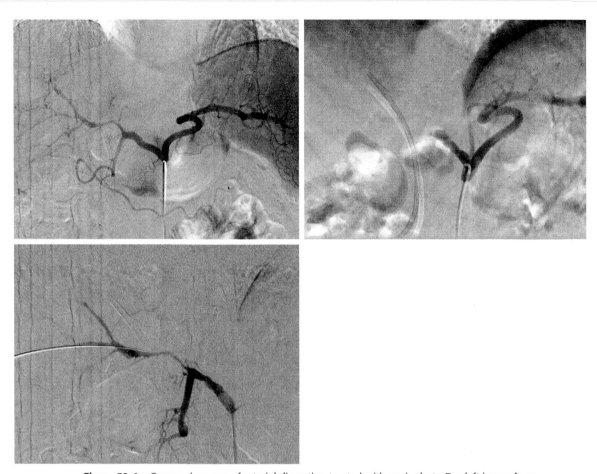

Figure 32-1   Companion case of arterial dissection treated with angioplasty. Top left image from celiac angiogram with widely patent branches. Top right image after failed attempt to select the proper hepatic artery with a microcatheter demonstrates occlusive dissection just proximal to the takeoff of the gastroduodenal artery (GDA). A wire is skillfully negotiated into the true lumen, and after balloon dilation (bottom left image), there is restoration of flow in both the GDA and proper hepatic artery. As seen in the presented cases, microcatheter navigation through small arteries can be a delicate work. The arteries can be even more fragile after exposure to certain systemic chemotherapeutic agents such as bevacizumab (Avastin).

References: Brown DB. Hepatic artery dissection in a patient on bevacizumab resulting in pseudoaneurysm formation. *Semin Intervent Radiol.* 2011;28(2):142-146.

Jung E, Shin JH, Kim JH, Yoon HK, Ko GY, Sung KB. Arterial dissections during transcatheter arterial chemoembolization for hepatocellular carcinoma: a 19-year clinical experience at a single medical institution. *Acta Radiol.* 2017;58(7):842-848.

Sakamoto I, Aso N, Nagaoki K, et al. Complications associated with transcatheter arterial embolization for hepatic tumors. *Radiographics.* 1998;18(3):605-619.

33   **Answer B.**   This is a very typical angiogram for hepatocellular cancer (HCC). One of the hallmarks of HCC is early arterial filling of the tumor. Although this is harder to depict on static images, observe the abnormal tumor vessels, which opacify before the normal liver parenchyma. On the more delayed phase image, the round tumor mass seemingly displaces the normal liver vessels. Hypervascularity, neovascularity, and arteriovenous shunting are features commonly seen with HCC. Traumatic injury may present as heterogeneous parenchymal filling, active extravasation, pseudoaneurysm formation, and/or arterioportal shunting. A cyst may demonstrate mass effect but is, by definition, avascular. Similar to the characteristic imaging features on CECT and MRI, liver hemangiomas display discontinuous peripheral nodular contrast accumulation with slow central fill-in.

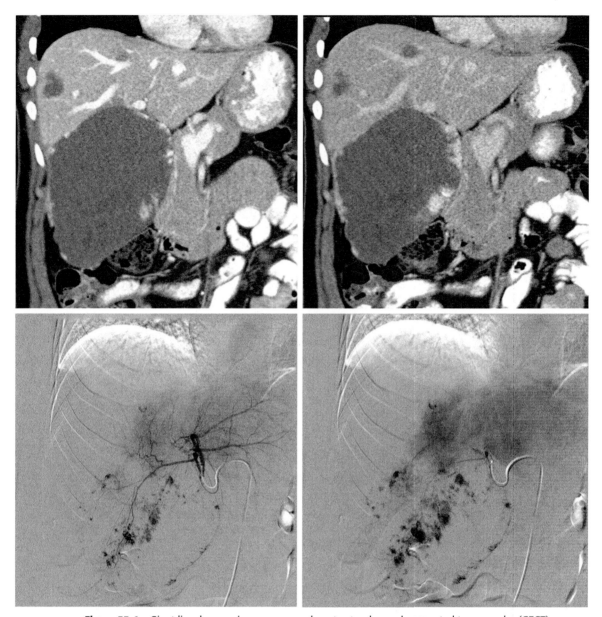

Figure 33-1   Giant liver hemangioma on coronal contrast-enhanced computed tomography (CECT) with corresponding hepatic arteriogram. Note the early (left) discontinuous peripheral nodular enhancement with gradual fill in on the delayed phase (right).

References: Fielding L. Current imaging strategies of primary and secondary neoplasms of the liver. *Semin Intervent Radiol.* 2006;23(1):3-12.

Watson RC, Baltaxe HA. The angiographic appearance of primary and secondary tumors of the liver. *Radiology.* 1971;101(3):539-548.

34   **Answer C.**   The angiographic images demonstrate an oval hypervascular mass encompassing and replacing the proximal left humerus. Certain cancers such as renal cell carcinoma have a predilection for the bone and can be quite hypervascular. Resection and reconstruction can be a daunting task for the surgeon in this scenario, with significant operative blood loss at stake. Preoperative angiography and embolization, often with particles and sometimes adjunctive coil occlusion of large feeders, can reduce the vascularity of the tumor and reduce operative blood loss. In many locations, treatment must be performed carefully with subsequent selection

of direct tumor feeders to prevent nontarget embolization of healthy tissue. In this case, inadvertent administration of particles and/or coils into the brachial artery would be catastrophic and almost certainly result in limb-threatening ischemia.

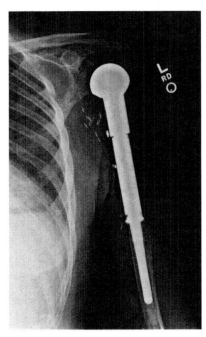

Figure 34-1 Radiograph following preoperative embolization, resection of bony metastasis, and reconstruction of the humerus. Operative blood loss was only 100 mL.

References: Chatziioannou AN, Johnson ME, Pneumaticos SG, Lawrence DD, Carrasco CH. Preoperative embolization of bone metastases from renal cell carcinoma. *Eur Radiol.* 2000;10(4):593-596.

Rilling WS, Chen GW. Preoperative embolization. *Semin Intervent Radiol.* 2004;21(1):3-9.

35 **Answer B.** NASCET demonstrated significant benefit to carotid endarterectomy in symptomatic patients with internal carotid artery stenosis measuring 70% to 99%. In this pivotal trial, a specific measurement of stenosis was used, and the method has been used in several additional key studies. The percent stenosis measured on the angiogram was defined as (1 − [internal carotid artery stenosis diameter/internal carotid artery normal diameter]) × 100. In the provided angiogram centered at the carotid arterial bifurcation, the external carotid artery is easily identified by its multiple side branches, whereas the cervical internal carotid artery has none. Based on the measurements provided, the percent stenosis is (1 − [1/4]) × 100 or 75%.

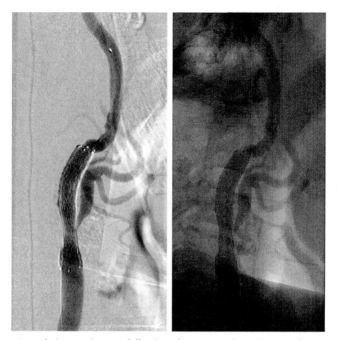

Figure 35-1 Completion angiogram following placement of a self-expanding uncovered stent across a severe stenosis in the proximal internal carotid artery (ICA). Note the embolic protection device in the distal segment of the ICA. The stent covers the ostium of the external carotid artery, which stills fills in antegrade fashion.

References: Barnett HJM, Taylor DW, Haynes RB, et al. Beneficial effect of carotid endarterectomy in symptomatic patients with high-grade carotid stenosis. *N Engl J Med.* 1991;325(7):445-453.

Cheng EM, Bravata DM, El-Saden S, et al. Carotid artery stenosis: wide variability in reporting formats–a review of 127 veterans affairs medical centers. *Radiology.* 2013;266(1):289-294.

36 **Answer D.**   While physicians who practice IR as a specialty pride themselves on problem-solving and creative solutions for patient care, one must know the benefits and indications of alternative methods of treatment. This case demonstrates a densely calcified atherosclerotic plaque throughout the proximal to mid common femoral artery that appears occlusive. The endovascular options here are limited, and surgical endarterectomy is the treatment of choice. Guidelines, such as the Trans-Atlantic inter-Society Consensus (TASC) II, exist to help with management decisions in the realm of peripheral arterial disease. Pathology is graded as level A, B, C, and D. For level A disease, endovascular treatment is strongly preferred; for level D disease, surgical treatment is strongly preferred.

Reference: Norgren L, Hiatt WR, Dormandy JA, et al. Inter-society consensus for the management of peripheral arterial disease (TASC II). *J Vasc Surg.* 2007;45(suppl S):S5-S67.

37 **Answer A.**   The arteriogram of the wrist and hand shows corkscrew collateral formation in the distribution of the first digit, as well as a distal ulnar artery occlusion. Note the intact deep and superficial palmar arches. These findings in a relatively young male are most characteristic of Buerger disease aka thromboangiitis obliterans. Small- and medium-sized arteries and veins of the extremities are most commonly affected. Tobacco use is ubiquitous in these patients, and cessation is arguably the most important treatment strategy. Although corkscrew collaterals are often associated with Buerger disease, they can be seen with other diseases affecting the small arteries of the extremities and have been demonstrated to represent hypertrophied vasa vasorum or vasa nervorum. The appearance of well-formed collateral vessels points to more chronic pathology, making an acute process such as septic emboli less likely. Atherosclerosis would be rare in a young person, and

is uncommon peripheral to the subclavian level. A more central atherosclerotic lesion near a great vessel origin can shower atheroemboli, producing downstream short-segment occlusions, often involving the digital arteries (not seen here). Raynaud disease can be primary (no underlying disease) or secondary (associated with underlying diseases such as scleroderma). Primary Raynaud disease often presents with a history of digital pallor or cyanosis with cold exposure or emotional stress followed by a reperfusion hyperemia. With severe Raynaud disease (often secondary), critical digital ischemia can occur and angiography may demonstrate a variety of findings including stenosis, occlusion, and vasospasm.

References: Bozlar U, Ogur T, Khaja MS, All J, Norton PT, Hagspiel KD. CT angiography of the upper extremity arterial system: part 2- clinical applications beyond trauma patients. *AJR Am J Roentgenol.* 2013;201(4):753-763.

Dimmick SJ, Goh AC, Cauzza E, et al. Imaging appearances of Buerger's disease complications in the upper and lower limbs. *Clin Radiol.* 2012;67(12):1207-1211.

Kim YH, Ng SW, Seo HS, Chang Ahn H. Classification of Raynaud's disease based on angiographic features. *J Plast Reconstr Aesthet Surg.* 2011;64(11):1503-1511.

Mcmahan ZH, Wigley FM. Raynaud's phenomenon and digital ischemia: a practical approach to risk stratification, diagnosis and management. *Int J Clin Rheumtol.* 2010;5(3):355-370.

38 **Answer C.** An abdominal aortic aneurysm is most commonly defined as aortic diameter >3.0 cm or diameter 1.5x normal. When considering abdominal aortic aneurysm treatment, cross-sectional imaging can evaluate a number of features that may affect the decision to treat with open or endovascular techniques.

- Aneurysm neck length, diameter, angulation, and atherosclerotic disease
  - The neck is critical for the attachment of the endograft to the aortic wall. A poor proximal seal can result in immediate or delayed type I endoleak, as well as stent graft migration.
- Accessory renal arteries
  - Although not a contraindication, coverage may infarct part of the kidney and can also provide a path for future endoleak.
- Small (<7 mm), diseased, and/or tortuous iliofemoral arterial system
  - Difficulty with access and device passage.
- Aneurysmal common or external iliac arteries
  - Difficulty with achieving a distal seal that may necessitate stent graft extensions.
- Occluded internal iliac arteries
  - Increased risk of buttock claudication and impotence after EVAR.
- Preexisting mesenteric arterial disease
  - Increased risk of mesenteric ischemia as IMA will be covered during EVAR.

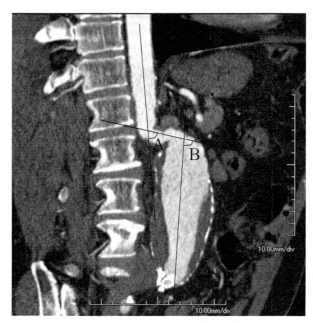

Figure 38-1   Reconstructed image from computed tomography angiography (CTA) performed to evaluate abdominal aortic aneurysm (AAA) demonstrating measurements for the aortic neck angulation (suprarenal angle, A; infrarenal angle, B). For routine endovascular aneurysm repair (EVAR), angle B is most relevant, with angles above 45° to 60° conferring an increased risk of post-EVAR complications. This case demonstrates severe (>60°) aortic neck angulation at both A and B.

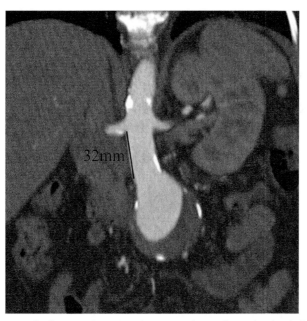

Figure 38-2   Coronal reformatted computed tomography angiography (CTA) demonstrating the infrarenal aortic neck measurement. Note the lack of neck tapering and paucity of underlying atherosclerotic disease. This neck will provide a good proximal seal between the endograft and aortic wall during endovascular aneurysm repair (EVAR).

References: Bryce Y, Rogoff P, Romanelli D, Reichle R. Endovascular repair of abdominal aortic aneurysms: vascular anatomy, device selection, procedure, and procedure-specific complications. *Radiographics*. 2015;35(2):593-615.

Kicska G, Litt H. Preprocedural planning for endovascular stent-graft placement. *Semin Intervent Radiol*. 2009;26(1):44-55.

Picel AC, Kansal N. Essentials of endovascular abdominal aortic aneurysm repair imaging: preprocedural assessment. *AJR Am J Roentgenol*. 2014;203(4):W347-W357.

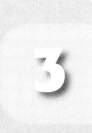
Venous Interventions

1 Which is a prophylactic indication for inferior vena cava (IVC) filter placement?

   A. Contraindication to anticoagulation in the setting of lower extremity deep vein thrombosis (DVT)
   B. Massive pulmonary embolism (PE) with residual lower extremity DVT
   C. Severe traumatic injury without known DVT
   D. Free floating iliac or femoral DVT
   E. Recurrent PE despite anticoagulation

2 A 35-year-old man presents with right leg swelling and is diagnosed with right lower extremity DVT involving the femoral and popliteal veins on duplex ultrasound. The left lower extremity demonstrates no deep vein thrombosis. A cavogram is performed before IVC filter placement. What is the most likely diagnosis?

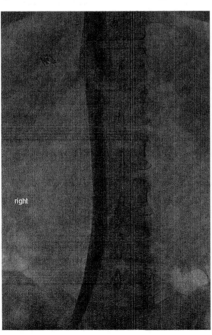
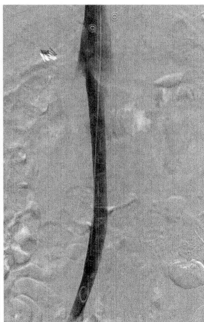

   A. Left iliac venous thrombosis
   B. May-Thurner syndrome
   C. Duplicated IVC
   D. Circumaortic left renal vein
   E. Azygous continuation of the IVC

3   With a duplicated IVC, where does the left-sided IVC drain?

A. Right atrium
B. Azygos vein
C. Left renal vein
D. Hemiazygos vein

4   If a patient with known duplicated IVC is in need of filter placement for lower extremity DVT, which of the following is the preferred approach?

A. No filter as it is contraindicated with this anatomy
B. Suprarenal IVC filter
C. Right infrarenal IVC filter
D. Superior vena cava filter

5   Which answer choice best summarizes the 2010 FDA Safety Communication (updated in 2014) regarding retrievable IVC filters?

A. Implanting physicians should not place retrievable IVC filters because of increased long-term risk of filter-associated complications when compared with permanent type filters
B. Implanting physicians should consider removing retrievable IVC filters when they are no longer medically needed for protection from PE.
C. Implanting physicians are responsible for following patients with retrievable IVC filters and are obligated to contact them regarding potential retrieval procedure
D. Implanting physicians should consider filter retrieval at 100 to 150 days from initial placement, as analysis of prior studies indicates that the risk/benefit profile begins to favor removal after this time period

6   Before central venous catheter placement, the radiology technologist asks you to look at the right internal jugular vein because it "looks funny." What is the diagnosis?

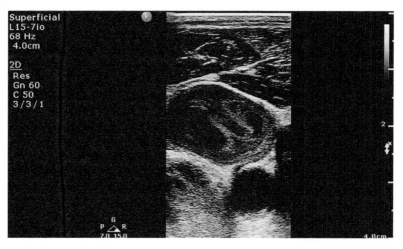

A. Slow flow
B. Acute thrombosis
C. Chronic occlusion
D. Air embolism

7 A patient on chronic hemodialysis presents for evaluation of a palpable subcutaneous nodule (arrows) just below the right clavicle. He has had several tunneled hemodialysis catheters in the past few years. What is the patient feeling on examination?

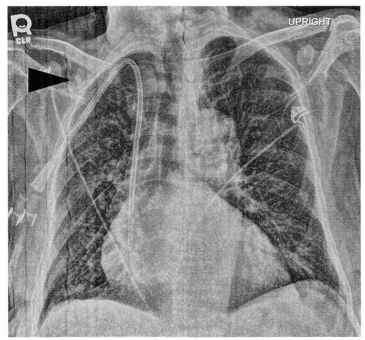
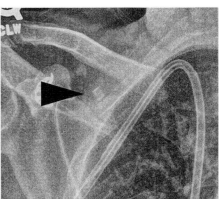

A. Retained cuff
B. Calciphylaxis
C. Calcified aneurysm
D. Fractured venous stent

8 Based on these images, which is the path a red blood cell will take in the right upper extremity of this patient with end-stage renal disease?

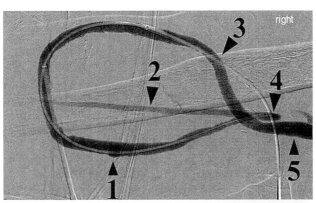
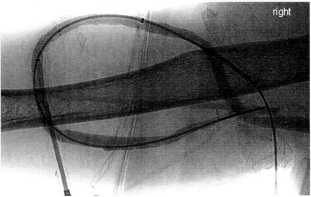

A. $2 \rightarrow 4 \rightarrow 3 \rightarrow 1 \rightarrow 5$
B. $4 \rightarrow 3 \rightarrow 1 \rightarrow 5$
C. $5 \rightarrow 3 \rightarrow 1 \rightarrow 4 \rightarrow 2$
D. $4 \rightarrow 1 \rightarrow 3 \rightarrow 5$

9   In this patient on hemodialysis with a left elbow brachiocephalic arteriovenous fistula, what physical examination finding will be encountered at the arrow?

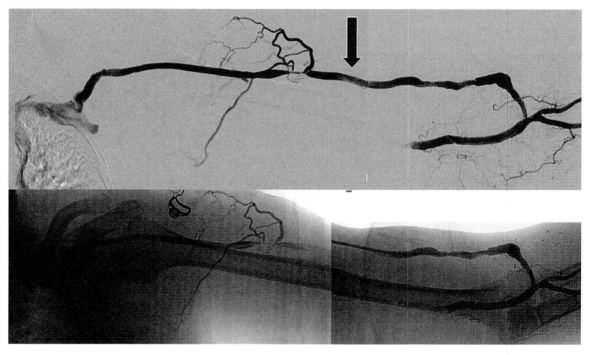

A. Nothing palpable
B. Nonpulsatile thrill
C. Pulsatile flow
D. Active bleeding

10   Which of these patients on hemodialysis would present with the indication of "prolonged bleeding" from their access after needle decannulation?

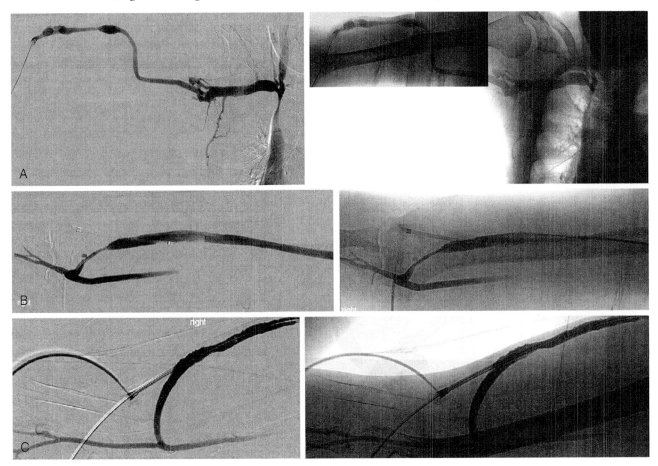

A. A
B. B
C. C

11   A 59-year-old man with a history of left lower extremity DVT involving the common femoral vein, femoral vein, and popliteal vein has been therapeutic with anticoagulation for 12 months. He now presents for evaluation of a new ulceration along the medial aspect of the left ankle with progressive swelling, pain, and skin hyperpigmentation in the distal leg. There is a palpable left dorsalis pedis pulse. A left lower extremity venous duplex shows complete recanalization of previously seen DVT and no evidence of an acute thrombus. There is insufficiency in the femoral vein. For which underlying condition should the patient be evaluated?

A. Right-sided heart failure
B. Iliac venous obstruction
C. Concomitant peripheral arterial disease
D. Duplicated IVC

12   A 28-year-old woman presents with progressive left lower extremity swelling, pain, and varicose veins. Venous duplex examination shows what pathology?

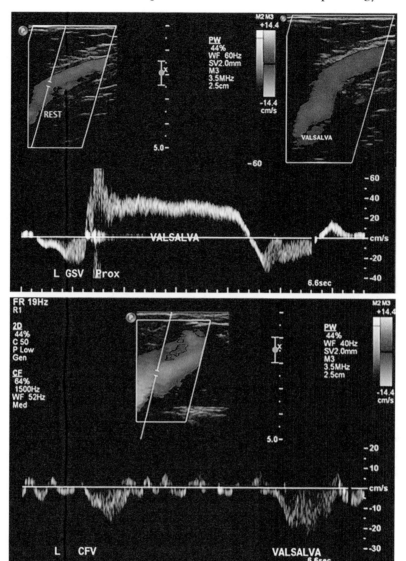

A. Deep venous insufficiency
B. Superficial venous insufficiency
C. Arteriovenous fistula
D. Pelvic venous obstruction

13   In a patient diagnosed with symptomatic left great saphenous venous insufficiency, which of the following is the preferred treatment?

A. Closure of the left great saphenous vein with endovenous ablation
B. Pelvic venogram with stenting
C. Coil embolization of the left great saphenous vein
D. Vein valve transplant

14   A man on chronic hemodialysis presents for evaluation of his femoral access. What
is the best description of the access type?

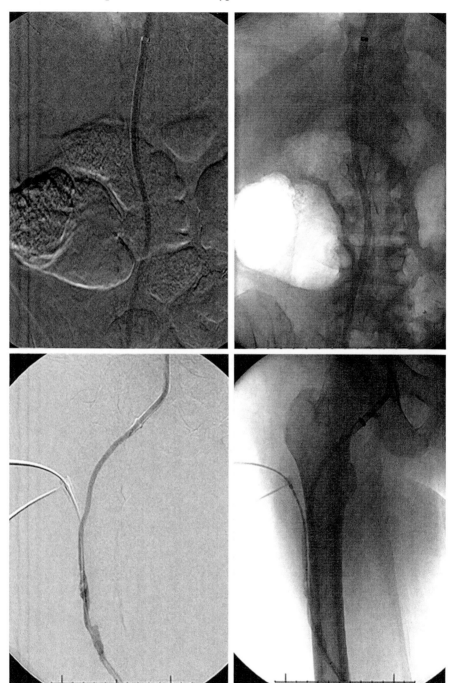

A. Tunneled hemodialysis catheter
B. Nontunneled hemodialysis catheter
C. Arteriovenous fistula with stented IVC
D. Hemodialysis reliable outflow (HeRO) graft

15   A thrombosed forearm loop AVG is successfully declotted. A diagnostic angiogram
of the graft is then performed to evaluate for underlying stenosis. What do the
regions of irregular increased caliber most likely represent (arrowheads)?

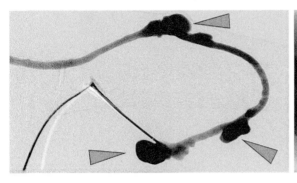 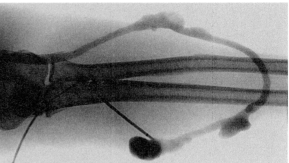

A. Mycotic aneurysm
B. Graft degeneration
C. Active extravasation
D. Collateral veins

16   A 44-year-old patient presents for evaluation of a dysfunctional arteriovenous
fistula. Angiography identifies a venous outflow stenosis in the upper arm, which is
treated with balloon angioplasty. Based on the sequential DSA images after angioplasty, what should be done next?

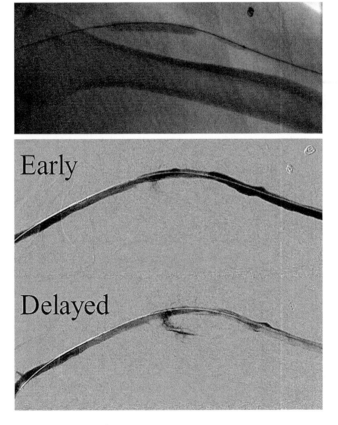

A. No intervention required
B. Coil embolization
C. Reinflate balloon
D. Emergent surgical revision

17 Which of the following measurements is consistent with a mature arteriovenous fistula for hemodialysis?

    A. Venous outflow flow rate of 800 mL/min

    B. Venous outflow diameter of 3.5 mm

    C. Venous outflow depth of 10 mm from the skin

    D. Venous outflow pressure of 6 mmHg

18 A patient new to hemodialysis presents for placement of a cuffed tunneled central venous catheter. Before prepping the access site, ultrasound of the neck demonstrates chronic occlusion of the right and left internal jugular veins. Which of the following is the next best access site?

    A. Right axillosubclavian vein

    B. Right common femoral vein

    C. Right external jugular vein

    D. Right hepatic vein

19 Which of the following IVC filters is a retrievable type?

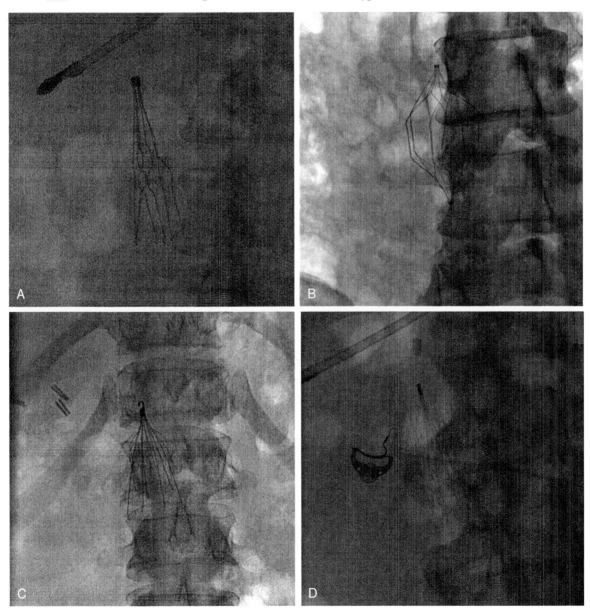

A. A
B. B
C. C
D. D

20   A 65-year-old man had an IVC filter placed for lower DVT in the setting of a contra-indication to anticoagulation. The contraindication has resolved in the last month, and he is now therapeutic on Coumadin for 3 weeks. He presents for filter retrieval, and a venogram is obtained. What is the next step in management?

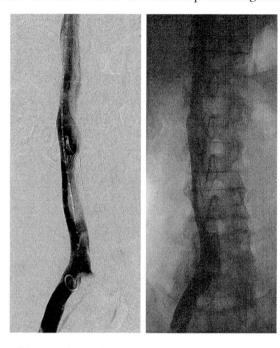

A. Retrieve the filter as planned
B. Continue anticoagulation and bring him back for a repeat venogram and possible retrieval in 2 months
C. Abort procedure and keep filter in for life
D. Place a suprarenal IVC filter

21   A 55-year-old patient presents for IVC filter placement. What abnormality is present on the venogram?

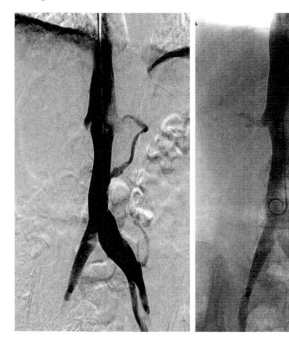

 A. Circumaortic renal vein
 B. Absent hepatic veins
 C. Aortocaval fistula
 D. Duplicated IVC

22   At what diameter is the IVC considered a "megacava"?

 A. 18 mm
 B. 28 mm
 C. 38 mm
 D. 48 mm

23   A left neck approach central venous catheter is placed by the ICU team. The catheter has intermittent difficulty with aspiration, and the IR team is asked to evaluate its position. Which is the best next step to determine management?

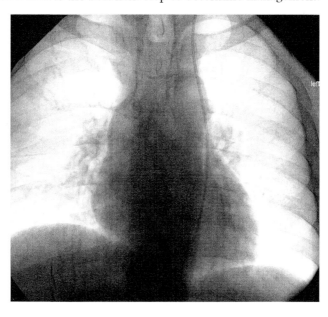

A. Catheter angiogram
B. CTA of the chest
C. Review old imaging studies
D. Ultrasound of accessed neck vessel

24   Describe the vascular course of this functioning tunneled central venous catheter.

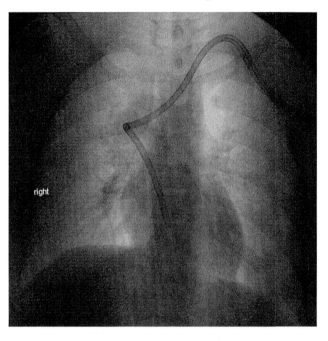

A. Left IJ vein >> left brachiocephalic vein >> SVC >> azygos vein
B. Left IJ vein >> left brachiocephalic vein >> SVC >> RA
C. Left IJ vein >> left brachiocephalic vein >> hemiazygos vein
D. Left IJ vein >> left brachiocephalic vein >> RA >> RV >> Main PA

25 A 65-year-old woman with end stage renal disease on hemodialysis presents for evaluation of a dysfunctional arteriovenous graft in the right upper extremity. What is the location of the culprit lesion?

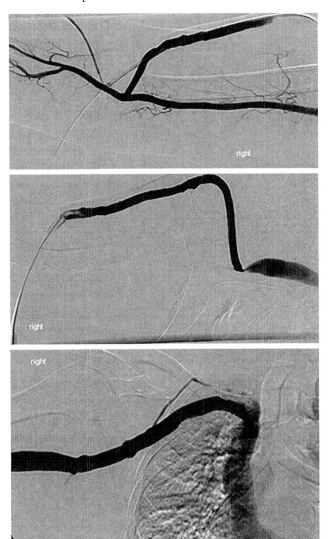

A. Arterial anastomosis
B. Mid-graft
C. Venous anastomosis
D. Central veins

26 The overnight radiology resident is consulted regarding a patient with "extreme" lower extremity DVT. Which of the following is the most critical piece of information that should be obtained to appropriately triage the care of this patient?

A. Unilateral versus bilateral lower extremity DVT
B. IVC involvement
C. Lower extremity pulse examination
D. Hypercoagulable history

27   An 18-year-old avid swimmer presents with 24 hours of a painful and swollen left arm. The following images are obtained as part of the same procedure. Which of the following is the next best step?

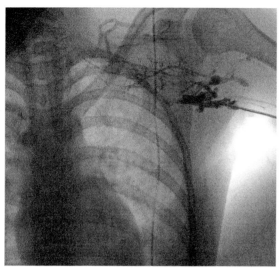 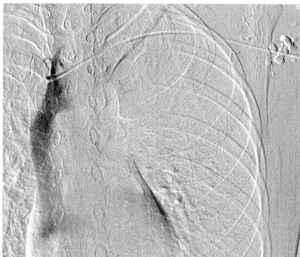

A. Coil embolization
B. Covered stent placement
C. Catheter-directed thrombolysis
D. SVC filter placement

28   A 2-year-old has a portacath placed for chemotherapy. A few months later, the patient presents for difficulty with access, and frontal and lateral radiographs are obtained. What is the most likely issue?

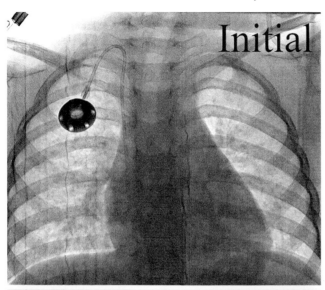

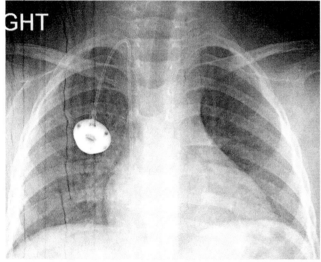

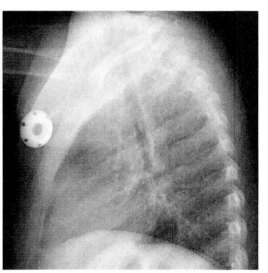

A. Catheter tip malpositioned
B. Reservoir detached from the catheter
C. Fibrin sheath
D. Reservoir malpositioned

29   A 33-year-old man presents with extensive venous thrombosis of the right lower extremity, extending from the popliteal vein to the common iliac vein. He is appropriately anticoagulated with intravenous heparin and then treated with adjunctive catheter-directed thrombolysis using tPA (tissue plasminogen activator). This is successful in clearing virtually all of the acute clot, and the swelling subsides quickly. His hospital course is prolonged by an acquired pneumonia, and during this time, he is continued on systemic heparin. Eight days after completion of his venous procedure, his right leg becomes swollen and extensive rethrombosis is confirmed on ultrasound.

Admission day labs	Rethrombosis day labs
Hemoglobin: 13.6 g/dL	Hemoglobin: 11.0 g/dL
WBC: 8.7 10e9/L	WBC: 13.2 10e9/L
Creatinine: 0.9 mg/dL	Creatinine: 1.5 mg/dL
Platelets: 380,000/µL	Platelets: 155,000/µL

Which lab value most likely explains his venous rethrombosis?

A. Hemoglobin
B. WBC
C. Creatinine
D. Platelets

30   Which of the following is the best approach to this finding?

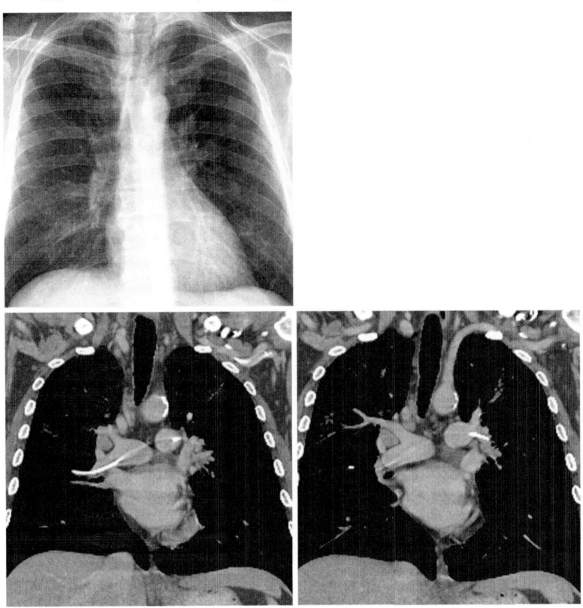

    A. Common femoral vein access for intervention
    B. Common femoral artery access for intervention
    C. Lifelong anticoagulation
    D. Surgical consult

ANSWERS AND EXPLANATIONS

1   **Answer C.**   Indications for IVC filter placement are categorized as "therapeutic" or "prophylactic." The clear difference here is that patients with a "therapeutic" indication have established venous thromboembolic (VTE) disease, whereas those for "prophylactic" are deemed at significant risk of a future event.

TABLE 1-1   Indications for IVC Filter Placement

Therapeutic	Prophylactic
• Contraindication to AC	• Severe traumatic injury
• Complication of AC	• Closed head injury
• Failure of AC (new DVT/PE despite AC)	• Spinal cord injury
• Inability to maintain/achieve adequate AC	• High-risk orthotrauma (long bone fracture, pelvic fracture)
• Massive PE with residual DVT	• Patients deemed high risk of VTE event (prolonged immobilization, etc.)
• DVT with low cardiopulmonary reserve	
• Free floating iliofemoral DVT or IVC thrombus	

Adapted from Caplin DM, Nikolic B, Kalva SP, et al. Quality improvement guidelines for the performance of inferior vena cava filter placement for the prevention of pulmonary embolism. *J Vasc Interv Radiol*. 2011;22(11):1499-1506.
AC, anticoagulation.

Reference: Caplin DM, Nikolic B, Kalva SP, et al. Quality improvement guidelines for the performance of inferior vena cava filter placement for the prevention of pulmonary embolism. *J Vasc Interv Radiol*. 2011;22(11):1499-1506.

2   **Answer C.**   Native and subtracted images from inferior venacavogram demonstrate a widely patent right common iliac vein that smoothly transitions to the infrarenal segment of the IVC. Notice that the caliber of the infrarenal IVC does not change significantly at the level of the presumed common iliac vein confluence. Also, there is no inflow of unopacified blood from the left common iliac vein. Together, these findings support the diagnosis of duplicated IVC. Left common iliac vein thrombosis can have a similar appearance; however, there is typically some irregularity of flow or even a partially visualized filling defect protruding from the vein ostium at the confluence. With normal anatomy, the infrarenal IVC usually has a larger caliber than depicted in the case example. May-Thurner syndrome is a vascular phenomenon classically occurring on the left because of pulsatile compression injury by the right common iliac artery on the left common iliac vein. It presents as left lower extremity swelling, and the affected vein may be thrombosed or demonstrate fenestrations and webs with collateral vein formation. Circumaortic left renal vein is the most common renal venous anomaly (reported prevalence up to 17% of patients) whereby the normal preaortic left renal vein is present in

addition to a retroaortic left renal vein. It is an important anomaly as filter placement between the left renal veins exposes a potential pathway for a thrombus to embolize to the heart and lungs from the lower extremities. Azygos continuation of the IVC is the absence of a normal intrahepatic IVC portion. There is normal position and appearance of the visualized suprarenal IVC excluding this option.

References: Al-Katib S, Shetty M, Jafri SM, Jafri SZ. Radiologic assessment of native renal vasculature: a multimodality review. *Radiographics*. 2017;37(1):136-156.

Smillie RP, Shetty M, Boyer AC, Madrazo B, Jafri SZ. Imaging evaluation of the inferior vena cava. *Radiographics*. 2015;35(2):578-592.

3 **Answer C.**   Duplicated IVC (prevalence 0.2%-0.3%) is due to persistence of both supracardinal veins forming right and left infrarenal IVC segments. The left infrarenal IVC segment classically drains into the left renal vein. The right infrarenal IVC receives the right and left renal veins, forming a normal suprarenal IVC.

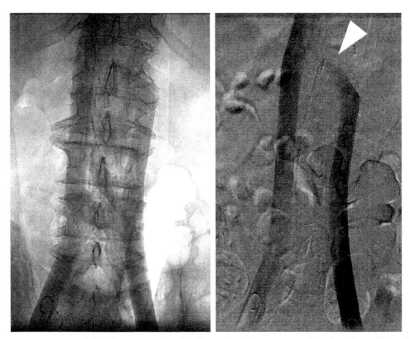

Figure 3-1 Venography demonstrating duplicated IVC anatomy. Notice that the caliber of the common iliac veins roughly matches the right and left infrarenal IVC segments. The left infrarenal IVC segment drains into the left renal vein (arrowhead) at the level of L1.

Reference: Smillie RP, Shetty M, Boyer AC, Madrazo B, Jafri SZ. Imaging evaluation of the inferior vena cava. *Radiographics*. 2015;35(2):578-592.

4 **Answer B.**   In the scenario of a duplicated IVC, there are traditionally 2 options. A single filter can be placed in a suprarenal location or separate filters can be deployed in each infrarenal moiety. Clearly, a filter placed in the superior vena cava will have no effect on the prevention of PE from lower extremity DVT.

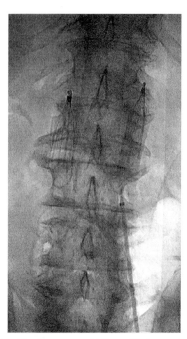

Figure 4-1 Duplicated IVC with placement of bilateral infrarenal IVC filters. Although many cases demonstrate completely separate infrarenal IVC segments, occasionally there can be venous connections between the infrarenal IVC segments.

References: Malgor RD, Oropallo A, Wood E, Natan K, Labropoulos N. Filter placement for duplicated cava. *Vasc Endovascular Surg.* 2011;45(3):269-273.

Smillie RP, Shetty M, Boyer AC, Madrazo B, Jafri SZ. Imaging evaluation of the inferior vena cava. *Radiographics.* 2015;35(2):578-592.

5   **Answer B.**   IVC filters come in 2 types: permanent and retrievable. Permanent filters are designed to be left in place and do not have features built into the design to facilitate easy removal. Retrievable filters are designed for both long-term (permanent) and short-term (temporary) usage. The filter design includes a hook at the apex of the filter (or some other feature to engage with a removal device) that can be secured with a snare or other device to allow for the filter to be safely and securely withdrawn into a sheath for complete removal. Over the past several years, there has been increasing attention within the medical and lay press regarding filter-associated complications, particularly among retrievable type filters. Complications seen include strut/leg penetration into surrounding structures, filter fracture and/or migration, and venous thrombosis. In 2010, the FDA produced a communication to medical professionals to help guide the care of patients with IVC filters. The communication is available online through the FDA website. Choice B accurately reflects the recommendation for implanting physicians. Choice A is incorrect as the communication does not prohibit the use of retrievable filters. The communication "encourages" both implanting physicians and responsible providers to consider the risks and benefits of filter removal for each patient. Obligatory communication is not delineated (choice C incorrect). The communication discusses that research suggests that the risk/benefit profile favors removal of an IVC filter between 29 and 54 days after implantation (choice D incorrect).

References: Morales JP, Li X, Irony TZ, Ibrahim NG, Moynahan M, Cavanaugh KJ. Decision analysis of retrievable inferior vena cava filters in patients without pulmonary embolism. *J Vasc Surg Venous Lymphat Disord.* 2013;1(4):376-384.

Wadhwa V, Trivedi PS, Chatterjee K, et al. Decreasing utilization of inferior vena cava filters in post-FDA warning era: insights from 2005 to 2014 nationwide inpatient sample. *J Am Coll Radiol.* 2017;14(9):1144-1150.

6   Answer A.   To interpret the ultrasound image, first identify the internal jugular vein. It is an ovoid structure situated between the superficial neck musculature and the deeper circular anechoic common carotid artery. The echotexture of the vein is heterogeneous with a swirled appearance. This appearance is not consistent with acute clot, which is more uniform in echotexture (most often hypoechoic) and produces venous distention. A chronically occluded jugular vein is diminutive in size, often difficult to find, and tends to have a hyperechoic thrombus. If there is a visible chronic thrombus, recanalization channels may be present. Also, prominent collaterals are often seen elsewhere in the neck. The sonographic appearance of slow flow (choice A correct) has been attributed to rouleaux red blood cell formation, whereby stacked or clumped red blood cells become sonographic reflectors producing curvilinear and swirling echoes as seen in the case image. The most important next step in evaluation is to perform compression ultrasound to obliterate the lumen and confirm patency, which was done next in this case. With intravenous air, mobile nondependent hyperechoic foci with shadowing will be present.

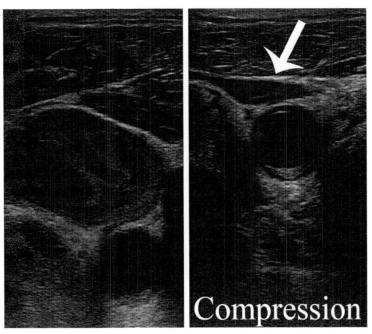

Figure 6-1   Images from the case example with compression show obliteration of the venous lumen (arrow) confirming patency. The finding of slow flow should not be ignored as this may be a hint that there is a central venous obstruction beyond the field of view.

References: Albertyn LE, Alcock MK. Diagnosis of internal jugular vein thrombosis. *Radiology.* 1987;162(2):505-508.

Blanco P, Volpicelli G. Common pitfalls in point-of-care ultrasound: a practical guide for emergency and critical care physicians. *Crit Ultrasound J.* 2016;8(1):15.

7   Answer A.   On radiography, the finding of interest is a calcium density with a rectangular shape just below the right clavicle. Given the history of multiple tunneled hemodialysis catheters, the abnormality most likely represents a calcified retained polyester cuff from a previous catheter. A retained cuff is not uncommon, but they do not always calcify. The rectangular shape is clearly not physiologic therefore cannot represent calciphylaxis or a calcified aneurysm. The size and shape is not consistent with a venous stent.

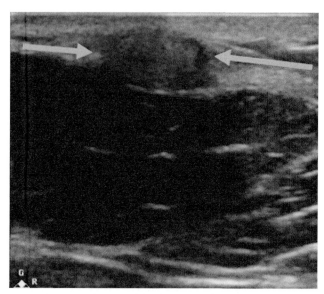

Figure 7-1   Companion case of a noncalcified retained dialysis catheter cuff (arrows) on grayscale ultrasonoghraphy.

References: Huang BK, Hubeny CM, Dogra VS. Sonographic appearance of a retained tunneled catheter cuff causing a foreign body reaction. *J Ultrasound Med*. 2009;28(2):245-248.

Kohli MD, Trerotola SO, Namyslowski J, et al. Outcome of polyester cuff retention following traction removal of tunneled central venous catheters. *Radiology*. 2001;219(3):651-654.

8   **Answer D.**   Dialysis access work is admittedly disorienting when first encountered. This case demonstrates a right upper extremity arteriovenous graft (AVG). With AVGs, there is an inflow artery anastomosed to a prosthetic tube graft. The graft is typically straight or looped, and then is anastomosed to a larger draining vein. The graft serves as a conduit for blood and dialysis needle insertion. In this case, there are 2 short vascular sheaths in the graft segment. There is a diagnostic catheter-directed retrograde (against the direction of flow) with its tip residing in the brachial artery just upstream from the arterial anastomosis at position #4. Blood will flow from the inflow artery into the graft (4 >> 1), travel through the graft (1 >> 3), and finally out of the graft into the venous outflow (3 >> 5). Position #2 represents the downstream brachial artery, which opacifies when contrast is injected near the arterial anastomosis and fills both parent artery and graft.

References: Quencer KB, Friedman T. Declotting the thrombosed access. *Tech Vasc Interv Radiol*. 2017;20(1):38-47.

Zaleski G. Declotting, maintenance, and avoiding procedural complications of native arteriovenous fistulae. *Semin Intervent Radiol*. 2004;21(2):83-93.

9   **Answer C.**   Physical examination is an important adjunct to the angiographic evaluation of the dysfunction hemodialysis access. The images demonstrate a patent arterial anastomosis between the brachial artery at the elbow and the cephalic vein. There is a short-segment severe stenosis in the mid-upper-arm cephalic vein, with collateral venous formation. As a result of increased resistance from the stenosis, there is upstream high pressure, which translates to pulsatile flow on examination at the designated location. If there was no such stenotic region, there would be a nonpulsatile thrill on examination. If there were nothing palpable, this would be most consistent with arteriovenous fistula thrombosis. The images show collateral formation, not active bleeding.

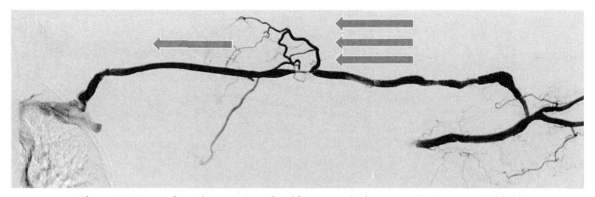

Figure 9-1 Image from the case example with pressure in the access circuit represented by the arrows.

References: Quencer KB, Arici M. Arteriovenous fistulas and their characteristic sites of stenosis. *AJR Am J Roentgenol.* 2015;205(4):726-734.

Quencer KB, Friedman T. Declotting the thrombosed access. *Tech Vasc Interv Radiol.* 2017;20(1):38-47.

Whittier WL. Surveillance of hemodialysis vascular access. *Semin Intervent Radiol.* 2009;26(2):130-138.

10 **Answer A.**   The provided indication for a hemodialysis access evaluation can often lead the IR physician to the site of pathology. If the dialysis unit or patient reports prolonged bleeding after needle decannulation, this implies that the pressure within the dialysis circuit is increased because of outflow obstruction. Other signs include reduced flow in the circuit and high return pressures on the dialysis machine. Images from choice A demonstrate a severe stenosis in the central veins, specifically the right innominate vein, with retrograde flow up the internal jugular vein. As this location is downstream from the needle cannulation sites, it will produce elevated pressures in the circuit, making it the best choice. Images from choice B demonstrate a severe stenosis just beyond the arterial anastomosis of a radiocephalic arteriovenous fistula. This lesion will produce diminished flow in the circuit and high negative inflow pressures on the dialysis machine and often reported clinically as "difficulty with cannulation." Images from choice C demonstrate the normal appearance of the arterial anastomosis of an AVG.

References: Quencer KB, Arici M. Arteriovenous fistulas and their characteristic sites of stenosis. *AJR Am J Roentgenol.* 2015;205(4):726-734.

Whittier WL. Surveillance of hemodialysis vascular access. *Semin Intervent Radiol.* 2009;26(2):130-138.

Zaleski G. Declotting, maintenance, and avoiding procedural complications of native arteriovenous fistulae. *Semin Intervent Radiol.* 2004;21(2):83-93.

11   **Answer B.**   The patient presents with signs and symptoms that are not congruent with the venous duplex findings, which should raise suspicion for unseen pathology. In this case, the patient had extensive left lower extremity femoropopliteal DVT with excellent recanalization. He had signs and symptoms of worsening post-thrombotic syndrome despite the duplex result. Lower extremity venous outflow obstruction can be difficult to evaluate on duplex examination and, if present, can lead to significant lower extremity symptoms. Abdominopelvic imaging is warranted. The clinical findings suggest ongoing venous pathology with no mention of right leg problems, making choice A less likely. Concomitant peripheral arterial disease is important to consider with nonhealing wounds, but the location of the ulcer and associated symptoms again support an underlying venous problem. Also, with a palpable pedal pulse, significant arterial obstruction is very unlikely.

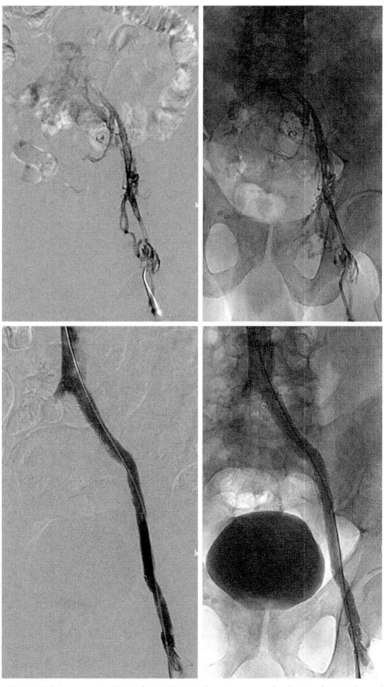

Figure 11-1   Pelvic venogram from the patient in the case example shows chronic thrombosis of the left external and common iliac veins with collateral formation and cross pelvic filling (top images). After recanalization and stenting, there is excellent in-line venous outflow for the left lower extremity (bottom images). The patient's ulcer healed in 1 month, and swelling was markedly improved.

At this point, it is good to review the entity of May-Thurner syndrome. There is a natural compression point in the body where the left common iliac vein travels between the more superficial right common iliac artery and deeper lumbar spine. Although this is normal anatomy, in a subset of people, pathologic changes in the vein can occur producing acute and chronic venous obstruction. At venography, different obliquities should be assessed to evaluate for stenosis, acute and chronic thrombus, webs and fenestrations, as well as collateral filling. Intravascular ultrasound (IVUS) is an important adjunct especially when the venogram appears normal.

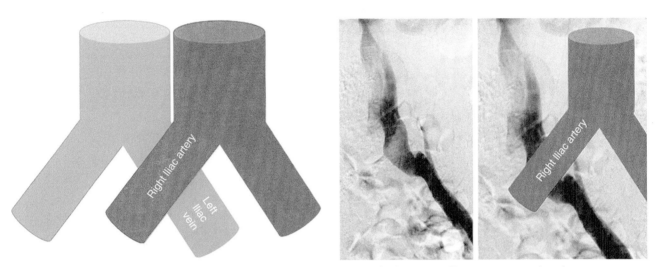

Figure 11-2   Diagrammatic and venographic appearance of right common iliac artery compression of the left common iliac vein. IVUS demonstrated >60% luminal narrowing in the left common iliac vein.

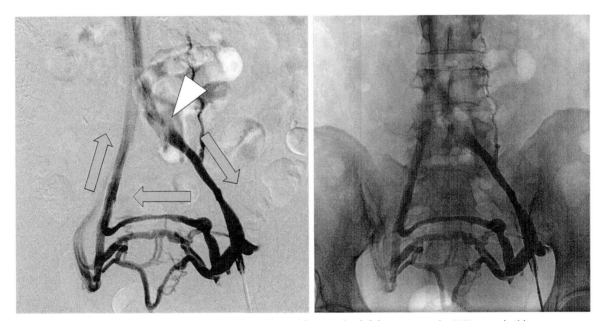

Figure 11-3   Companion case of a patient with extensive left lower extremity DVT treated with catheter-directed lysis. Image obtained after excellent result with tPA reveals an underlying May-Thurner lesion (white arrowhead) in the left common iliac vein, which was subsequently treated with balloon angioplasty and stenting. Preexisting collateral veins (blue arrows) circumvent the obstruction with left-to-right cross pelvic venous drainage.

References: Knuttinen MG, Naidu S, Oklu R, et al. May-Thurner: diagnosis and endovascular management. *Cardiovasc Diagn Ther*. 2017;7(suppl 3):S159-S164.

Neglén P. Chronic deep venous obstruction: definition, prevalence, diagnosis, management. *Phlebology*. 2008;23(4):149-157.

12   Answer B.   The patient presents with signs and symptoms of lower extremity venous disease and is appropriately assessed with venous duplex ultrasound. The top image shows a spectral Doppler assessment of the left great saphenous vein (L GSV). Note the color scale, angle of interrogation, and spectral tracing. During Valsalva, the blood flow is above the zero line on the spectral tracing for several seconds. According to the adjacent numerical scale, flow above the zero line is a positive number. When correlated to the color duplex scale of the interrogated vein, we see that positive numbers on the color scale (red) correspond to flow toward the transducer, whereas negative numbers on the color scale (blue) correspond to flow away from the transducer. Anatomically, the transducer is pointed to the left or toward the patient's head. This would indicate several seconds of reversed flow, down the leg, in the left great saphenous vein. Diagnostic criteria for reflux in the superficial system is >0.5 seconds of reversed flow (choice B correct). The bottom image shows a spectral Doppler assessment of the left common femoral vein (L CFV). On the spectral tracing, flow is mostly below the zero line with brief periods of reversal. When correlated to the color duplex scale of the interrogated vein, we see that negative numbers on the color scale correspond to flow away from the transducer. This would indicate normal deep venous blood flow out of the leg toward the heart with short periods of reversal (normal finding due to time for valve closure). Diagnostic criterion for reflux in the deep system is >1.0 second of reversed flow. An arteriovenous fistula on spectral duplex of the vein would show regular arterial pulses on the waveform. If the vein is imaged downstream of the fistula, there will also be continuous high diastolic flow. Pelvic venous obstruction presents as loss of respiratory phasicity in the venous waveform and diminished augmentation with Valsalva.

Reference: Khilnani NM, Grassi CJ, Kundu S, et al. Multi-society consensus quality improvement guidelines for the treatment of lower-extremity superficial venous insufficiency with endovenous thermal ablation from the Society of Interventional Radiology, Cardiovascular Interventional Radiological Society of Europe, American College of Phlebology and Canadian Interventional Radiology Association. *J Vasc Interv Radiol.* 2010;21(1):14-31.

13   Answer A.   Venous insufficiency can lead to several clinical issues, ranging from mild swelling and varicose veins to nonhealing ulcers. When seeing patients, we utilize a classification scheme that evaluates the clinical, anatomic, etiologic, and pathophysiologic (CEAP) features of the disease. Venous duplex is critical to the initial evaluation. In many patients, symptomatic insufficiency of the superficial (great or small saphenous) veins is present. Conservative treatment includes maintaining a healthy weight, exercise as tolerated, elevation of the affected extremity, and wearing a graded compression stocking daily. Many patients have incomplete relief, and invasive treatment is pursued. With superficial venous insufficiency, the primary goal of the procedure is to eliminate blood flow into the dilated refluxing saphenous vein. This was previously accomplished with high ligation of the saphenous vein and/or surgical stripping. In modern practice, the overwhelmingly majority of saphenous treatment involves a minimally invasive procedure known as "closure," which is accomplished by introducing a small catheter into the great or small saphenous vein and ablating it throughout its course with radiofrequency energy, laser energy, or glue.

References: Khilnani NM, Grassi CJ, Kundu S, et al. Multi-society consensus quality improvement guidelines for the treatment of lower-extremity superficial venous insufficiency with endovenous thermal ablation from the Society of Interventional Radiology, Cardiovascular Interventional Radiological Society of Europe, American College of Phlebology and Canadian Interventional Radiology Association. *J Vasc Interv Radiol.* 2010;21(1):14-31.

Sydnor M, Mavropoulos J, Slobodnik N, Wolfe L, Strife B, Komorowski D. A randomized prospective long-term (>1 year) clinical trial comparing the efficacy and safety of radiofrequency ablation to 980 nm laser ablation of the great saphenous vein. *Phlebology.* 2017;32(6):415-424.

14   Answer D.   The case images demonstrate a surgically created HeRO graft for hemodialysis. This access type consists of 2 parts. The first segment is a prosthetic conduit, which is anastomosed to an inflow artery, much like a standard arteriovenous graft. Instead of normal venous outflow, the graft drains via a specialized catheter that is placed into the central veins, which ends at or near the right atrium. The entire access is subcutaneous or intravenous (no exposed catheter). Although not common, it is important to recognize this access type in order to intervene appropriately. The characteristic radiodense titanium attachment between the 2 components and distal marker band are clues.

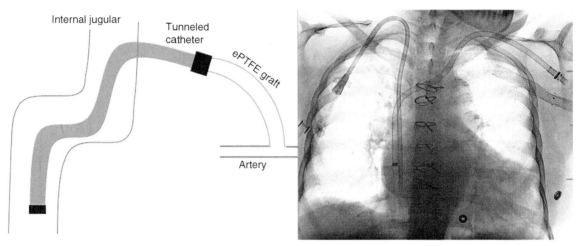

Figure 14-1   Diagrammatic and fluoroscopic depiction of a left-sided HeRO graft. The patient also has a right-sided tunneled hemodialysis catheter for comparison. Notice the external ports and lack of radiodense bands on the tunneled catheter for differentiation.

Reference: Al Shakarchi J, Houston JG, Jones RG, Inston N. A review on the hemodialysis reliable outflow (HeRO) graft for haemodialysis vascular access. *Eur J Vasc Endovasc Surg.* 2015;50(1):108-113.

15   Answer B.   Arteriovenous grafts for hemodialysis are synthetic conduits created from expanded polytetrafluoroethylene (ePTFE) or a similar product. Although durable, they are not completely immune to damage, especially in the setting of large gauge needle access multiple times a week. If the graft breaks down at a site of repeated access, a focal contained outpouching can develop (likely contained by surrounding scar tissue), which is termed graft degeneration or pseudoaneurysm formation. The National Kidney Foundation Kidney Disease Outcomes Quality Initiative (KDOQI) recommends intervention when the following features are present:

- The pseudoaneurysm size or number limits available needle cannulation sites
- The pseudoaneurysm threatens viability of the overlying skin
- The pseudoaneurysm causes pain
- There is evidence of associated infection

Traditionally, graft degeneration is treated surgically with revision or repair; however, endovascular stent grafting can be appropriate in certain situations. An infected graft with aneurysm formation (choice A) may present with local signs of infection overlying the graft (pain, redness, draining sinus tract, or exposed graft material), repeated graft thrombosis, or systemic illness from bacteremia and septic emboli. Angiography is not sensitive or specific for graft infection. With active extravasation, the more delayed image should show an enlarging pool of contrast rather than clearing. No veins are present on the case images.

References: Pandolfe LR, Malamis AP, Pierce K, Borge MA. Treatment of hemodialysis graft pseudo-aneurysms with stent grafts: institutional experience and review of the literature. *Semin Intervent Radiol.* 2009;26(2):89-95.

Sequeira A, Naljayan M, Vachharajani TJ. Vascular access guidelines: summary, rationale, and controversies. *Tech Vasc Interv Radiol.* 2017;20(1):2-8.

16   **Answer C.**   Angioplasty is by definition a form of controlled vessel injury. Following balloon dilatation of a stenosis, there is a small risk of vessel wall disruption and extraluminal extravasation. This is more often seen when treating a tight stenosis in a large parent vessel without performing gradual serial dilatation. In the case example, there is focal rupture of the outflow vein with active extravasation. While the pressure and flow in an arteriovenous fistula are higher than a normal vein, conservative treatment measures are often successful. The most appropriate first step is to reinflate the balloon across the site of rupture to tamponade the bleed. After a few minutes of balloon inflation, the problem is often fixed. If bleeding continues, serial reinflation or ultimately placement of a stent (often a covered self-expanding type) can be performed. Performing no intervention in this circumstance (choice A) will result in an expanding hematoma at the site of rupture, which is an unacceptable outcome that can compromise the access. Coil embolization (choice B) will cause occlusion of the entire dialysis access circuit and is reserved for a catastrophic rupture that cannot be treated with balloon tamponade or a stent. Similarly, emergent surgery is unnecessary for this type of complication. Of note, this case is a good opportunity to stress the importance of maintaining wire access across any lesion that has been intervened upon. If the wire is pulled back before evaluating the result of angioplasty with a completion angiogram, there is a chance that the operator will no longer be able to cross the lesion (because of restenosis, spasm, massive injury) to address the resultant extravasation with angioplasty or stenting. In this case, loss of wire access could have led to loss of the dialysis access. In other scenarios, such as with complex iliac artery recanalization, loss of wire access across a treated lesion can be fatal.

Reference: Zaleski G. Declotting, maintenance, and avoiding procedural complications of native arteriovenous fistulae. *Semin Intervent Radiol.* 2004;21(2):83-93.

17   **Answer A.**   The "rule of 6s" is an easy way to assess an arteriovenous fistula for readiness to cannulate. Following a period of maturation (typically 6-8 wk), the fistula venous outflow should have a flow rate of >600 mL/min, achieve a diameter of >6 mm, and travel <6 mm from the skin surface. Essentially, a large, high-flow conduit is easy to access with large gauge needles multiple times a week. Certainly, not all working fistulas meet or exceed these criteria. With choice B or inadequate venous outflow caliber, a diagnostic ultrasound and/or fistulogram can be useful to identify underlying inflow or outflow stenosis as well as competing outflow veins. When the vein is too deep (choice C), successful needle access and achieving hemostasis after decannulation becomes challenging; this issue is best addressed with surgical revision. Regarding choice D, venous pressure measurements are not routinely used to evaluate access maturity.

Reference: Clinical practice guidelines for vascular access. *Am J Kidney Dis.* 2006;48(suppl 1): S176-S247.

18 **Answer C.**   Many options are available for venous access when placing a cuffed tunneled central venous catheter for hemodialysis. The right internal jugular vein is established as the best initial option. Beyond this, there is no universally accepted order. The order of venous access used at our institution is (1) right internal jugular vein (2) left internal jugular vein (3) right external jugular vein (4) left external jugular vein (5) unnamed right or left neck collateral vein that drains centrally. Essentially, stay in the neck if possible. This is in line with practice guidelines from the KDOQI and others. Beyond this, the access site depends on the patient's candidacy for future upper extremity, lower extremity, or chest wall arteriovenous conduit. Options include axillosubclavian, femoral, translumbar, transhepatic, transrenal, and transthoracic approaches. Each has advantages and disadvantages. The access plan should be individualized to the patient. As most patients will eventually get an upper extremity AVF or AVG, we avoid the axillosubclavian approach in patients new to HD, given its high association with venous stenosis and/or thrombosis.

References: Clinical practice guidelines for vascular access. *Am J Kidney Dis.* 2006;48(suppl 1): S176-S247.

Patel AA, Tuite CM, Trerotola SO. K/DOQI guidelines: what should an interventionalist know? *Semin Intervent Radiol.* 2004;21(2):119-124.

Sequeira A, Naljayan M, Vachharajani TJ. Vascular access guidelines: summary, rationale, and controversies. *Tech Vasc Interv Radiol.* 2017;20(1):2-8.

19 **Answer C.**   There are 2 major types of IVC filters: permanent and retrievable (for completeness, there are convertible filters on the market). Both carry an indication for long-term placement; however, the latter is designed to facilitate easy retrieval. Most retrievable filters have a hook at the filter apex (choice C) that can be secured with a loop snare or other device. The filter is then withdrawn into a larger sheath for complete removal. Some retrievable type filters do not have a formal hook at the apex; however, those that do are all retrievable types. In modern IR practice, retrievable filters are removed when no longer clinically indicated or if there is a filter-associated complication. Most filter retrieval procedures are quick and straightforward, as long the apex and/or filter struts are not embedded or penetrated into the wall of the IVC. Even if this occurs, advanced techniques have been developed such as wire slings, laser-tipped sheaths, and the use of rigid bronchial forceps (the favored technique of the authors) that ensure a very high rate of safe retrieval.

References: Desai KR, Pandhi MB, Seedial SM, et al. Retrievable IVC filters: comprehensive review of device-related complications and advanced retrieval techniques. *Radiographics.* 2017;37(4):1236-1245.

Iliescu B, Haskal ZJ. Advanced techniques for removal of retrievable inferior vena cava filters. *Cardiovasc Intervent Radiol.* 2012;35(4):741-750.

20 **Answer B.**   A venogram should always be performed before filter retrieval to evaluate the position of the filter and to ensure there is no thrombus in the IVC or the filter itself, which could immediately embolize during or after retrieval. The venogram from the case example demonstrates a large wall-adherent thrombus inferior to and within the filter (choice A is incorrect). The next step in management should be in keeping with the goal of temporary filtration and not expose the patient to significant additional risk. As the patient has recently started therapeutic anticoagulation following a temporary contraindication, he should continue with treatment and return for a repeat venogram no sooner than 1 month. If there is significant clot resolution, the filter can then be safely removed. Abandoning all hope of filter retrieval (choice C) at this point is premature. A suprarenal filter (choice D) will not confer additional benefit, as there is no thrombus extending above the filter.

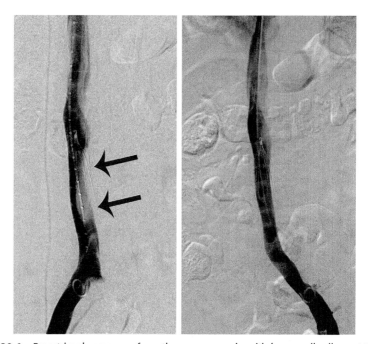

Figure 20-1 Preretrieval venogram from the case example with large wall-adherent thrombus (arrows) extending throughout the infrarenal IVC and into the filter itself. The clot does not extend cephalad to the filter. The patient was continued on therapeutic anticoagulation for another 3 months and repeat venogram (right) showed complete clot resolution, and the filter was then removed.

Reference: Teo TK, Angle JF, Shipp JI, et al. Incidence and management of inferior vena cava filter thrombus detected at time of filter retrieval. *J Vasc Interv Radiol.* 2011;22(11):1514-1520.

21   **Answer A.**   A cavogram is virtually always performed before placing an IVC filter in order to (1) identify renal vein location; (2) identify anomalous venous anatomy; (3) assess the diameter of the IVC; and (4) evaluate for thrombus in the IVC. The case images demonstrate a circumaortic left renal vein, with classic configuration of a renal vein in the normal location (level L1-L2), and a second moiety draining caudally to the lower IVC segment (sometimes to the iliac veins). This anomaly is important to identify as the venous pathway can serve as a potential channel for clot to circumvent a filter placed just below the main renal vein at L1-L2. Filter position is more optimally located below the lower left renal vein or suprarenal. Although the hepatic veins are not visualized, this does not indicate absence, as flow is out of the liver for most of the cardiac cycle. Aortocaval fistula is a rare complication mainly seen in the setting of penetrating trauma or an abdominal aortic aneurysm. It is easily identified on an arteriogram, rather than a venogram, because of the direction of blood flow.

References: Bass JE, Redwine MD, Kramer LA, Huynh PT, Harris JH. Spectrum of congenital anomalies of the inferior vena cava: cross-sectional imaging findings. *Radiographics.* 2000;20(3):639-652.

Funaki B. Inferior vena cava filter insertion. *Semin Intervent Radiol.* 2006;23(4):357-360.

22   **Answer B.**   Megacava is defined by an IVC diameter >28 mm. In practice, this becomes important as the instructions for use (IFU) of most available filters indicate that placement is appropriate for IVC diameter up to 28 mm. If megacava is present, one must place a specially designed filter (such as a Cook Bird's Nest) or consider placing traditional filters in the common iliac veins.

Reference: Doe C, Ryu RK. Anatomic and technical considerations: inferior vena cava filter placement. *Semin Intervent Radiol.* 2016;33(2):88-92.

23   **Answer C.**   There are 4 possibilities to explain the catheter position: (1) extravascular catheter; (2) intra-arterial placement; (3) intravenous placement but incorrect venous pathway; and (4) intravenous placement but variant venous anatomy. In this example, a quick look at old imaging demonstrates a known left-sided SVC. A persistent left-sided superior vena cava (PLSVC) is an incidental finding in <0.5% of the general population. It is typically found as a duplication system with a right SVC present and an absent left brachiocephalic vein. Drainage of the left SVC is nearly always into a coronary sinus, with drainage into the left atrium being rare (except in known cardiac anomalies).

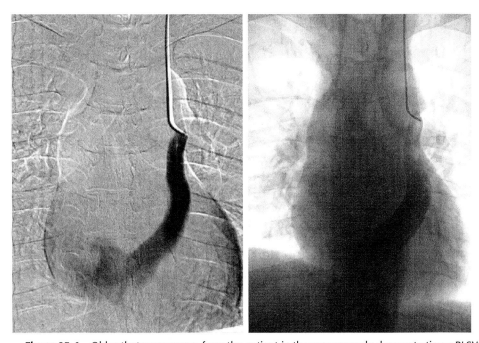

Figure 23-1   Old catheter venogram from the patient in the case example demonstrating a PLSVC. The central venous catheter present on the initial case images had difficulty with aspiration as it was positioned very deep and was sucking up against the wall of the left SVC. The catheter was retracted a few centimeters and worked well thereafter.

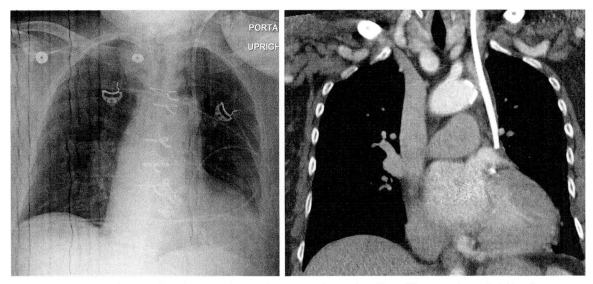

Figure 23-2   Left neck approach central venous catheter placed in a different patient mimicking the course seen with a PLSVC. The distal segment of the catheter was kinked. Old imaging showed no venous anomalies. CT chest was performed demonstrating a transvenous catheter traversing the left innominate vein with catheter tip in the mediastinal fat. Treatment was uneventful. In a hybrid endovascular/OR suite, the catheter was removed with simultaneous balloon tamponade of the transvenous catheter tract. Completion venogram showed no extravasation or other evidence of injury.

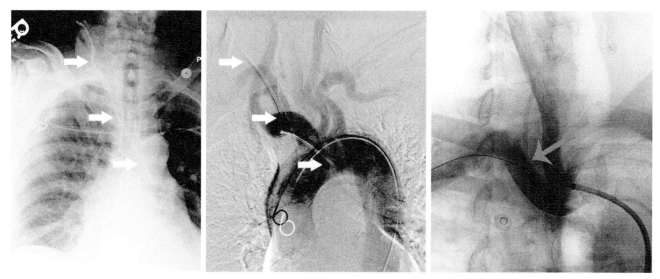

Figure 23-3   Companion case of malpositioned central venous catheter placed in the ICU. Chest X-ray shows right neck approach catheter (white arrows) crossing midline from right to left, suspicious for either extravascular placement or arterial placement. A venous pathway would not produce this catheter course. Arterial waveforms were obtained when the catheter lumen was transduced. Angiography at the time of removal showed a transjugular catheter entering the subclavian artery with catheter tip in the aortic arch. The injury was treated by placing a balloon expandable covered stent across the arterial entry site (red arrow) as the catheter was removed from the neck.

References: Bhutta ST, Culp WC. Evaluation and management of central venous access complications. *Tech Vasc Interv Radiol.* 2011;14(4):217-224.

Demos TC, Posniak HV, Pierce KL, Olson MC, Muscato M. Venous anomalies of the thorax. *AJR Am J Roentgenol.* 2004;182(5):1139-1150.

Povoski SP, Khabiri H. Persistent left superior vena cava: review of the literature, clinical implications, and relevance of alterations in thoracic central venous anatomy as pertaining to the general principles of central venous access device placement and venography in cancer patients. *World J Surg Oncol.* 2011;9:173.

24   Answer A.   Knowledge of radiographic landmarks and the basic technique for tunneled central venous catheter placement is needed to answer this question. In the case image, just cephalad to the right mainstem bronchus, the catheter deviates medially rather than straight down the SVC to the right atrium. This course is classic for azygos vein positioning. In this particular case, the tunneled hemodialysis catheter was purposefully placed in the azygos vein as the SVC was chronically occluded. Azygos vein catheter positioning in the routine patient should be avoided because of increased complications, namely vessel perforation and catheter dysfunction. Following central venous catheter placement, if there is concern for inadvertent azygos vein positioning, a lateral image can demonstrate the classic posterior deviation of the catheter.

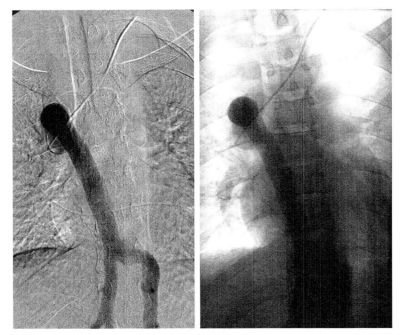

Figure 24-1 Catheter angiogram from the patient in the case example demonstrating the absence of the SVC due to chronic occlusion and massively hypertrophied azygos vein draining the upper extremities, head and neck. When intentionally placing a catheter in the azygos vein, we routinely perform a venogram to evaluate the size and course of the vein.

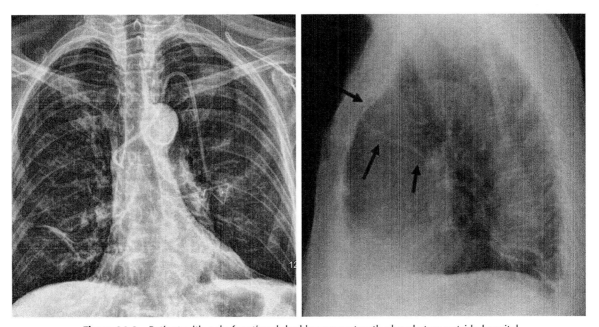

Figure 24-2 Patient with a dysfunctional dual lumen portacath placed at an outside hospital. The frontal radiograph shows abnormal course of the distal catheter segment, and overall catheter length appears too short. The lateral radiograph shows several centimeters of catheter coursing posteriorly (arrows), classic for azygos vein positioning. Note the reservoir was relatively low lying over the third anterior rib on the left chest. The patient had pendulous breasts, and the portacath reservoir was excessively mobile. The revision procedure involved suturing the reservoir in place and using a flush pigtail catheter to ensnare the malpositioned distal segment and mobilize it back to the upper cavoatrial junction.

References: Gibson F, Bodenham A. Misplaced central venous catheters: applied anatomy and practical management. *Br J Anaesth.* 2013;110(3):333-346.

Wong JJ, Kinney TB. Azygos tip placement for hemodialysis catheters in patients with superior vena cava occlusion. *Cardiovasc Intervent Radiol.* 2006;29(1):143-146.

25   Answer C.   An AVG is a common access type for patients on hemodialysis. The graft, a prosthetic tube, is sewn to an inflow artery (arterial anastomosis) and an outflow vein (venous anastomosis) and serves as a conduit for blood flow and needle cannulation. The orientation of the graft can be variable. The graft may be straight, as demonstrated in the case example, or looped. It can be placed in the forearm, upper arm, chest wall, or groin. When evaluating a dysfunctional AVG, the complete circuit from the arterial anastomosis to the right atrium should be evaluated. In this particular case, the angiographic images demonstrate that the graft is tied into the brachial artery at the level of the elbow. The graft itself is widely patent with no apparent stenosis. Note the uniform caliber of the graft segment with smooth walls and lack of venous branches, differentiating it from the outflow vein of an arteriovenous fistula. At the venous anastomosis, there is a severe focal stenosis. The central veins are widely patent. AVG dysfunction is most commonly due to stenosis at the venous anastomosis (80%-85% of lesions). According the KDOQI guidelines, the initial treatment of dialysis access stenosis (minimum stenosis of 50%) is balloon angioplasty. While this is true for virtually all flow limiting lesions in the access circuit, randomized data exist, which support primary placement of self-expanding covered stents for stenosis at the venous anastomosis in failing upper extremity AVGs. When compared with balloon angioplasty alone, primary stenting demonstrated almost a twofold increase in access patency at 6 months in a randomized study.

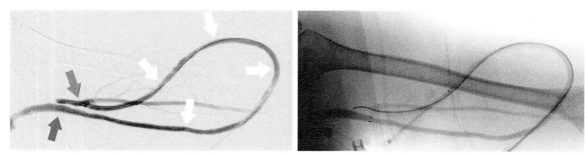

Figure 25-1   Upper arm loop graft configuration. Arterial anastomosis, red arrow; graft, white arrows; stented venous anastomosis, blue arrow.

References: Dariushnia SR, Walker TG, Silberzweig JE, et al. Quality improvement guidelines for percutaneous image-guided management of the thrombosed or dysfunctional dialysis circuit. *J Vasc Interv Radiol.* 2016;27(10):1518-1530.

Haskal ZJ, Trerotola S, Dolmatch B, et al. Stent graft versus balloon angioplasty for failing dialysis-access grafts. *N Engl J Med.* 2010;362(6):494-503.

Vesely T, Davanzo W, Behrend T, Dwyer A, Aruny J. Balloon angioplasty versus Viabahn stent graft for treatment of failing or thrombosed prosthetic hemodialysis grafts. *J Vasc Surg.* 2016;64(5):1400-1410.e1.

26 Answer C. There exists an uncommon but critical vascular condition termed phlegmasia cerulea dolens. When the degree of acute thrombotic venous obstruction in an extremity is so great that outflow of fluid is nearly completely blocked, the interstitial pressure rises, arterial perfusion is compromised, and essentially a compartment syndrome occurs with resultant tissue ischemia. The clinical presentation consists of a markedly swollen extremity, which is discolored and exquisitely tender to palpation. This is an emergency, and the condition can result in limb loss or fatality if not treated aggressively. In addition to prompt recognition and initiation of anticoagulation, endovascular venous thrombectomy is often the first option in contemporary practice with surgical venous thrombectomy still performed first at certain centers. All of the other choices from this question are data points that are good to know when working up a venous thrombosis case, but not as critical as the extremity pulse examination.

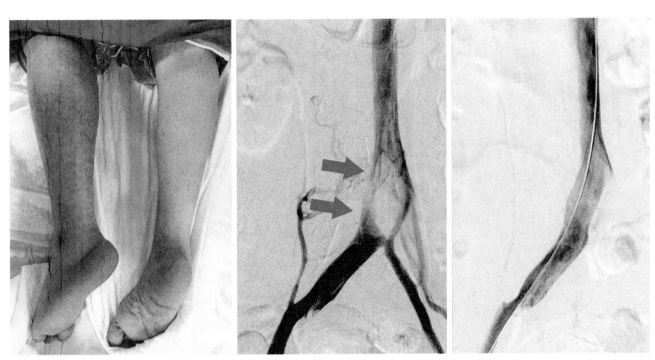

Figure 26-1 A 54-year-old woman with no history of prior venous thrombotic events presents with a swollen, diffusely tender, and discolored left leg. Arterial pulses in the left foot are not palpable, and the pedal Doppler signals are weak. Motor and sensory is intact. A CT scan is performed in the ED, which shows acute thrombosis of the left lower extremity from the popliteal vein through the left common iliac vein. Anticoagulation is initiated, and endovascular thrombectomy is promptly performed. After acute clot lysis, venography identified the culprit May-Thurner lesion (arrows) in the left common iliac vein, which is treated with a self-expanding stent. Clinical improvement is rapid with near complete resolution of swelling and discoloration within 48 hours of admission.

References: Chinsakchai K, Ten Duis K, Moll FL, de Borst GJ. Trends in management of phlegmasia cerulea dolens. *Vasc Endovascular Surg.* 2011;45(1):5-14.

Oguzkurt L, Ozkan U, Demirturk OS, Gur S. Endovascular treatment of phlegmasia cerulea dolens with impending venous gangrene: manual aspiration thrombectomy as the first-line thrombus removal method. *Cardiovasc Intervent Radiol.* 2011;34(6):1214-1221.

27 **Answer C.**   This is a classic example of Paget-Schroetter syndrome, also known as venous thoracic outlet syndrome (TOS) or effort thrombosis of the axillosubclavian vein. In these patients, there is chronic repetitive injury to the vein as it traverses the thoracic outlet. The trauma to the endothelium causes activation of the clotting cascade and ultimately venous thrombosis. There is often an underlying anatomic abnormality such as a cervical rib and/or occupational risk factor that involves vigorous use of the upper extremity (swimmers, baseball pitchers). Underlying coagulopathy may also play a role. Different management algorithms exist, but if the clot is acute and there is no contraindication, catheter-directed thrombolytic therapy is often the first step. Once venous patency is restored, surgical decompression of the thoracic outlet is performed. Occasionally, despite decompression, there may be chronic venous stenosis, which can subsequently be treated with balloon angioplasty. An alternative approach with similar outcomes is anticoagulation alone followed by surgical decompression of the thoracic outlet, avoiding the risks of tPA.

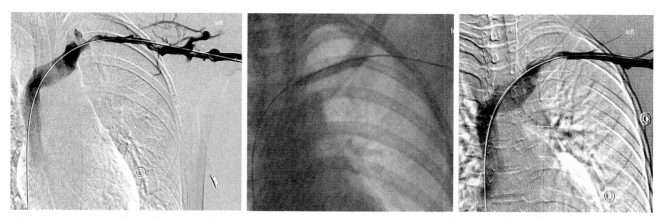

Figure 27-1   Procedural images from the patient in the case example. After overnight thrombolytic therapy with catheter-directed tPA, venous patency is restored revealing a narrowed subclavian vein (left). Following balloon angioplasty, there is significantly improved flow with the disappearance of collateral venous filling (right). As the underlying vein was still at risk from the underlying pathologic process, first rib resection is subsequently performed.

Stenting is generally avoided in venous TOS, with or without surgical decompression. Long-term patency of central venous stents in this location is relatively poor, and many of these patients are young at presentation. The other answer choices are not appropriate to treat acute venous thrombosis. Notably, although SVC filter placement has been described for the prevention of PE from upper extremity clot, there is not a device approved for this location. Operators have used IVC filters off-label in the SVC; however, unique complications can occur such as pneumothorax and pericardial perforation with cardiac tamponade.

References: Guzzo JL, Chang K, Demos J, Black JH, Freischlag JA. Preoperative thrombolysis and venoplasty affords no benefit in patency following first rib resection and scalenectomy for subacute and chronic subclavian vein thrombosis. *J Vasc Surg.* 2010;52(3):658-662.

Owens CA, Bui JT, Knuttinen MG, Gaba RC, Carrillo TC. Pulmonary embolism from upper extremity deep vein thrombosis and the role of superior vena cava filters: a review of the literature. *J Vasc Interv Radiol.* 2010; 21(6):779-787.

Sheeran SR, Hallisey MJ, Murphy TP, Faberman RS, Sherman S. Local thrombolytic therapy as part of a multidisciplinary approach to acute axillosubclavian vein thrombosis (Paget-Schroetter syndrome). *J Vasc Interv Radiol.* 1997;8(2):253-260.

28 Answer D. There is a clear difference in the orientation of the portacath reservoir between the initial placement and the images obtained months later. The lateral image is quite useful as the lucent silicone septum (the part of the port that is accessed with a needle) is pointed posteriorly in relation to the base of the port, indicating it has flipped. Because there are many different makes and models of portacaths, it is not always easy to look at a frontal image and identify a flipped port, especially if prior imaging is not available. One can always attempt live fluoroscopic-guided needle access and use rotational fluoroscopy to truly determine if it is flipped.

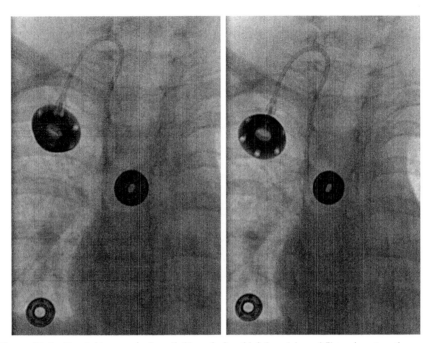

Figure 28-1   Frontal images before (left) and after (right) revision of flipped portacath reservoir from the patient in the case example.

Reference: Etezadi V, Trerotola SO. Comparison of inversion ("flipping") rates among different port designs: a single-center experience. *Cardiovasc Intervent Radiol.* 2017;40(4):553-559.

29 Answer D. Unexpected or unexplained vascular thrombosis in the setting of recent heparin exposure should raise the suspicion for heparin-induced thrombocytopenia (HIT). In short, HIT is an immune-mediated reaction caused by recent heparin exposure (typically in the preceding 5-10 days). Platelet level decrease is the hallmark of the condition. Importantly, the level need not drop below 150,000/μL; a drop to <50% of preheparin exposure levels is concerning. Skin lesions at injection sites and systemic reactions after heparin administration are also suspicious clinical clues. The anti-PF4 antibodies that form activate platelets and can cause potentially catastrophic venous or arterial thrombosis. Once HIT is suspected, providers should discontinue all forms of heparin and switch to an alternative anticoagulation such as bivalirudin. An antibody test can confirm the condition.

References: Resnick SB, Resnick SH, Weintraub JL, Kothary N. Heparin in interventional radiology: a therapy in evolution. *Semin Intervent Radiol.* 2005;22(2):95-107.

Warkentin TE, Greinacher A. Management of heparin-induced thrombocytopenia. *Curr Opin Hematol.* 2016;23(5):462-470.

30   Answer A.   The provided images demonstrate a catheter fragment straddling the right and left pulmonary arteries. Luckily, endovascular foreign object retrieval is typically a straightforward process averting surgical intervention. In order to access the pulmonary arterial tree, venous access is required, often the common femoral or internal jugular vein. There are preshaped catheters that aid in maneuvering into the pulmonary arterial system. Typically, a long sheath is positioned close to the foreign body. If possible, we use a sheath of adequate internal diameter to accommodate the object being retrieved. Most retrievals involve using a snare, of which there are several models and configurations. A single wire loop snare is the most simple design and works well for catheter and wire retrievals. Once the loop is passed over the foreign body, the wire is retracted to cinch down on the object for secure capture. The catheter and snare are retracted together under countertension, pulling the foreign object into the sheath for safe removal. In addition to a single wire loop snare, more complex snares, lassos, balloons, wires, and forceps may be necessary for object retrieval.

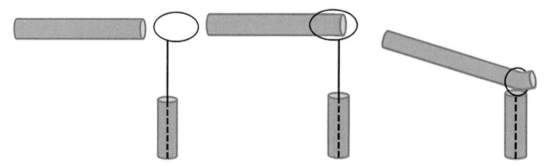

Figure 31-1   Diagrammatic representation of using a single wire loop snare to secure an object.

Reference: Woodhouse JB, Uberoi R. Techniques for intravascular foreign body retrieval. *Cardiovasc Intervent Radiol*. 2013;36(4):888-897.

4 Thoracic

1 What is the least common finding on bronchial artery angiography performed for massive hemoptysis?

   A. Neovascularity
   B. Hypervascularity
   C. Arteriovenous shunting
   D. Dilated and tortuous bronchial arteries
   E. Active bleeding

2 What is the most commonly used first-line embolic agent in bronchial artery embolization for hemoptysis?

   A. Coils
   B. nBCA (N-butyl cyanoacrylate) glue
   C. Gelfoam slurry
   D. Permanent particles
   E. Amplatzer vascular plug

3 What is the most common cause of pulmonary artery pseudoaneurysm?

   A. Iatrogenic
   B. Penetrating trauma
   C. Congenital
   D. Infection
   E. Collagen vascular disease

4   A 48-year-old woman with multiple myeloma and preexisting left chest portacath presents for placement of a dual-lumen tunneled central venous catheter for apheresis. Following placement, the new catheter only aspirates a small amount of clear fluid. The patient complains of chest pain and becomes tachycardic and hypotensive. What are you most concerned about?

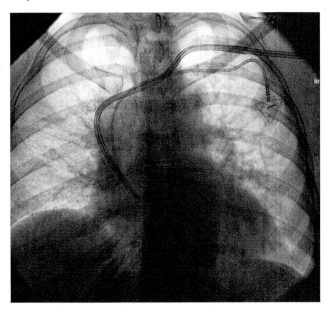

A. Tension pneumothorax
B. Cardiac tamponade
C. Vena cava laceration with hemorrhagic shock
D. Adverse reaction to intravenous sedation

5   Patients with cardiac tamponade demonstrate which of the following?

A. Collapse of the internal jugular vein on physical examination
B. Mediastinal shift to the left on radiography
C. Cardiac chamber collapse on echosonography
D. High-voltage QRS complexes on the electrocardiogram

6   A 38-year-old man is found unconscious by the side of a road, apparently ejected from a nearby vehicle that had crashed into a telephone pole. He is brought to the ED (emergency department) and a CTA (computed tomography angiography) of the chest is performed. What is the most likely diagnosis?

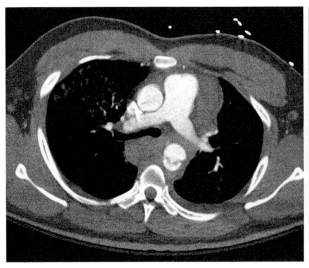 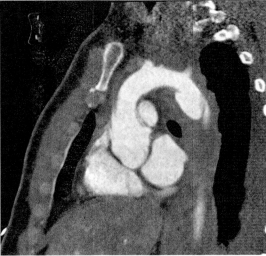

A. Acute traumatic aortic injury (ATAI)
B. Chronic aortic dissection with aneurysm formation
C. Aortitis
D. Motion artifact

7   An adult with a grade III descending thoracic aortic injury due to blunt trauma is admitted to the ICU. The patient is hemodynamically stable. What is the treatment of choice for this type of traumatic aortic injury?

A. Immediate surgery with excision and placement of an interposition graft
B. Medical management with blood pressure control
C. Urgent thoracic endovascular aortic repair (TEVAR) before discharge
D. Elective TEVAR after discharge

8   What best explains the preserved in-line flow to the left upper extremity in this patient immediately after TEVAR for descending thoracic aortic dissection? The image is an LAO (left anterior oblique) thoracic aortogram.

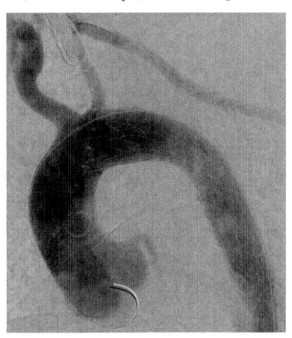

A. Normal arterial variant
B. Surgical bypass
C. Arteriovenous fistula
D. In-line flow is not preserved

9   A patient undergoes placement of a single lumen portacath by a local surgeon. She presents for evaluation of chest and neck swelling after receiving a chemotherapy infusion through the portacath. A portacath study with iodinated contrast is performed. What is the diagnosis?

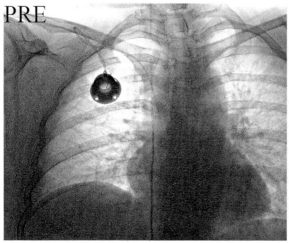
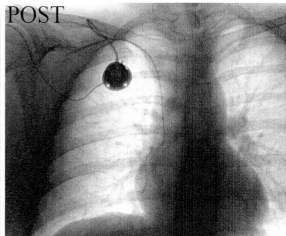

PRE   POST

   A. Fibrin sheath
   B. Clotted portacath reservoir
   C. Pinch-off syndrome with extravasation
   D. Normal portacath

10   A 55-year-old woman on chronic hemodialysis presents for evaluation of a dysfunctional tunneled dialysis catheter. The catheter will flush but not aspirate. The scout image (left) demonstrates appropriate positioning with tip of the catheter at the superior cavoatrial junction. The catheter is freed up and retracted several centimeters. Injection of contrast through the catheter (right) demonstrates what pathology?

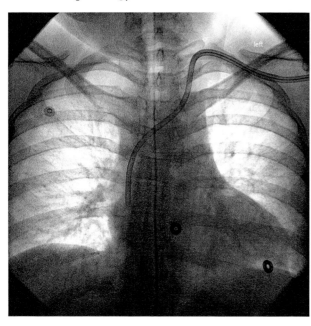
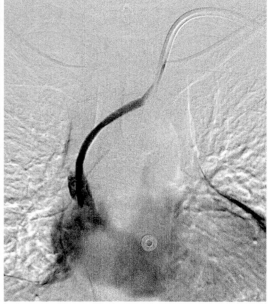

   A. Normal finding
   B. Venous perforation with extravasation
   C. Fibrin sheath formation
   D. Thrombosis of the left innominate vein and superior vena cava

11 Which of the following is a durable treatment for catheter-associated fibrin sheath formation?

    A. Balloon fragmentation

    B. Anticoagulation

    C. Catheter exchange over the wire

    D. Reversing the lines during hemodialysis

12 An 18-year-old woman on oral contraceptive therapy presents to the ED with chest pain and shortness of breath. What is the diagnosis?

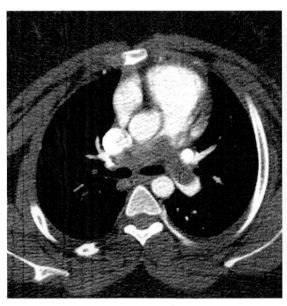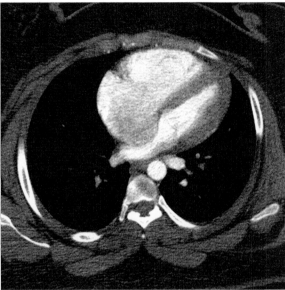

    A. Aortic dissection

    B. Pulmonary embolism

    C. Pulmonary angiosarcoma

    D. Lymphoma

13 What is the minimum RV:LV ratio to diagnose right heart strain in patients with acute pulmonary embolism (PE)?

    A. >0.5

    B. >0.9

    C. >1.5

    D. >2.0

14 A patient presents with a large pulmonary embolus occluding the main left pulmonary artery. There is right heart strain on the CTA. She is tachycardic to 130 bpm, and her blood pressure is 83/48. What is the clinical category of PE in this patient?

    A. Low-risk PE

    B. Intermediate-risk (submassive) PE

    C. High-risk (massive) PE

15 Which of the following is the most appropriate treatment for a patient with massive PE?

    A. IVC filter placement

    B. Catheter-directed PE intervention

    C. Systemic anticoagulation alone

16   A 53-year-old woman with a history of stroke presents to the ED with chest pain.
Chest CTA is performed with images given below. What is the most likely diagnosis?

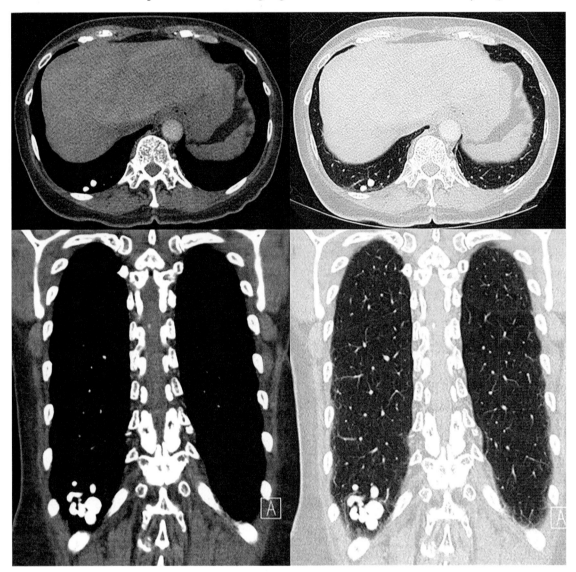

A. Pulmonary arteriovenous malformation
B. Primary lung carcinoma
C. Pulmonary artery pseudoaneurysm
D. Pulmonary varix

17   What underlying condition is often present in patients with a pulmonary arteriovenous malformation (PAVM)?

A. Klippel-Trenaunay
B. Hereditary hemorrhagic telangiectasia
C. Tuberous sclerosis
D. Sturge-Weber

18   Which accurately reflects current recommendations for PAVM embolization in
adults?

A. Treat when PAVM is symptomatic; observe asymptomatic patients
B. Treat when PAVM feeding artery diameter is >5 mm, or when draining vein is
>10 mm
C. Treat when PAVM feeding artery diameter is >3 mm, treatment may be appropri-
ate when feeding artery diameter is <3 mm

19   Which of the following is the preferred embolic agent for the treatment of PAVM?

   A. Fibered coil
   B. Permanent particles
   C. nBCA glue
   D. Gelfoam slurry

20   A 43-year-old man with a history of treated lymphoma presents with a 3-day history of dizziness, chest pain, and swelling of the head and neck. A chest radiograph is obtained. Which of the following are you most concerned for?

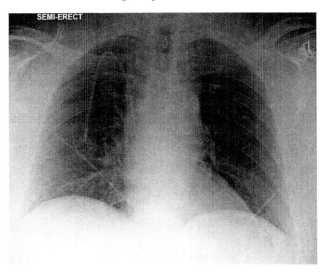

   A. Thoracic aortic aneurysm with rupture
   B. Pericardial effusion with tamponade
   C. Recurrent thoracic lymphoma
   D. Occlusion of the superior vena cava (SVC)

21   Which of the following is the feared complication in this patient?

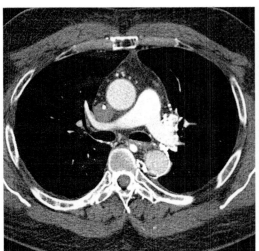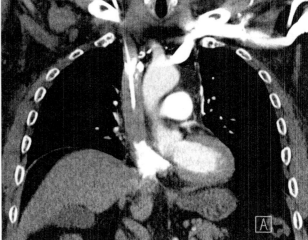

   A. Airway compromise
   B. Cardiac tamponade
   C. Hemomediastinum
   D. Stroke

22   A 61-year-old man with a known squamous cell cancer eroding into the left axilla was treated with palliative radiation. He presents with brisk external bleeding from the treated site that is not controlled by a pressure dressing. He is taken emergently to interventional radiology, and diagnostic angiography is performed. Based on the sequential images given below, what is the best endovascular treatment for the abnormality (the pathology is directly from the axillary artery, not from a side-branch)?

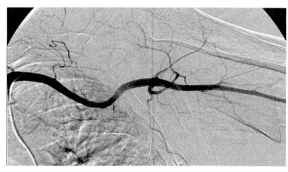 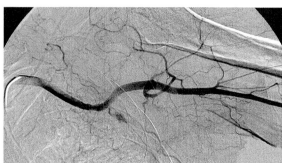

A. Placement of a covered stent
B. Embolization with coils
C. Embolization with particles
D. Embolization with nBCA glue

23   Based on the sequential angiographic images, what is the most likely clinical presentation of this patient?

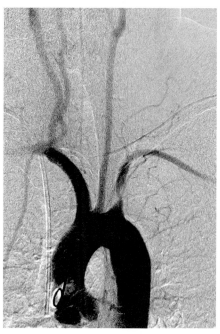 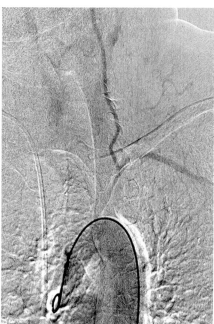

A. Syncope
B. Left arm claudication
C. Ataxia
D. Diplopia
E. Stroke

24   Which of the following is an indication to treat a left subclavian artery stenosis?

A. Reversal of flow in the left vertebral artery
B. Peak systolic velocity > 300 cm/s
C. End diastolic velocity > 140 cm/s
D. Planning for a left coronary artery bypass graft using the internal thoracic artery

25 Which is the optimal catheter tip position for a portacath?

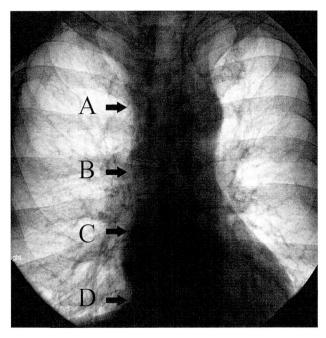

A. A
B. B
C. C
D. D

26 Which of the following qualifies a type B thoracic aortic dissection as complicated?

A. Compromised kidney perfusion
B. Aortic diameter 3.3 cm
C. Thrombosis of the false lumen
D. False lumen:true lumen ratio > 1.0

27 This artery (arrow) shares watershed territory most directly with which of the following vessels?

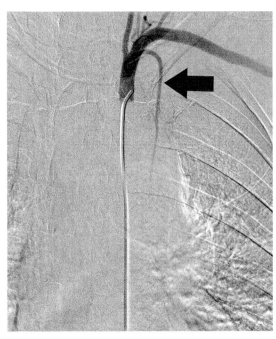

A. Left inferior epigastric artery
B. Left pulmonary artery
C. Left inferior phrenic artery
D. L2 lumbar artery

28   Which is the best route for percutaneous core needle biopsy of this lung nodule?

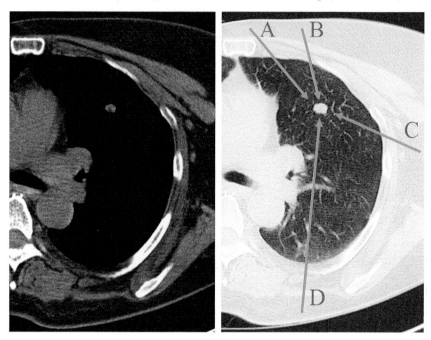

A. A
B. B
C. C
D. D

29   Which of the following is an indication for chest tube placement for a pneumothorax after a CT-guided lung lesion biopsy?

A. Pneumothorax >10% thoracic volume
B. All pneumothoraces, which are large enough to accommodate a tube
C. Patient with shortness of breath
D. Oxygen saturation <94%

30   Which is the best approach for IR (interventional radiology) management of an adult with a lung abscess?

A. Percutaneous drainage is an option if the patient is not a candidate for surgery
B. Contraindicated, given the high risk of bronchopleural fistula
C. If tube is <10 Fr, it can be placed without concern
D. It is the preferred treatment if there is underlying malignancy

31   A 45-year-old woman presents for bilateral thoracentesis as well as CT-guided drainage catheter placement into 2 separate abdominal fluid collections. As the patient is short of breath at baseline, bilateral thoracentesis is performed first.

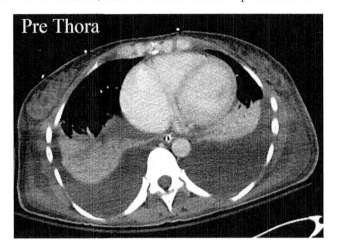

Bilateral thoracentesis is performed with just over 1 L of fluid removed from each pleural space. The patient is then positioned supine, and a scout CT is performed before abdominal drain placement.

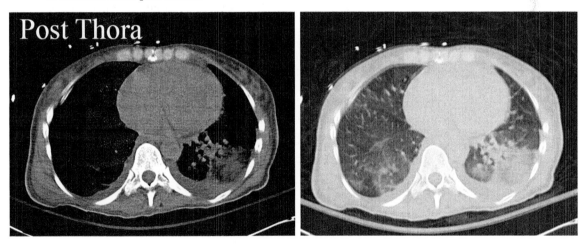

Her respiratory status begins to worsen rather than improve, and final CT images are acquired after abdominal drain placement.

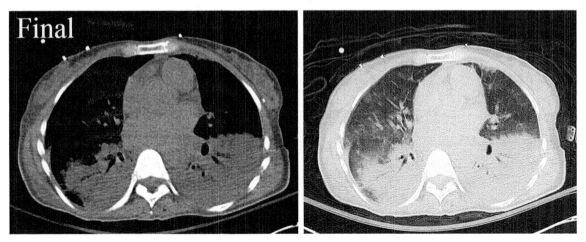

Which condition explains the changes on imaging and clinical deterioration?

A. Acute myocardial infarction

B. Hemothorax

C. Underlying malignancy

D. Reexpansion pulmonary edema

32a A 56-year-old man with prior left pacemaker placement has marked left arm enlargement. There is a subtle thrill on palpation of the upper arm and an underlying arteriovenous fistula (AVF) is suspected. Given the findings on the initial upper arm arteriogram, what is the next step in evaluation?

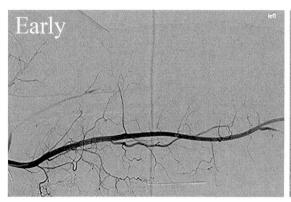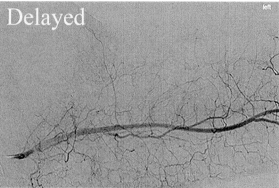

A. More selective (distal) catheter position

B. Less selective (proximal) catheter position

C. Carbon dioxide angiography from the same catheter position

D. Give intra-arterial nitroglycerin and then repeat the angiogram

32b The catheter is pulled back into a more proximal position. Based on these sequential images from left subclavian arteriography, what is the diagnosis?

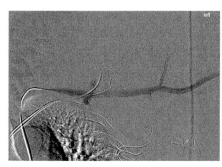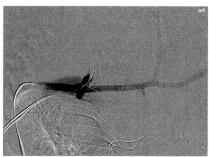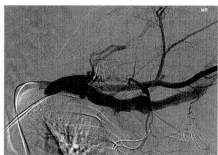

A. Arteriovenous fistula

B. Normal variant

C. Tumor vascularity

D. Active extravasation

33   In the absence of any recent trauma or intervention, what is the most likely pathology?

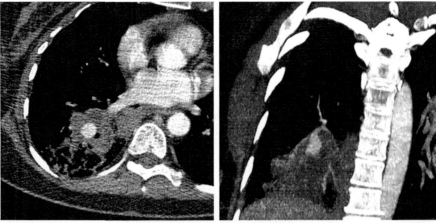

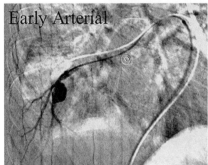 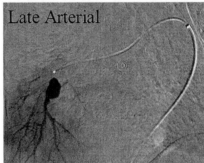 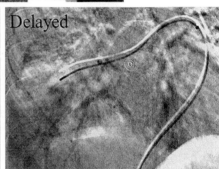

A. Pulmonary artery active extravasation
B. Pulmonary AVF
C. Pulmonary artery mycotic aneurysm
D. Hypervascular tumor

34   A 41-year-old man presents for a percutaneous lung nodule biopsy. Immediately after the biopsy, the patient has large-volume hemoptysis and decreasing oxygen saturation. Which of the following is the best next step in management?

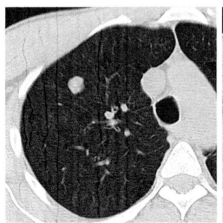 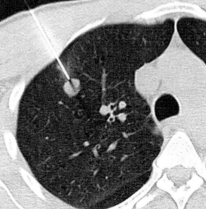 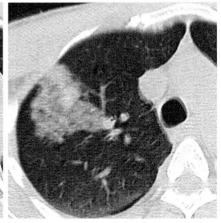

A. Place a right chest tube
B. Position the patient right-side down
C. Position the patient in reverse Trendelenburg
D. Transport to IR for immediate embolization

35   Which of the following is true regarding percutaneous image-guided thermal abla-
      tion of lung malignancy?

      A. Bronchopleural fistula is a frequent complication
      B. Percutaneous thermal ablation is preferable to surgery as first-line therapy when
         possible
      C. Microwave (as opposed to radiofrequency or cryo) thermal ablation cannot be
         used within the lung parenchyma
      D. It is an appropriate treatment option for both primary and metastatic lesions

36   A 57-year-old woman presents for CT-guided biopsy of a right lower lobe lung nod-
      ule. Based on the images, what is the patient at risk for?

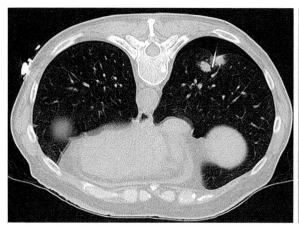 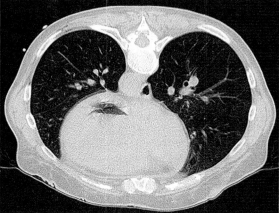

      A. Stroke
      B. Tumor seeding
      C. Cardiac tamponade
      D. Empyema

ANSWERS AND EXPLANATIONS

1   **Answer E.**   Massive hemoptysis is a term with varying definitions; however, in practice, it roughly equates to an expelled quantity of at least 300 mL blood in 24 hours. The typical patient has a history of chronic lung disease such as cystic fibrosis or sarcoidosis, chronic infection such as fungal or mycobacterial, or malignancy such as primary lung carcinoma. Although the blood loss from hemoptysis virtually never results in hemodynamic instability, it remains life-threatening because of potential airway and lung parenchyma compromise. Initial management includes airway protection with dependent positioning of the bleeding lung, and often intubation and placement of a bronchial blocker on the affected side. Angiography with embolization has an increasing role among the different strategies to control lung hemorrhage. In the IR suite, catheterization of the bronchial arteries, which often arise from the descending thoracic aorta at level T5-T6, is the primary objective. The arteries may be enlarged and tortuous. Dense networks of neo- and hypervascularity are often seen in the affected lung segments. Frank shunting to the pulmonary veins or arteries may be present and does not represent a contraindication to embolization, although the technique may be adjusted. Active bleeding is virtually never seen angiographically, and embolization should be performed in its absence. Additionally, in patients who have undergone prior embolization or those with long-standing chronic lung diseases, extensive parasitization may occur with feeding arteries emanating from the intercostals, inferior phrenics, internal thoracics, and costo- and thyrocervical trunks, among others.

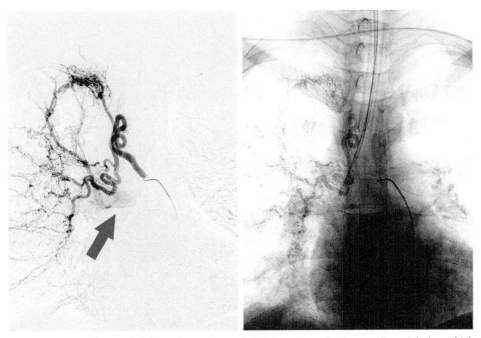

Figure 1-1 Subtracted (left) and unsubtracted (right) angiographic images from right bronchial artery catheterization demonstrate a tortuous and dilated bronchial artery, neovascularity, hypervascularity, and shunting to the superior pulmonary vein (arrow) in the right lung. Note the bronchial blocker in the right mainstem bronchus. The patient has cystic fibrosis and presented with massive hemoptysis.

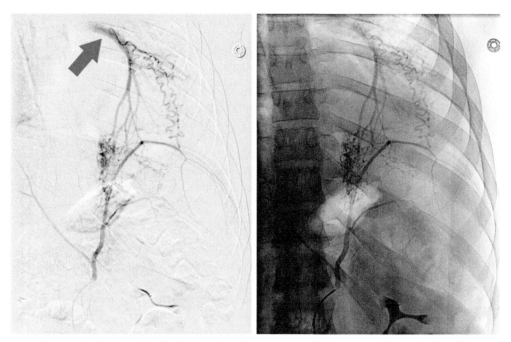

Figure 1-2   Patient with allergic bronchopulmonary aspergillosis and multiple episodes of hemoptysis treated with bronchial artery embolization. Thoracic angiography demonstrated no further filling of bronchial arteries. Angiography from the left inferior phrenic artery showed parasitization to the left lung with neo- and hypervascularity as well as shunting to the left pulmonary artery (arrow).

References: Lorenz J, Sheth D, Patel J. Bronchial artery embolization. *Semin Intervent Radiol.* 2012;29(3):155-160.

Yoon W, Kim JK, Kim YH, Chung TW, Kang HK. Bronchial and nonbronchial systemic artery embolization for life-threatening hemoptysis: a comprehensive review. *Radiographics.* 2002;22(6):1395-1409.

2   **Answer D.**   Bronchial artery embolization in the setting of hemoptysis relies on selective catheterization of the bronchial arteries, which arise from the descending thoracic aorta. Various anatomic configurations exist including right and left bronchial arteries, and intercostobronchial artery trunks. Once a bronchial artery is selected, the diagnostic catheter, or more often a coaxially introduced microcatheter, is advanced to a stable position to ensure delivery of an embolic agent to the intended territory. Nontarget embolization can occur to the spinal artery if present, as well as to the aorta and its downstream branches. Ideally, the embolic agent produces distal arterial occlusion, but not so distal that tissue devascularization and infarction can occur. Particles are the ideal agent, as they can be sized accordingly, delivered in precise amounts, and mixed with iodinated contrast for visualization. Permanent particles, such as polyvinyl alcohol (PVA) and tris-acryl gelatin microspheres (TAGM), are commonly used. Temporary agents such as gelfoam slurry are less desirable, as early recanalization can occur leading to rebleeding. Because hemoptysis often occurs in the setting of chronic lung diseases, future rebleeding should be anticipated. Coils and plugs are avoided, as they would produce permanent proximal arterial occlusion and eliminate the pathway for future catheterizations if (when) rebleeding occurs. Glue, a liquid embolic, can be difficult to control and can produce such distal occlusion that tissue infarction can occur.

References: Lorenz J, Sheth D, Patel J. Bronchial artery embolization. *Semin Intervent Radiol.* 2012;29(3):155-160.

Yoon W, Kim JK, Kim YH, Chung TW, Kang HK. Bronchial and nonbronchial systemic artery embolization for life-threatening hemoptysis: a comprehensive review. *Radiographics.* 2002;22(6):1395-1409.

3   **Answer A.**   Pulmonary artery catheterization for the purposes of physiologic monitoring and cardiopulmonary evaluation represents the most common etiology for pulmonary artery pseudoaneurysm. During catheter manipulation, or balloon inflation or deflation, a pulmonary artery branch may develop a contained perforation resulting in a pseudoaneurysm. Endovascular treatment consists of selective catheterization of the feeding pulmonary artery branch, and ideally occlusion of the branch distal and proximal to the pseudoaneurysm, effectively excluding it from the circulation. Coils or plugs work well in this application. Penetrating trauma, congenital, infection, and collagen vascular disease are more rare etiologies.

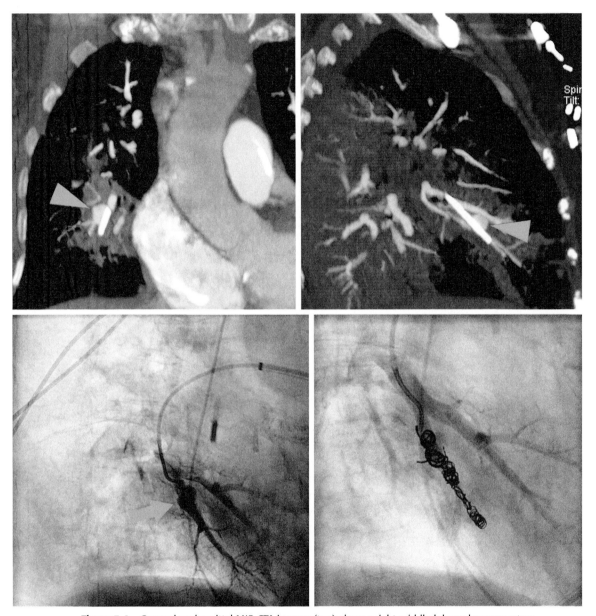

Figure 3-1   Coronal and sagittal MIP CTA images (top) show a right middle lobe pulmonary artery branch with indwelling Swan-Ganz catheter and associated pseudoaneurysm (arrowheads). There is extensive surrounding parenchymal consolidation from episodic hemorrhage. Subsequent selective catheterization and coil embolization (bottom) distal and proximal to the pseudoaneurysm (arrow) is performed, effectively excluding it from the circulation and eliminating the risk of future rupture.

Reference: Lafita V, Borge MA, Demos TC. Pulmonary artery pseudoaneurysm: etiology, presentation, diagnosis, and treatment. *Semin Intervent Radiol.* 2007;24(1):119-123.

4 **Answer B.**   Placement of central venous catheters is one of the most basic IR procedures; however, complications from the procedure, albeit uncommon, can be fatal. The case image shows a left chest portacath and a larger-caliber tunneled central venous catheter. Note the right lateral course of the tunneled catheter outside the expected region of the superior vena cava, concerning for extravascular position. The completion radiograph shows no large pneumothorax, hemothorax, or widened mediastinum, eliminating choices A and C. Reactions to intravenous sedation more commonly cause slowed breathing with hypoxia, bradycardia, as well as hypotension. One must keep in mind that the pericardial reflections extend well beyond the cardiac chambers, encompassing portions of the superior vena cava, inferior vena cava, main pulmonary artery, ascending aorta, and pulmonary veins. In the case example, a right lateral wall perforation of the lower superior vena cava occurred, allowing blood under venous pressure to fill the pericardial space. Ultimately, the injury was treated using a combination of endovascular balloon tamponade over the SVC perforation as well as a placement of a subxiphoid pericardial drain.

References: Gibson F, Bodenham A. Misplaced central venous catheters: applied anatomy and practical management. *Br J Anaesth*. 2013;110(3):333-346.

Mitchell SE, Clark RA. Complications of central venous catheterization. *AJR Am J Roentgenol*. 1979;133(3):467-476.

5 **Answer C.**   On physical examination, patients in cardiac tamponade often demonstrate jugular venous distention, diminished heart sounds, tachycardia, pulsus paradoxus, and altered mental status. Radiography is often normal or may show an enlarged cardiac silhouette because of the accumulation of pericardial fluid (more common with chronic effusions). On electrocardiogram, sinus tachycardia, electrical alternans, and low-voltage QRS complexes can be seen. On echosonography, pericardial fluid is present in variable quantities depending on the rate of accumulation. Additionally, the cardiac chambers demonstrate impaired diastolic filling and collapse, often the right-sided chambers first, as the pericardial pressure exceeds intracardiac pressure.

References: Bayer O, Schummer C, Richter K, Fröber R, Schummer W. Implication of the anatomy of the pericardial reflection on positioning of central venous catheters. *J Cardiothorac Vasc Anesth*. 2006;20(6):777-780.

Spodick DH. Acute cardiac tamponade. *N Engl J Med*. 2003;349(7):684-690.

6 **Answer A.**   ATAI includes minimal intimal injury (grade I), intramural hematoma (grade II), pseudoaneurysm formation (grade III), and transection with active bleeding (grade IV). ATAIs classically occur at the 3 fixation points: (1) aortic root, (2) aortic isthmus, and (3) diaphragmatic hiatus. Injuries at the isthmus represent the overwhelming majority of those seen in practice, whereas aortic root injuries are rarely encountered because of the high lethality of the injury location. The images in the case example show abnormal contour of the descending thoracic aorta with focal fusiform dilatation, as well as periaortic and mediastinal hematoma. Choices B and C are incorrect given the history, CT appearance, and secondary findings such as periaortic hematoma and pulmonary contusions.

References: Lee WA, Matsumura JS, Mitchell RS, et al. Endovascular repair of traumatic thoracic aortic injury: clinical practice guidelines of the Society for Vascular Surgery. *J Vasc Surg*. 2011;53(1):187-192.

Raptis CA, Hammer MM, Raman KG, Mellnick VM, Bhalla S. Acute traumatic aortic injury: practical considerations for the diagnostic radiologist. *J Thorac Imaging*. 2015;30(3):202-213.

7 **Answer C.** Clinical practice guidelines from the Society of Vascular Surgery recommend TEVAR over open surgery and over expectant medical management for aortic injury grades II through IV. Additionally, TEVAR should be performed within 24 hours of diagnosis or before discharge in selected patients. Type I injuries can be managed expectantly with serial cross-sectional imaging.

Reference: Lee WA, Matsumura JS, Mitchell RS, et al. Endovascular repair of traumatic thoracic aortic injury: clinical practice guidelines of the Society for Vascular Surgery. *J Vasc Surg.* 2011;53(1):187-192.

8 **Answer B.** The normal branching of the thoracic aorta arch is right brachiocephalic artery, left common carotid artery, and most distal, the left subclavian artery. With thoracic aorta endograft placement, it is sometimes necessary to cover/exclude the left subclavian artery in order to fully treat the pathology and have an adequate landing zone for the device. In the case example, the right brachiocephalic artery and left common carotid artery are visualized; however, the native left subclavian artery is not filling. Instead, a left common carotid to left subclavian arterial bypass with a synthetic graft has been performed with preservation of in-line flow to the left upper extremity. This is easily distinguished from a normal variant, given the orthogonal takeoff of the bypass graft from the left common carotid artery (end-to-side anastomosis), as well as lack of visualized branches off the section of bypass graft. There is no venous filling to indicate an AVF, nor would this preserve flow to the left arm.

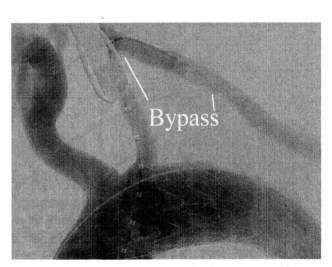

Figure 8-1 Angiographic appearance of left carotid-subclavian arterial bypass with synthetic graft.

Reference: Morgan TA, Steenburg SD, Siegel EL, Mirvis SE. Acute traumatic aortic injuries: posttherapy multidetector CT findings. *Radiographics.* 2010;30(4):851-867.

9 **Answer C.** The case images show a right axillosubclavian approach single lumen portacath with tip in the superior vena cava. Following injection of contrast through the access needle, there is appropriate opacification of the reservoir and catheter tubing. However, there is a jet of contrast extending laterally in the infraclavicular region that appears to arise from the catheter as it courses by the lateral border of the right first rib (Figure 9-1, red arrow).

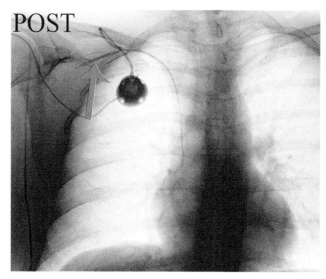

Figure 9-1   Portacath dye study showing "pinch-off syndrome" with catheter perforation and extravasation into the soft tissues (arrow).

The findings are consistent with "pinch-off syndrome." This occurs when the vein is accessed medial to the lateral border of the first rib at the time of porta-cath placement. The catheter becomes trapped between the overlying clavicle and underlying first rib, resulting in repetitive trauma and catheter injury. Findings can vary from subtle kink in the catheter to complete transection with catheter frag-ment embolization to the right heart chambers and pulmonary arteries. Portacath revision is recommended when pinch-off is identified. Axial CT image from the patient in the case example (Figure 9-2) shows extreme medial venous access in the subclavian vein. In the Instructions for Use (IFU), many manufacturers explicitly state venous access medial to the lateral border of the first rib is contraindicated when placing infraclavicular portacaths.

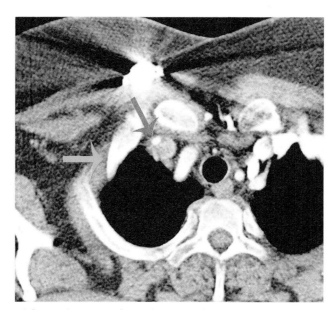

Figure 9-2   Axial CECT (contrast-enhanced computed tomography) image from the patient in the case example shows the venous entry (red arrow) of the catheter quite medial to the lateral border of the first rib (blue arrow).

Reference: Hinke DH, Zandt-Stastny DA, Goodman LR, Quebbeman EJ, Krzywda EA, Andris DA. Pinch-off syndrome: a complication of implantable subclavian venous access devices. *Radiology*. 1990;177(2):353-356.

10 **Answer C.**   The scout image shows a normally positioned tunneled hemodialysis catheter. Injection of contrast through the retracted catheter shows a long, thin tube filling with contrast extending from the left innominate vein into the superior vena cava, instead of the normal large-caliber central veins. Notice the double density in the caudal segment of the superior vena cava, where there is contrast filling the fibrin sheath and opacifying the normal vessel. Long-term indwelling central venous catheters are prone to the development of a fibrin sheath that forms along the catheter tubing and may ultimately obstruct some or all of the catheter lumens. A clue to its presence is a history of difficulty with aspiration. As negative pressure is applied to the catheter lumen, the fibrin sheath obstructs the end- or sideholes causing obstruction (similar to a one-way valve). Often, the catheter will flush appropriately.

Reference: Janne d'Othée B, Tham JC, Sheiman RG. Restoration of patency in failing tunneled hemodialysis catheters: a comparison of catheter exchange, exchange and balloon disruption of the fibrin sheath, and femoral stripping. *J Vasc Interv Radiol.* 2006;17(6):1011-1015.

11 **Answer A.**   Catheter-associated fibrin sheath formation can be treated in several ways. Studies have shown short-duration tPA infusion through the catheter, catheter stripping, and balloon fragmentation of the sheath to be effective in restoring catheter function. Anticoagulation for 3 months is appropriate treatment for catheter-associated venous thrombosis, but unlikely to affect a fibrin sheath. If the catheter is exchanged over a wire, the new catheter will still reside within the sheath and quickly become dysfunctional. Our patient underwent balloon fragmentation with repeat venogram showing disruption of the sheath with filling of normal central veins (see Figure 11-1).

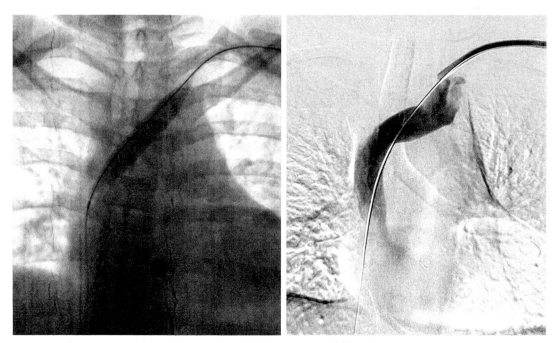

Figure 11-1   Balloon fragmentation of catheter-associated fibrin sheath (see pretreatment image from question 10). The new catheter remained functional for 9 months after this intervention.

References: Janne d'Othée B, Tham JC, Sheiman RG. Restoration of patency in failing tunneled hemodialysis catheters: a comparison of catheter exchange, exchange and balloon disruption of the fibrin sheath, and femoral stripping. *J Vasc Interv Radiol.* 2006;17(6):1011-1015.

Savader SJ, Ehrman KO, Porter DJ, Haikal LC, Oteham AC. Treatment of hemodialysis catheter-associated fibrin sheaths by rt-PA infusion: critical analysis of 124 procedures. *J Vasc Interv Radiol.* 2001;12(6):711-715.

12 Answer B. The CTA images demonstrate a relatively uniform low-density filling defect straddling the main pulmonary artery bifurcation, extending into the right and left pulmonary arteries. The filling defect conforms to the vessel, without extension beyond. There are additional filling defects in the peripheral pulmonary artery branches. The right atrium and ventricle are abnormally dilated, and the left atrium and ventricle appear collapsed. With the patient history provided, the findings are consistent with acute pulmonary embolism (with severe right heart strain). The aorta appears normal. Pulmonary angiosarcoma is a rare tumor, which can arise in the pulmonary artery wall. The tumor is locally aggressive and often produces an irregular, lobulated, avidly enhancing soft tissue mass that fills the pulmonary artery (similar to clot) and can invade adjacent structures.

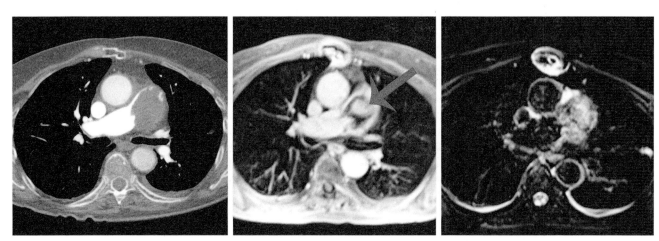

Figure 12-1 Companion case of presumptive pulmonary embolism. Axial CTA image (left) shows a large central filling defect in the main pulmonary artery. Although enhancement of clot is not evident, there are no distal emboli, and MRI is recommended for further evaluation. Axial postcontrast T1 VIBE (middle) shows avid central enhancement (arrow) of the filling defect, which is hyperintense on T2 FS (right). These CT and MRI features are consistent with tumor, and biopsy confirmed pulmonary angiosarcoma.

References: Liu M, Luo C, Wang Y, et al. Multiparametric MRI in differentiating pulmonary artery sarcoma and pulmonary thromboembolism: a preliminary experience. *Diagn Interv Radiol.* 2017;23(1):15-21.

Wittram C, Maher MM, Yoo AJ, Kalra MK, Shepard JA, Mcloud TC. CT angiography of pulmonary embolism: diagnostic criteria and causes of misdiagnosis. *Radiographics.* 2004;24(5):1219-1238.

13 **Answer B.** The RV:LV ratio is a comparison of the short-axis diameter measured on an axial or reformatted cross-sectional images. Normal is < 0.9. Anything > 0.9 is considered right heart strain.

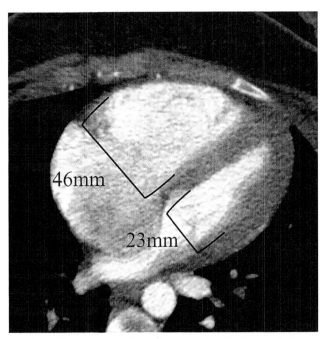

Figure 13-1 Patient with acute PE and right heart strain. RV:LV ratio of 2.0 measured on an axial CTA image. The measured short axis diameter is the maximum distance from the interventricular septum to the endocardial border perpendicular to the long axis of the heart.

References: Kamel EM, Schmidt S, Doenz F, Adler-etechami G, Schnyder P, Qanadli SD. Computed tomographic angiography in acute pulmonary embolism: do we need multiplanar reconstructions to evaluate the right ventricular dysfunction? *J Comput Assist Tomogr.* 2008;32(3):438-443.

Kumamaru KK, George E, Ghosh N, et al. Normal ventricular diameter ratio on CT provides adequate assessment for critical right ventricular strain among patients with acute pulmonary embolism. *Int J Cardiovasc Imaging.* 2016;32(7):1153-1161.

14 **Answer C.** The patient from the case example is hemodynamically unstable (hypotension or shock) with acute PE placing her in the high-risk or massive PE category. Hemodynamically stable patients with acute PE, positive biomarkers (troponin or BNP elevation), and/or imaging evidence of right heart strain are considered intermediate-risk or submassive PE. Hemodynamically stable patients with acute PE but no evidence of right heart strain are considered low-risk PE. The quantity and/or location of clot is not typically used in this classification.

References: Konstantinides SV, Barco S, Lankeit M, Meyer G. Management of pulmonary embolism: an update. *J Am Coll Cardiol.* 2016;67(8):976-990.

Piazza G, Goldhaber SZ. Management of submassive pulmonary embolism. *Circulation.* 2010;122(11):1124-1129.

15 **Answer B.** Current national guidelines support treatment beyond anticoagulation alone when patients present with high-risk or massive PE. This condition, if left untreated, has a high mortality. Options for treatment include systemic fibrinolysis with intravenous tPA (or its equivalent), catheter-directed intervention, or surgical embolectomy. An IVC filter may be a useful adjunct in this situation when there is extensive residual lower extremity clot; however, it is not primary therapy. Notably, management of intermediate-risk (submassive) PE is in flux with treatment ranging from solely anticoagulation to surgical embolectomy.

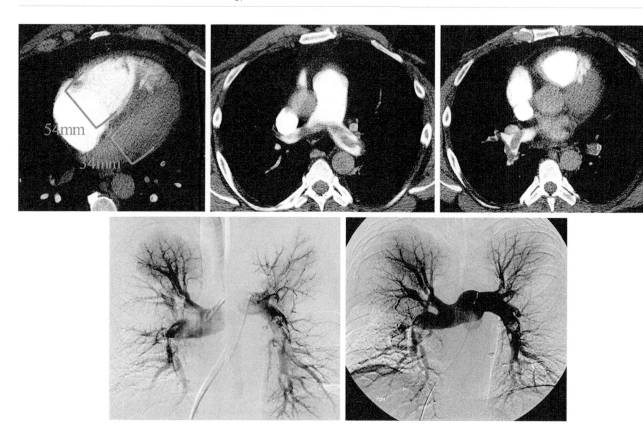

Figure 15-1 Example of a patient with massive PE. Initial chest CTA (top images) shows a saddle embolus with extensive bilateral lower lobe emboli. The RV:LV ratio is 1.5. He is hypotensive and has a contraindication to systemic tPA. Initial pulmonary angiogram (bottom left) shows the significant embolic burden and overall poor filling of both lungs. He is treated with rotary pigtail catheter clot fragmentation and clot aspiration, and he undergoes 24 hours of low-dose tPA infusion through multi-sidehole catheters draped into each lower lobe pulmonary artery. His hypotension resolves quickly, and repeat pulmonary angiogram the following day (bottom right) shows significant clot resolution and overall markedly improved perfusion to both lungs.

References: Kearon C, Akl EA, Comerota AJ, et al. Antithrombotic therapy for VTE disease: antithrombotic therapy and prevention of thrombosis, 9th ed. American College of Chest Physicians Evidence-Based Clinical Practice Guidelines. *Chest*. 2012;141(2 suppl):e419S-e496S.

Xue X, Sista AK. Catheter-directed thrombolysis for pulmonary embolism: the state of practice. *Tech Vasc Interv Radiol*. 2018;21(2):78-84.

16   **Answer A.** The axial CTA images demonstrate 2 enlarged vessels in the periphery of the right lower lobe. On the coronal images, there is a tangle of blood vessels clumped together at the right lung base. With the patient's history, this is most consistent with a PAVM. The enlarged vessels represent the hypertrophied feeding pulmonary artery and draining pulmonary vein (slightly larger than the artery), and the tangle of vessels represents the dilated venous sac(s). PAVM represents a right to left shunt, putting the patient at risk for paradoxical embolism, as well as infections such as brain abscess. Pulmonary artery pseudoaneurysm and pulmonary varix, while vascular abnormalities, do not have an enlarged feeding artery and vein, although they may look similar to the venous sac of a PAVM. All pseudoaneurysms should be treated, whereas pulmonary varix is classically asymptomatic and not a danger to the patient. Choice B is a soft tissue tumor, not a vascular abnormality.

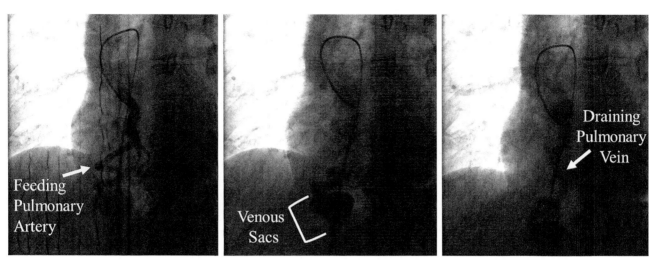

Figure 16-1 Unsubtracted images from right lower lobe selective pulmonary artery catheterization. Arterial phase image on the left shows single 6 mm feeding pulmonary artery branch coursing inferiorly with filling of lobulated venous sacs. On the delayed image (right), the draining pulmonary vein is visualized. This is a simple type PAVM with single inflow artery, well-formed venous sacs, and single draining vein. PAVMs are characterized as complex when there are multiple feeding arteries and/or draining veins, or when there is more diffuse involvement of a segment or lobe of the lung.

Reference: Gill SS, Roddie ME, Shovlin CL, Jackson JE. Pulmonary arteriovenous malformations and their mimics. *Clin Radiol.* 2015;70(1):96-110.

17 **Answer B.** Hereditary hemorrhagic telangiectasia (HHT) or Osler-Weber-Rendu is an inherited condition, autosomal dominant, characterized by recurrent and spontaneous nosebleeds (from mucosal telangiectasias), multiple telangiectasias on the skin and within the GI tract, and arteriovenous malformations of the internal organs (commonly lung, liver, brain). There are several HHT Centers of Excellence in the United States that specialize in the diagnosis and treatment of patients with HHT. The Curaçao criteria assist practitioners in evaluating patients with suspected HHT.

Klippel-Trenaunay is a vascular malformation syndrome characterized by the presence of a capillary malformation, venous malformation, limb growth abnormality, and often a lymphatic malformation. Patients with Klippel-Trenaunay frequently have mutations in the PIK3CA gene. Tuberous sclerosis is a complex genetic disorder (genetic mutation on chromosome 9 or 16) in which affected patients can develop benign tumors and cysts in the central nervous system, skin, lungs, kidneys, heart, eyes, and pancreas. Sturge-Weber is a genetic disorder manifested at or soon after birth by a facial capillary malformation. Associated intracranial leptomeningeal vascular abnormalities result in cerebral ischemia, producing developmental delay, seizures, and other neurologic symptoms.

Reference: Faughnan ME, Palda VA, Garcia-tsao G, et al. International guidelines for the diagnosis and management of hereditary haemorrhagic telangiectasia. *J Med Genet.* 2011;48(2):73-87.

18 **Answer A.** For years, it was accepted practice that only PAVMs with feeding artery size >3 mm needed to be embolized. This guideline was based on limited data, and the technology for embolization has greatly improved in the last few years. Complications from PAVM with smaller feeding arteries have been reported, and successful embolizations are now being performed in this cohort. Current HHT guidelines recommend embolization of PAVMs in adults whether symptomatic or asymptomatic. Selection of a PAVM for embolization continues to be based on feeding artery diameter, with 3 mm as a generally accepted threshold for considering embolization. However, operators may consider embolization when the feeding artery diameter is 2 to 3 mm.

References: Narsinh KH, Ramaswamy R, Kinney TB. Management of pulmonary arteriovenous malformations in hereditary hemorrhagic telangiectasia patients. *Semin Intervent Radiol.* 2013;30(4):408-412.

Trerotola SO, Pyeritz RE. PAVM embolization: an update. *AJR Am J Roentgenol.* 2010;195(4):837-845.

19 **Answer A.** As a PAVM represents a right to left shunt, the embolization procedure and selected embolic agent need to be carefully controlled to avoid nontarget embolization to the systemic arteries. Additionally, the embolization should be permanent with low rate of recanalization. Coils (both pushable and detachable) can be delivered through selective diagnostic and microcatheters. Good technique is necessary to minimize the risk of coil migration or maldeployment into the pulmonary venous system. Uncovered (Amplatzer Vascular Plug) and covered (Micro Vascular Plug) detachable plugs have also been used with good success, sometimes with adjunctive coils to reduce future recanalization.

Particles are much smaller than the pathologic artery to vein connection of a PAVM, and if used will shunt directly to the pulmonary vein and subsequently the systemic arteries. Glue, a liquid embolic, is difficult to control and also is likely to immediately shunt through to the draining pulmonary vein, which could be catastrophic. Gelfoam slurry is not only considered a temporary embolic agent with relatively fast recanalization, its embolic size is highly variable and shunting to the draining pulmonary vein is assured.

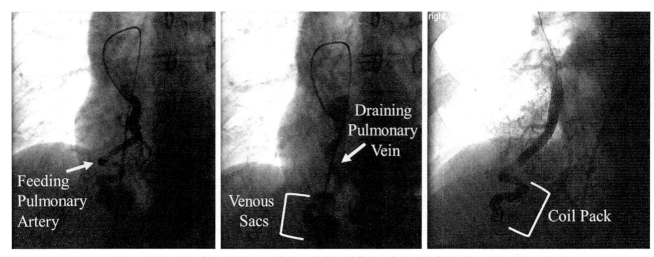

Figure 19-1 Unsubtracted images before (left, middle) and after (right) coil embolization of a simple PAVM. Following embolization with multiple pushable and detachable coils, there is no further filling of the venous sacs or draining vein. Factors associated with future recanalization of the coil pack include large feeding artery, use of single coil, coil oversizing, and positioning of coils too far from the venous sac (>1 cm).

References: Narsinh KH, Ramaswamy R, Kinney TB. Management of pulmonary arteriovenous malformations in hereditary hemorrhagic telangiectasia patients. *Semin Intervent Radiol.* 2013;30(4):408-412.

Trerotola SO, Pyeritz RE. PAVM embolization: an update. *AJR Am J Roentgenol.* 2010;195(4):837-845.

20   **Answer D.**   The chest radiograph demonstrates a normal cardiac silhouette, and the presence of a right internal jugular vein approach single lumen portacath with catheter tip near the superior cavoatrial junction. With choices A, B, or C you would expect some abnormality such as mediastinal widening, hilar masses, pleural effusion, or enlargement of the cardiac silhouette. The history supports a diagnosis of acute SVC occlusion.

References: Rachapalli V, Boucher LM. Superior vena cava syndrome: role of the interventionalist. *Can Assoc Radiol J.* 2014;65(2):168-176.

Shaikh I, Berg K, Kman N. Thrombogenic catheter-associated superior vena cava syndrome. *Case Rep Emerg Med.* 2013;2013:793054.

21   **Answer A.**   The CECT images demonstrate injection of contrast through a left upper extremity peripheral venous access. Note the dense opacification of the left-sided central veins, but also contrast in the right atrium, right ventricle, pulmonary artery, and thoracic aorta. The only structure not opacified is the superior vena cava. The portacath catheter is visualized and surrounded by low attenuation that fills the entire superior vena cava, consistent with an acute thrombus. If the central venous obstruction is severe and sudden, adequate venous collaterals will not have developed and SVC syndrome will occur. The patient will present with marked head, neck, and upper extremity swelling, plethoric facies, and respiratory compromise. The following (Figure 21-1) is an example from a different patient with acute SVC thrombosis who required urgent intubation.

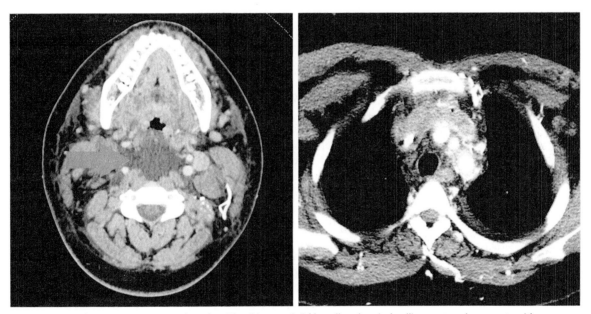

Figure 21-1   A young female with a history of sickle cell and an indwelling portacath presents with abrupt onset head and neck swelling. CECT imaging of the neck and chest shows massive retropharyngeal edema (arrow) with airway narrowing, as well as acute left innominate vein and SVC thrombosis (right image). Note the paucity of collateral vein formation. She is intubated for impending airway compromise and successfully treated with catheter-directed intervention over the next 2 days.

The treatment for acute catheter-associated thrombosis includes anticoagulation and consideration of removing the inciting catheter. If the patient is significantly symptomatic, more aggressive treatments such as catheter-directed intervention (tPA infusion, suction thrombectomy/aspiration) may be necessary. It is important to distinguish acute thrombosis of the superior vena cava (acute benign SVC syndrome) from malignant obstruction, as the treatment for malignant SVC syndrome is often external radiation therapy, chemotherapy, and/or endovascular recanalization with stenting. Malignant SVC syndrome often results from extrinsic compression of the SVC by lymphadenopathy, or mediastinal invasion from tumors such as bronchogenic carcinoma. In chronic benign occlusion of the SVC, often seen with long-standing hemodialysis catheters, the vessel will be absent/nonopacified with occasional calcification and tremendous collateral vein formation in the neck and chest.

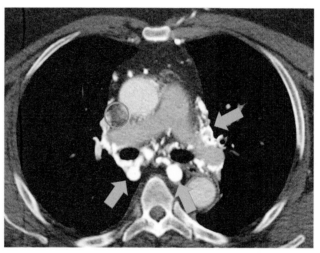

Figure 21-2 Example of chronic benign occlusion of the SVC in a patient with ESRD (end-stage renal disease) and multiple prior hemodialysis catheters. In the expected location of the SVC (orange circle), there is no visualized vein. There is compensatory dilation of mediastinal, azygous, and hemiazygous collaterals (arrows) to compensate for the central venous occlusion.

References: Rachapalli V, Boucher LM. Superior vena cava syndrome: role of the interventionalist. *Can Assoc Radiol J.* 2014;65(2):168-176.

Shaikh I, Berg K, Kman N. Thrombogenic catheter-associated superior vena cava syndrome. *Case Rep Emerg Med.* 2013;2013:793054.

22 **Answer A.** The patient is presenting with "vascular blowout" from the left axillary artery. This condition typically affects patients with advanced malignancies that have been previously treated with surgery, radiation, and/or chemotherapy. The involved vessels become friable or frankly invaded by tumor and over time can become exposed putting the patient at risk for catastrophic hemorrhage. The 3 clinical categories of vascular blowout include threatened (vessel exposed, involved with tumor, or pseudoaneurysm), impending (sentinel bleed controlled with local measures), and acute (uncontrolled bleeding). With endovascular treatment of hemorrhage, the operator must consider whether flow preservation is necessary (to prevent end organ damage) or that the bleeding artery can be sacrificed. In this case, if one were to coil embolize the axillary artery across the site of bleeding, the

arm would certainly be threatened. Particles such as PVA or TAGM could extravasate at the site of bleeding and treat the injury; however, most of the embolic would travel down the arm and lodge in the distal arteries producing limb ischemia. Glue would have the same issues and likely produce both proximal and distal arterial occlusion resulting in a threatened limb. A covered stent placed across the injury excludes the bleeding arterial rent and also maintains blood flow to the arm. If there is significant exposure of the artery, a potential complication that must be considered is stent infection. In addition to local measures such as pressure dressing, surgical bypass and surgical ligation may be appropriate in certain instances.

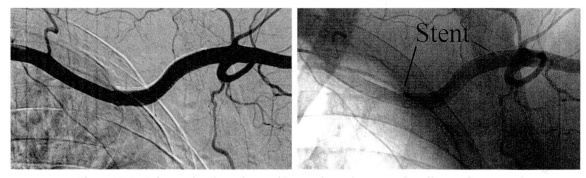

Figure 22-1 Subtracted and unsubtracted images from placement of a self-expanding covered stent across the actively bleeding left axillary artery from the case example. The stent was slightly oversized compared with the artery in order get a proximal and distal seal.

References: Huntress LA, Kogan S, Nagarsheth K, Nassiri N. Palliative endovascular techniques for management of peripheral vascular blowout syndrome in end-stage malignancies. *Vasc Endovascular Surg.* 2017;51(6):394-399.

Mousa A, Chong B, Aburahma AF. Endovascular repair of subclavian/axillary artery injury with a covered stent. A case report and review of literature. *Vascular.* 2013;21(6):400-404.

23 **Answer B.**   The case images show the early and delayed phase of an LAO thoracic aortogram. The initial image demonstrates an irregular, moderate to severe narrowing just beyond the origin of the left subclavian artery. On the delayed phase, contrast has washed out the aorta and proximal branch vessels, yet the left vertebral artery is now well opacified. This is due to retrograde filling from the cranial circulation aka subclavian steal. Although this physiology is often asymptomatic, patients can present with chronic left arm claudication, and less commonly posterior circulation symptoms such as syncope, ataxia, and diplopia.

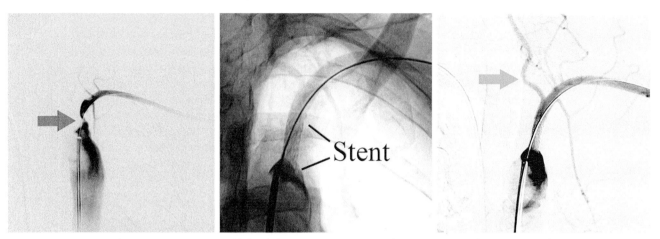

Figure 23-1 Treatment of left subclavian artery stenosis with stenting. Once the stenosis (red arrow) is crossed with a wire, a balloon expandable stent is deployed, landing well above and below the lesion. On the completion angiogram, there is now antegrade filling of the left vertebral artery (blue arrow). Interestingly, restoration of antegrade vertebral flow typically occurs at a variable (not immediate) time after treatment.

References: Potter BJ, Pinto DS. Subclavian steal syndrome. *Circulation*. 2014;129(22):2320-2323.

Wholey MH, Wholey MH. The supraaortic and vertebral endovascular interventions. *Tech Vasc Interv Radiol*. 2004;7(4):215-225.

24   **Answer D.**   Subclavian steal physiology is often asymptomatic. The reversal of flow in the vertebral artery alone (choice A) is not an indication for intervention. Unlike the carotid arterial system, there are no velocity parameters to act as guidelines for intervention. Symptoms such as arm claudication or vertebrobasilar insufficiency are indications for intervention. Additional indications include planned ipsilateral internal thoracic (mammary) artery to coronary artery bypass or existing bypass, which is adversely affected by the proximal stenosis.

References: Ochoa VM, Yeghiazarians Y. Subclavian artery stenosis: a review for the vascular medicine practitioner. *Vasc Med*. 2011;16(1):29-34.

Patel SN, White CJ, Collins TJ, et al. Catheter-based treatment of the subclavian and innominate arteries. *Catheter Cardiovasc Interv*. 2008;71(7):963-968.

25   **Answer C.**   There is debate regarding the ideal location of a central venous catheter tip, but it is widely accepted that it should be at or quite near the upper cavoatrial junction. Fluoroscopically, this lies 2 vertebral bodies below the carina.

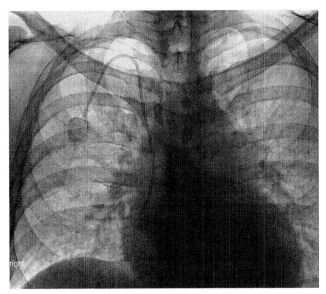

Figure 25-1   Completion fluoroscopic spot image after single lumen portacath placement. The reservoir sits over the second anterior rib in the midclavicular line. The venous access is low in the neck. The catheter tip lies 2 vertebral bodies below the carina. At the authors' institution, this is the desired positioning of a portacath.

If the catheter is too short, it can lead to fibrin sheath formation, malposition of the tip, venous stenosis, and/or venous thrombosis. The following (Figures 25-2 and 25-3) are examples of portacaths with the tip positioned in the mid-SVC that became dysfunctional over time. If a catheter is positioned very deep into the right atrium, complications such as dysrhythmia, thrombus formation, and catheter dysfunction can occur (see Figure 25-4).

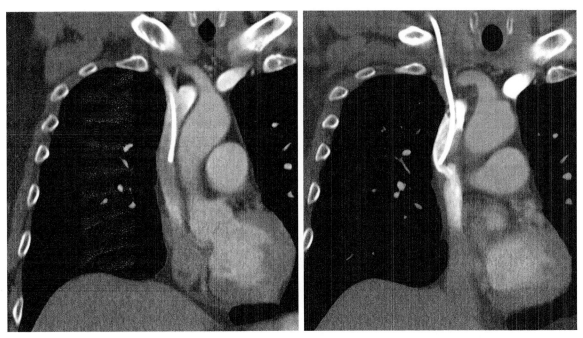

Figure 25-2   Chest CT immediately (left) and 12 months (right) after single lumen portacath placement. The catheter tip was in the mid-SVC, which appeared widely patent at first. Over time, the catheter became dysfunctional, because of progressive stenosis and deformity of the SVC at the catheter tip. The stenosis was treated with balloon angioplasty, and the portacath revised such that the tip was located in the upper right atrium.

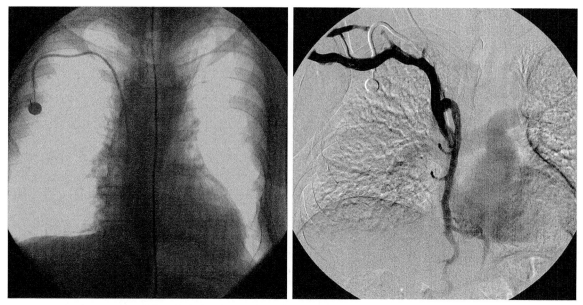

Figure 25-3   Right subclavian approach single lumen portacath was placed with the catheter tip in the mid-SVC (left). Years later, the patient presented with portacath dysfunction. Venography showed chronic occlusion of the SVC at the level of the catheter tip with retrograde filling of an enlarged azygos vein (right). The occlusion was traversed with a catheter and wire and treated with balloon angioplasty alone.

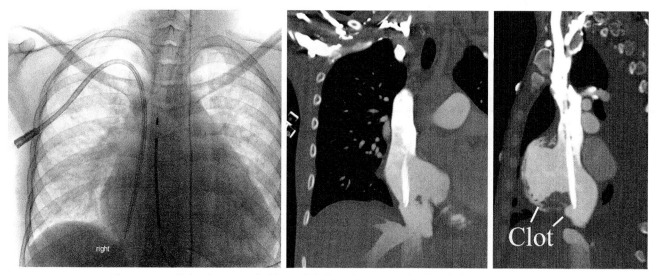

Figure 25-4   Right chest tunneled hemodialysis catheter was placed with the catheter at the lower cavoatrial junction, likely in contact with atrial wall (left). Five months later, the patient presented with acute onset shortness of breath and chest CTA demonstrated extensive pulmonary emboli as well as a large thrombus associated with the catheter tip deep in the atrium (coronal image, middle; sagittal image, right). The patient was treated with systemic anticoagulation and atrial clot removal using a large bore suction catheter system.

References: Baskin KM, Jimenez RM, Cahill AM, Jawad AF, Towbin RB. Cavoatrial junction and central venous anatomy: implications for central venous access tip position. *J Vasc Interv Radiol.* 2008;19(3):359-365.

Vesely TM. Central venous catheter tip position: a continuing controversy. *J Vasc Interv Radiol.* 2003;14(5):527-534.

26 **Answer A.**   The management of acute type B aortic dissections continues to evolve. Dissections can be classified as complicated or uncomplicated. Uncomplicated dissections are typically managed medically. Complicated dissections are often managed with an intervention, be it thoracic endovascular aortic repair (TEVAR) with a covered stent or open surgery. Complicated dissections are defined as those with impending rupture or malperfusion of organs such as the spinal cord, viscera, kidneys, or lower extremities. Refractory chest pain is a clinical sign of impending rupture and qualifies as complicated. The in-hospital survival for complicated type B dissection patients is approximately 50%, while about 90% of uncomplicated patients survive until discharge. The remaining choices are features of interest in evaluating a dissection; however, they do not define one as complicated.

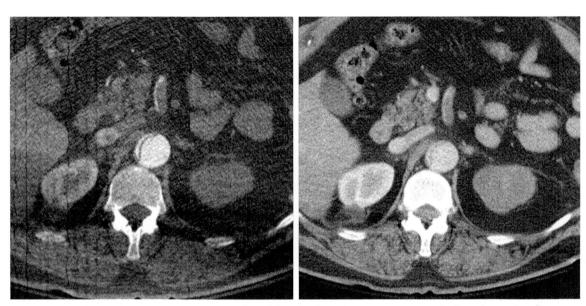

Figure 26-1   CTA images (arterial, left; delayed, right) of an acute type B aortic dissection with evolving left renal ischemia/infarction. Notice the involvement of the proximal SMA (superior mesenteric artery) as well. This case is in contradistinction to Q35 of noninvasive imaging, whereby a chronic type B dissection causes delayed enhancement of an adequately perfused left kidney (it just takes longer for the contrast to get there).

References: Nauta FJ, Trimarchi S, Kamman AV, et al. Update in the management of type B aortic dissection. *Vasc Med.* 2016;21(3):251-263.

Scott AJ, Bicknell CD. Contemporary management of acute type B dissection. *Eur J Vasc Endovasc Surg.* 2016;51(3):452-459.

27   **Answer A.**   The catheter is positioned in the origin of the left subclavian artery. The marked vessel is the left internal thoracic (mammary) artery, which is one of the first vessels to arise from the subclavian artery, almost directly opposite the cephalad coursing vertebral artery. The internal thoracic artery descends just lateral to the sternum and continues as the superior epigastric artery, ultimately meeting up with branches of the inferior epigastric artery (which arises from the external iliac artery) in the anterior abdominal wall. This pathway (subclavian >> internal thoracic >> superior epigastric >> inferior epigastric >> external iliac), termed Winslow pathway (see Figure 27-1), can hypertrophy in the setting of aortic occlusive disease, allowing for continued perfusion to the pelvis and lower extremities.

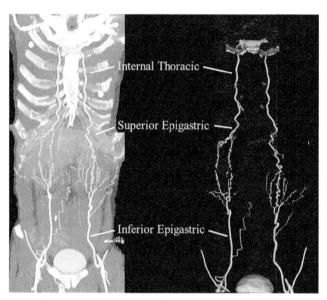

Figure 27-1   Coronal MIP (left) and 3D VR (right) CTA images in a male smoker with a chronic infrarenal aortic occlusion and resultant hypertrophy of Winslow pathway.

The pathway is also germane to patients with bleeding from the abdominal wall, which is occasionally seen with anticoagulation, after paracentesis, and following surgery or trauma. If the bleeding occurs lower on the abdomen, the inferior epigastric artery can be selected and embolized as close to the injury as possible. In some cases, particularly if the injury is in the watershed territory, bleeding may persist or recur, as collateral pathways from above allow for continued perfusion to the injured vessel. The following case (Figure 27-2) shows continued bleeding in the abdominal wall despite prior embolization of the inferior epigastric artery.

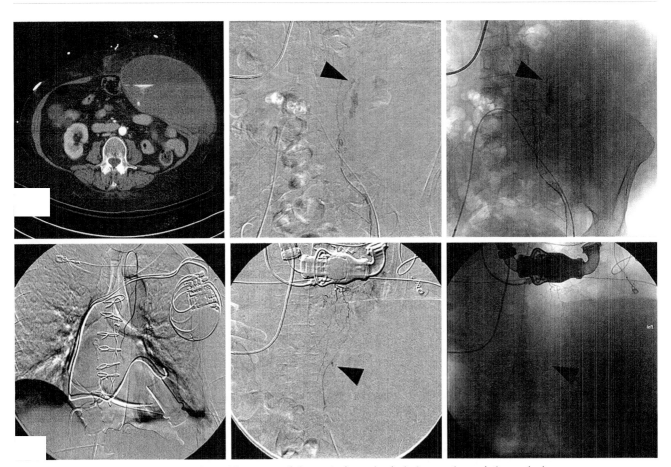

Figure 27-2 Patient with an LVAD (left ventricular assist device) on anticoagulation and a large hemoglobin drop. The CECT image shows large left rectus hematoma with active bleeding around the level of the umbilicus. After selection of the left inferior epigastric artery (top images), angiography shows brisk active bleeding (arrowheads) from a distal branch near the watershed territory. The bleed is treated with gelfoam slurry and coil embolization. Two days later, there is further drop in the hemoglobin level. Repeat angiography from above after selection of the left internal thoracic artery (bottom images) shows recurrent bleeding from the same site, being fed from the superior epigastric artery branches. The bleed is treated with gelfoam slurry and coil embolization with no recurrence.

Reference: Hardman RL, Lopera JE, Cardan RA, Trimmer CK, Josephs SC. Common and rare collateral pathways in aortoiliac occlusive disease: a pictorial essay. *AJR Am J Roentgenol.* 2011;197(3):W519-W524.

28 **Answer B.** With percutaneous lung lesion biopsy, there are often several acceptable needle paths. Some approaches have been shown to have a higher complication rate than others. Choice A intersects the internal thoracic artery. It also crosses the pleural surface at an oblique angle, which increases the risk of pneumothorax. Choice C intersects the lateral thoracic artery, crosses the pleural surface at an oblique angle, and would require decubitus positioning. Choice D requires crossing a major fissure and necessitates a long needle tract, both increasing the risk of pneumothorax. Choice B is best as it requires the shortest needle path with no intervening arteries, large pulmonary vessels, or pulmonary fissures. It crosses the pleural surface as close to perpendicular as possible. Other factors shown to increase the risk of postbiopsy pneumothorax are operator inexperience, lesion size <2 cm, and the presence of underlying chronic obstructive pulmonary disease.

References: Tsai IC, Tsai WL, Chen MC, et al. CT-guided core biopsy of lung lesions: a primer. *AJR Am J Roentgenol.* 2009;193(5):1228-1235.

Winokur RS, Pua BB, Sullivan BW, Madoff DC. Percutaneous lung biopsy: technique, efficacy, and complications. *Semin Intervent Radiol.* 2013;30(2):121-127.

29   **Answer C.**   Pneumothorax after percutaneous lung biopsy is the most common complication with rates reported between 17% and 26%. Fortunately, the majority of these will be self-limited and require no invasive treatment. A typical postprocedure regimen includes close clinical monitoring of the patient and a chest X-ray 2 hours postbiopsy. If there is a growing pneumothorax or a symptomatic pneumothorax, a chest tube is indicated. The size or volume of the pneumothorax is often difficult to accurately quantify and not an indication for tube placement. Oxygen saturation could help in the triage of these patients if there is a change in status, but O_2 saturation <94% may be the patient's baseline and alone is not a criterion for a chest tube.

References: Winokur RS, Pua BB, Sullivan BW, Madoff DC. Percutaneous lung biopsy: technique, efficacy, and complications. *Semin Intervent Radiol.* 2013;30(2):121-127.

Wu CC, Maher MM, Shepard JA. Complications of CT-guided percutaneous needle biopsy of the chest: prevention and management. *AJR Am J Roentgenol.* 2011;196(6):W678-W682.

30   **Answer A.**   Lung abscess is often seen in patients with alcohol dependence, altered mental status, gastroesophageal reflux, and/or poor dentition. Up to 90% can be managed conservatively with antibiotics alone. For refractory cases, intervention is required. Traditionally this has been the realm of thoracic surgery, but recently percutaneous or even endobronchial drainage have become acceptable options. There is a real risk of bronchopleural fistula with percutaneous drainage; therefore preprocedural consultation with thoracic surgery is strongly recommended. The risk does not constitute an absolute contraindication; therefore choice B is incorrect. The size of the percutaneous drain may logically correlate with the risk of bleeding, pneumothorax, or fistula; however, there is no specified size threshold. Additionally, the presence of an underlying malignancy plays no clear role in the treatment algorithm. Choice A is the best option. In addition to improved abscess resolution with percutaneous drainage, an equally important benefit is fluid sampling at the time of catheter placement. Direct fluid sampling has been shown to have a higher rate of culture growth compared with peripheral blood, bronchoscopic or sputum cultures. In one series, the results of direct fluid sampling changed antibiotic management in >50% of patients.

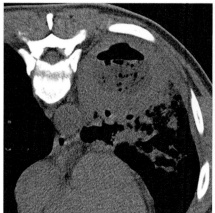 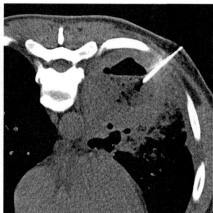 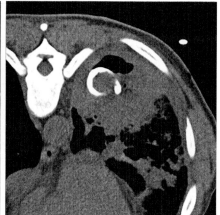

Figure 30-1   CT-guided placement of a 10 Fr pigtail drainage catheter into a persistent left lower lobe lung abscess.

References: Duncan C, Nadolski GJ, Gade T, Hunt S. Understanding the lung abscess microbiome: outcomes of percutaneous lung parenchymal abscess drainage with microbiologic correlation. *Cardiovasc Intervent Radiol.* 2017;40(6):902-906.

Klein JS, Schultz S, Heffner JE. Interventional radiology of the chest: image-guided percutaneous drainage of pleural effusions, lung abscess, and pneumothorax. *AJR Am J Roentgenol.* 1995;164(3):581-588.

31 Answer D.   Reexpansion pulmonary edema is an uncommon complication with a reported incidence of <1% after the drainage of pleural effusions. Unfortunately, the mortality can be as high as 20%. The pathophysiology is not completely understood. Symptoms typically occur within an hour of pleural drainage of either fluid and/or air. There may be a relationship with the volume of fluid/air removed; however, a consensus on volume removal limits does not exist. The images from this case demonstrate dependent ground glass opacities progressing to consolidation, which is typically described. Hemothorax is an accumulation of blood in the pleural space and is not shown in the provided images. Underlying malignancy would not explain the rapid change in CT appearance. An acute myocardial infarction could cause flash pulmonary edema, but this case presentation is temporally associated with bilateral thoracentesis, making choice D most likely.

References: Dias OM, Teixeira LR, Vargas FS. Reexpansion pulmonary edema after therapeutic thoracentesis. *Clinics (Sao Paulo)*. 2010;65(12):1387-1389.

Verhagen M, Van Buijtenen JM, Geeraedts LM. Reexpansion pulmonary edema after chest drainage for pneumothorax: a case report and literature overview. *Respir Med Case Rep*. 2015;14:10-12.

32a Answer B.   In the provided images, the catheter is positioned in the proximal brachial artery and there is opacification of only arteries. There is no early venous filling to indicate an AVF in the upper arm (or distally for that matter). The historical clue of previous pacemaker placement suggests that the pathology may be more centrally located. The catheter is likely positioned beyond the fistula and should be pulled back to a less selective position (choice B). More selective catheter positioning is often helpful in looking for a subtle bleed or identifying the exact feeding branch of an AVF. Carbon dioxide gas angiography is a good technique for ferreting out occult pathology, but often as a last resort, and would not be clearly beneficial in this circumstance. If there was evidence for vasospasm, which might mask the pathology, intra-arterial nitroglycerin can be administered. There is no evidence of spasm on the images.

References: Kumins NH, Tober JC, Love CJ, et al. Arteriovenous fistulae complicating cardiac pacemaker lead extraction: recognition, evaluation, and management. *J Vasc Surg*. 2000;32(6):1225-1228.

O'Connor DJ, Gross J, King B, Suggs WD, Gargiulo NJ, Lipsitz EC. Endovascular management of multiple arteriovenous fistulae following failed laser-assisted pacemaker lead extraction. *J Vasc Surg*. 2010;51(6):1517-1520.

32b Answer A.   With the catheter tip in the left subclavian artery, the angiogram shows initial arterial filling followed immediately by early opacification of the left subclavian and axillary veins due to an AVF. Interestingly, the contrast fills the left arm veins from central to peripheral, which is due to an underlying central venous occlusion at the level of the left innominate vein. This unfortunate combination of a large acquired AVF with concomitant central venous occlusion led to the patient's massive arm swelling. The thoracoacromial arterial trunk was the site of fistula formation, which was occluded with multiple precisely placed coils.

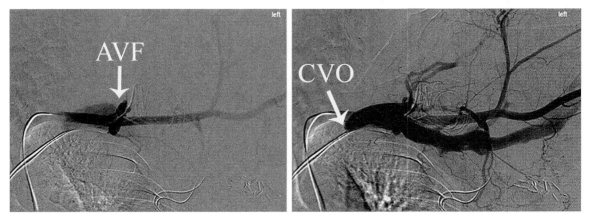

Figure 32b-1   DSA images from left subclavian arteriography with arteriovenous fistula (AVF) between the thoracoacromial trunk and the left subclavian vein. Because of the underlying central venous occlusion (CVO), the veins of the arm filled in retrograde fashion. Ultimately, the contrast filled large chest and neck collaterals, which drained back to the superior vena cava (not shown). This combination of vascular complications, both from pacemaker lead placement, was a source of tremendous patient morbidity. Following embolization, the left upper arm circumference went from 58 cm down to 25 cm, with no appreciable asymmetry when compared with the right arm.

References: Kumins NH, Tober JC, Love CJ, et al. Arteriovenous fistulae complicating cardiac pacemaker lead extraction: recognition, evaluation, and management. *J Vasc Surg.* 2000;32(6):1225-1228.

O'Connor DJ, Gross J, King B, Suggs WD, Gargiulo NJ, Lipsitz EC. Endovascular management of multiple arteriovenous fistulae following failed laser-assisted pacemaker lead extraction. *J Vasc Surg.* 2010;51(6):1517-1520.

33   Answer C.   The CECT images demonstrate an ovoid lesion in the right lower lobe of the lung with similar attenuation to the visualized vasculature. There is surrounding pulmonary consolidation. The pulmonary arteriogram demonstrates a well-defined, ovoid, contrast-filled structure in contiguity with a right pulmonary artery branch, which washes out over time. This appearance is consistent with a mycotic aneurysm (more accurate to call it a pseudoaneurysm). As there is no early filling of a draining pulmonary vein, this does not represent an AVF or AVM. The contrast remains contained in the pseudoaneurysm with delayed washout and no pooling to indicate active extravasation. This patient presented with hemoptysis in the setting of pneumonia. Mycotic aneurysm (pseudoaneurysm) formation is most commonly seen with *Staphylococcus* and *Streptococcus* species and develops as the infectious arteritis destroys the arterial wall resulting in contained rupture. They can enlarge rapidly and cause catastrophic hemorrhage. A similar entity with a recent resurgence is a Rasmussen aneurysm, which is a pulmonary artery pseudoaneurysm arising specifically in the setting of a mycobacterial cavitary lesion.

Regarding treatment, placing a covered stent would be challenging in this location. The parent artery is small, which limits stent selection and translates to low patency rates. Also, because of the extensive branching nature of the pulmonary arterial system, clean landing zones would be difficult to achieve. The endovascular treatment chosen here was coil embolization. Although it seems to be a large territory of pulmonary artery to embolize, it was tolerated quite well with long-term follow-up imaging demonstrating a small sliver of scar tissue peripherally to the coil pack.

References: Keeling AN, Costello R, Lee MJ. Rasmussen's aneurysm: a forgotten entity? *Cardiovasc Intervent Radiol.* 2008;31(1):196-200.

Lee WK, Mossop PJ, Little AF, et al. Infected (mycotic) aneurysms: spectrum of imaging appearances and management. *Radiographics.* 2008;28(7):1853-1868.

34 **Answer B.**   The CT images from the biopsy procedure demonstrate new extensive ground glass in the path of the biopsy needle and surrounding the nodule. This is consistent with pulmonary hemorrhage and explains the onset of hemoptysis. The best initial step is to position the patient biopsy side down. This position will spare the contralateral lung from aspirated blood, which could further compromise lung aeration and gas exchange. As the pathology is intraparenchymal and not intrapleural, a chest tube would not be of use. Reverse Trendelenburg or "head up" might help by keeping the hemorrhage dependent; however, it will not optimally protect the unaffected contralateral lung. Immediate embolization is not appropriate. Management of airway and breathing is paramount. If the bleeding does not stop and there is pulmonary compromise, intubation and bronchial blockade may be necessary. Angiography with embolization can then be considered but is rarely necessary in this scenario.

Reference: Khankan A, Sirhan S, Aris F. Common complications of nonvascular percutaneous thoracic interventions: diagnosis and management. *Semin Intervent Radiol.* 2015;32(2): 174-181.

35 **Answer D.**   Surgery is first-line therapy for both primary and oligometastatic lung malignancy, when possible. If surgery is not feasible, options include stereotactic body radiotherapy (SBRT) and percutaneous thermal ablation. Cryo, radiofrequency, and microwave thermal ablation have all been utilized in practice. Complication rates vary, with a pneumothorax being a regular occurrence (10 to 50%). Development of a bronchopleural fistula is relatively uncommon (<1%). Local tumor control correlates inversely with increasing size of the target tumor.

References: Egashira Y, Singh S, Bandula S, Illing R. Percutaneous high-energy microwave ablation for the treatment of pulmonary tumors: a retrospective single-center experience. *J Vasc Interv Radiol.* 2016;27(4):474-479.

Healey TT, March BT, Baird G, Dupuy DE. Microwave ablation for lung neoplasms: a retrospective analysis of long-term results. *J Vasc Interv Radiol.* 2017;28(2):206-211.

Mouli SK, Kurilova I, Sofocleous CT, Lewandowski RJ. The role of percutaneous image-guided thermal ablation for the treatment of pulmonary malignancies. *AJR Am J Roentgenol.* 2017;209(4):740-751.

Rose SC, Thistlethwaite PA, Sewell PE, Vance RB. Lung cancer and radiofrequency ablation. *J Vasc Interv Radiol.* 2006;17(6):927-951.

36 **Answer A.**   The intraprocedural CT images for this prone patient demonstrate a small right pneumothorax and nondependent air within the left ventricle. The most important step is early recognition of this complication. It is easy to get tunnel vision during the procedure and remain only focused on getting the biopsy needle into the target lesion. The reported incidence of systemic air embolism from percutaneous lung biopsy is 0.02% to 0.07% and can be associated with significant morbidity and mortality. As little as 2 cc air into the cerebral vasculature can be fatal, and 0.5 to 1 cc air in the pulmonary veins can cause cardiac arrest from coronary embolism. Altered mental status is often a presenting symptom. Once recognized, the procedure should be aborted and the needle removed to minimize any further air introduction. Regarding patient positioning, some advocate for Trendelenburg to prevent air embolus to the brain. Right lateral decubitus can theoretically trap the air in the left ventricle apex, but at least one case has been reported where left lateral decubitus was advantageous to trap the air in the left atrium. Flow rates in the left heart may be too fast to reliably trap air with any position. Hyperbaric oxygen therapy is an adjunctive treatment available in some centers. The high concentration of O_2 in the blood forces nitrogen out of the intravascular air, reducing the air bubble volume and associated inflammatory response from the embolus.

References: Kok HK, Leong S, Salati U, Torreggiani WC, Govender P. Left atrial and systemic air embolism after lung biopsy: importance of treatment positioning. *J Vasc Interv Radiol.* 2013;24(10):1587-1588.

Ramaswamy R, Narsinh KH, Tuan A, Kinney TB. Systemic air embolism following percutaneous lung biopsy. *Semin Intervent Radiol.* 2014;31(4):375-377.

5 Gastrointestinal

1   Which of the following is considered a potentially curative treatment for hepato-cellular carcinoma (HCC)?

   A. Thermal ablation
   B. Conventional transarterial chemoembolization (cTACE)
   C. Drug-eluting beads transarterial chemoembolization (DEBTACE)
   D. Sorafenib

2   What complication is depicted on these fluoroscopic images from a gastrostomy tube study?

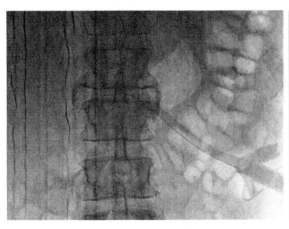 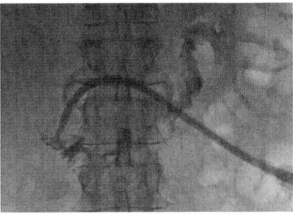

   A. Gastrostomy tube is clogged
   B. Internal fixation balloon is malpositioned
   C. Contrast extravasation into the lesser sac
   D. Contrast extravasation along the tube tract

3   How should interventional radiology best triage a gastrostomy tube placement request in a patient with ascites?

   A. Refer to gastroenterology as endoscopic placement is the only safe option
   B. Deny request as ascites is an absolute contraindication for gastrostomy tube placement
   C. Perform percutaneous gastrostomy tube placement with preprocedure paracentesis
   D. Perform percutaneous gastrostomy tube placement with ascites untouched to keep sterile

4   Which is the best approach for percutaneous cholecystostomy tube placement in this patient?

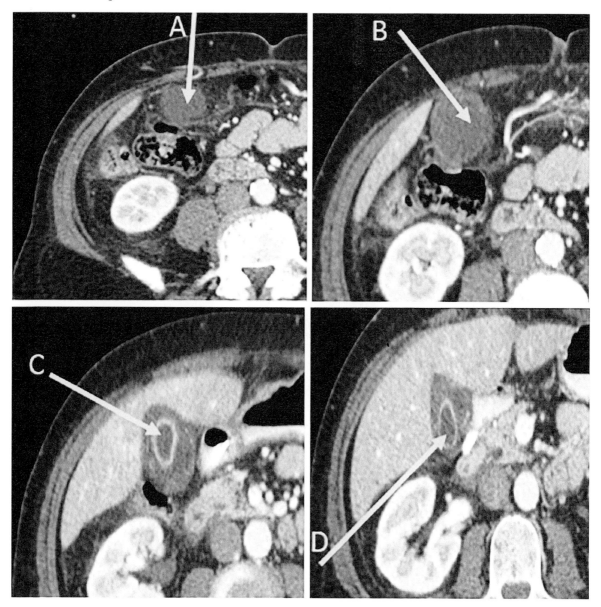

A. A
B. B
C. C
D. D

5   What is the most likely etiology of this finding (arrow) on antegrade cholangiography?

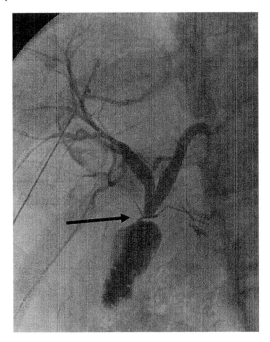

A. Benign stricture
B. Mirizzi syndrome
C. Choledochal cyst
D. Primary sclerosing cholangitis (PSC)

6   What is the standard technique for transjugular liver biopsy (TJLB)? Biopsy device positioned in the:

A. Left hepatic vein directed anteriorly
B. Left hepatic vein directed posteriorly
C. Right hepatic vein directed anteriorly
D. Right hepatic vein directed posteriorly

7   Which of the following is the most useful prognosticating factor for mortality following elective transjugular intrahepatic portosystemic shunt (TIPS)?

A. MELD score
B. Presence or absence of hepatocellular carcinoma
C. Presence or absence of ascites
D. Preprocedure portal vein pressure

8   Which of the following is the best intervention for this patient with liver failure and refractory ascites? Both images are hepatic venograms.

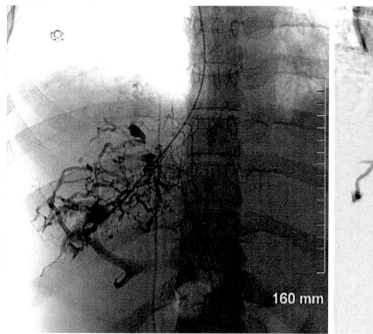
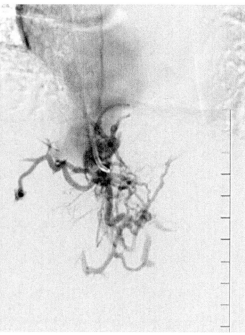

A. Balloon angioplasty
B. Catheter-directed tPA infusion
C. Transjugular intrahepatic portosystemic shunt creation
D. Systemic anticoagulation

9   A TIPS procedure involves the creation of a tract between an intrahepatic portal vein and a hepatic vein. What is the standard method to keep the tract open?

A. High-pressure balloon angioplasty
B. Drug-coated balloon angioplasty
C. Uncovered self-expanding stent
D. Covered self-expanding stent
E. Hybrid covered and uncovered self-expanding stent

10   Based on the DSA images what is the most likely diagnosis?

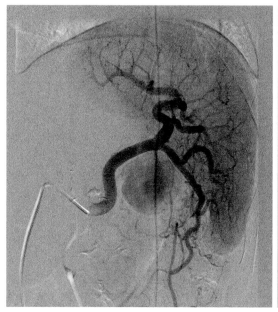
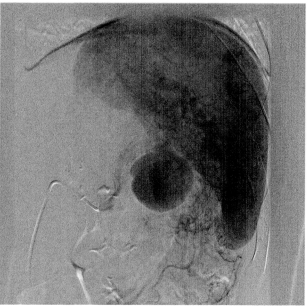

A. Arteriovenous fistula
B. Active arterial extravasation
C. Active venous extravasation
D. Aneurysm

11   What is the most commonly held threshold for treating a true aneurysm of the splenic artery in a healthy asymptomatic male patient?

A. >0.5 cm
B. >1 to 1.5 cm
C. >2 to 2.5 cm
D. >3 to 3.5 cm

12   Which artery (arrowheads) provides collateral flow to the spleen after this embolization?

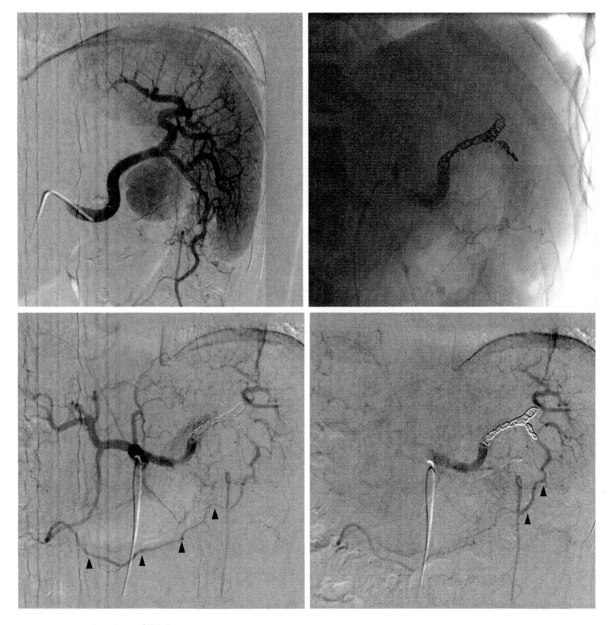

A. Arc of Riolan
B. Marginal artery of Drummond
C. Dorsal pancreatic artery
D. Gastroepiploic artery

13   The following angiographic images demonstrate a chronic pathology. Which of the following would be the most likely clinical presentation?

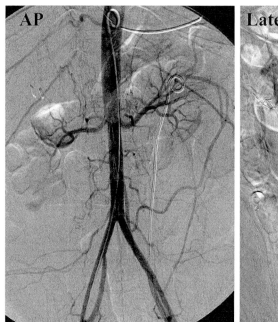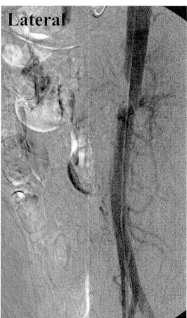

A. Threatened bowel
B. Transaminitis
C. Weight loss
D. Chronic kidney disease

14   Following liver transplant, a patient presents for evaluation. Where is the pathology located on these DSA images from celiac angiography (2 projections of the same process)?

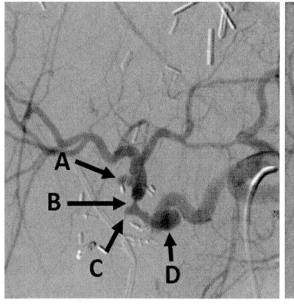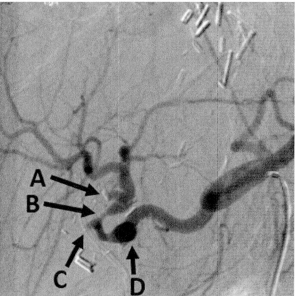

A. A
B. B
C. C
D. D

15 The following intravascular pressure measurements were obtained in 3 different patients. Which would most likely benefit from a TIPS?

A. Free hepatic vein 18 mmHg; wedged hepatic vein 25 mmHg
B. Free hepatic vein 6 mmHg; wedged hepatic vein 22 mmHg
C. Free hepatic vein 6 mmHg; wedged hepatic vein 9 mmHg

16 In the setting of a TIPS performed for bleeding gastroesophageal varices, which of the following is an appropriate posttreatment portosystemic pressure gradient?

A. 2 mmHg
B. 8 mmHg
C. 16 mmHg
D. 24 mmHg

17 Which of the following is an indication to constrain a TIPS?

A. Portosystemic gradient of 14 mmHg
B. Ascites recurrence
C. Refractory encephalopathy
D. New hepatocellular carcinoma

18 What is the indication for the procedure demonstrated?

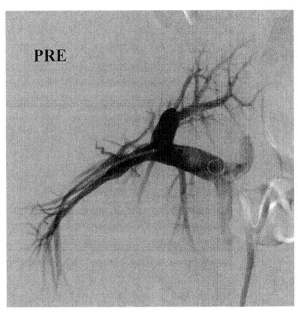
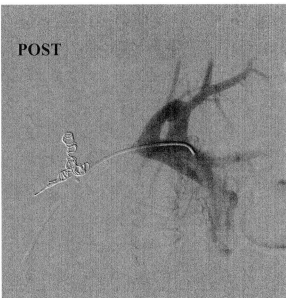

A. Preoperative for right lobe hepatocellular carcinoma
B. Uncontrolled right hepatic bile duct leak
C. Portal hypertension
D. Budd-Chiari syndrome

19 A cholecystostomy tube is placed for presumed cholecystitis in a critically ill patient. The patient eventually makes a complete recovery. Which of the following is the most critical step before cholecystostomy tube removal?

A. Fluoroscopic cholecystogram to confirm the absence of gallstones
B. Fluoroscopic cholecystogram to confirm patency of cystic duct and common bile duct
C. Confirm output of drain is <10 cc a day
D. Scintigraphy to confirm no bile leak

20   A patient presents with suspected mesenteric ischemia. Based on this angiographic image, what is the most likely etiology?

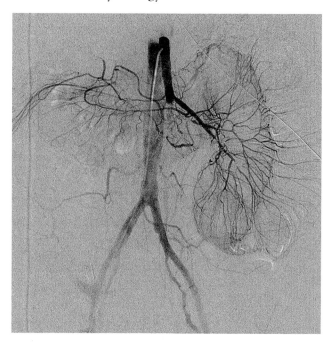

    A. Atherosclerosis with in situ thrombosis
    B. Embolus
    C. Nonocclusive mesenteric ischemia
    D. Venous thrombosis

21   A 49-year-old man with colorectal cancer metastatic to the liver presents for consideration of staged lobar treatments with yttrium-90 microspheres. What is the accepted total bilirubin cutoff for considering lobar radioembolization?

    A. 0.2 mg/dL
    B. 1.0 mg/dL
    C. 2.0 mg/dL
    D. 8.0 mg/dL

22   A patient with multifocal HCC undergoes yttrium-90 radioembolization to the right and left lobe of the liver (lobar treatments separated by 4 wk). Preprocedurally, the bilirubin was 2.0 mg/dL. Eight weeks after completing treatment, he presents at follow-up with significant fatigue and a total bilirubin of 12 mg/dL (normal <1.3 mg/dL). What is the best interpretation of this scenario?

    A. Bacterial cholangitis
    B. Radioembolization-induced liver disease
    C. Hepatic artery thrombosis
    D. Expected course

23   A patient with biopsy proven pancreatic cancer presents for management of biliary obstruction. The underlying anatomy is normal. What is the next step in treatment?

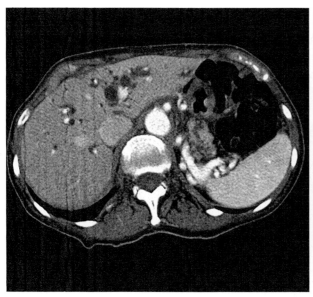 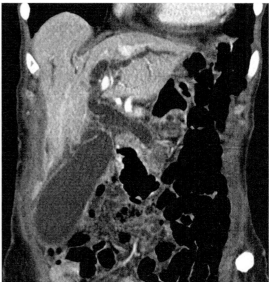

    A. Endoscopy with stent placement
    B. Percutaneous cholangiogram with stent placement
    C. Open surgical biliary decompression with hepaticojejunostomy
    D. Arterial embolization to shrink the obstructing mass

24   A 54-year-old man with Childs-Pugh A cirrhosis and a solitary mass in the right lobe of the liver is presented at multidisciplinary tumor board for consideration of treatment. Because of medical comorbidities, he is not a candidate for open surgery. Based on the CECT images given below, what is the preferred treatment?

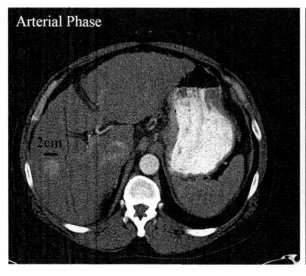 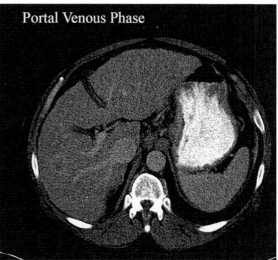

    A. Drug-eluting beads chemoembolization
    B. Yttrium-90 radioembolization
    C. Microwave thermal ablation
    D. Sorafenib

25   What is the recommended minimum ablative margin for HCC?

A. 1 mm
B. 5 mm
C. 15 mm
D. 30 mm

26   Immediately following microwave thermal ablation of a solitary right lobe HCC, a CECT in the arterial and portal venous phases is performed to evaluate which of the following? Portal venous phase image given below.

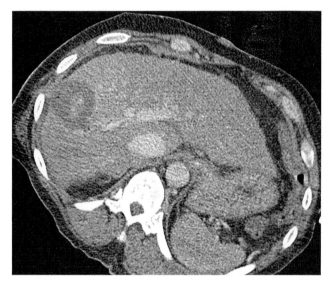

A. Local tumor progression
B. Extrahepatic malignancy
C. Ablative margin
D. Confirm portal vein still patent

27   What do the gas bubbles in the liver represent in this patient scanned with CECT immediately post microwave thermal ablation of right lobe HCC?

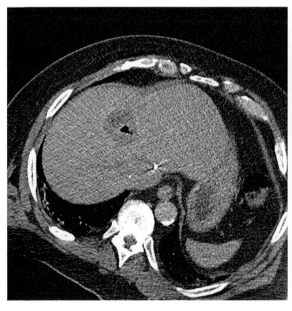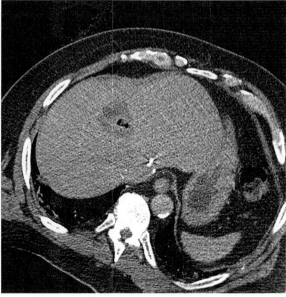

A. Hepatic abscess formation
B. Bowel perforation from ablation probes
C. Injury to the biliary tree
D. Expected finding immediately following microwave thermal ablation

28 A 52-year-old woman with known cirrhosis is admitted several times over a period of 6 months for confusion and forgetfulness. No precipitating event can be identified. Workup is unrevealing for other neuropsychiatric causes. She is treated with full-dose lactulose and rifaximin with some improvement. Despite strict adherence to medical treatment, she continues to have these symptoms resulting in additional hospitalizations. What is the most likely underlying abnormality?

A. Biliary obstruction
B. Hepatic hydrothorax
C. Portosystemic shunt

29 Immediately after embolization of a portosystemic shunt for refractory encephalopathy, which of the following will occur?

A. Portal venous pressure decreases
B. Portal venous pressure unchanged
C. Portal venous pressure increases

30 A 25-year-old woman with abdominal pain presents to the emergency department. A three-phase CECT scan is performed. What is the most likely diagnosis?

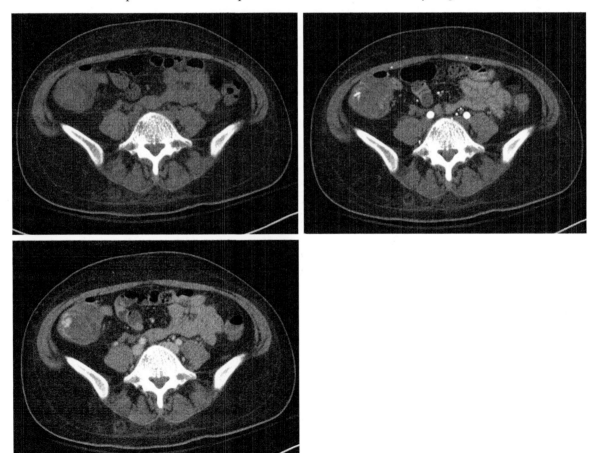

A. Active gastrointestinal bleeding
B. Ischemic necrosis of the cecum
C. Right lower quadrant abscess formation
D. Ectopic varices

31   A patient with a history of diverticulosis is hypotensive and a hemoglobin level is measured at 4 g/dL (normal 12-15 g/dL). Resuscitation begins promptly with intravenous fluids and blood products. She is transported to interventional radiology for emergent angiography. To evaluate a suspected right colon bleed, what artery should be selected first?

A. Celiac artery
B. Superior mesenteric artery
C. Inferior mesenteric artery
D. Internal iliac artery

32   The SMA is selected, and angiography is performed. Active bleeding is seen from the cecum. At what level should microcoil embolization be performed to stop the bleeding (arrow)?

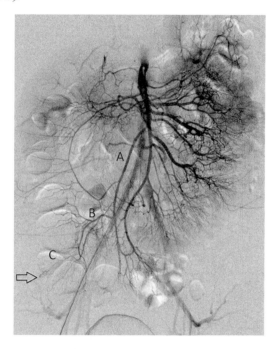

A. A
B. B
C. C

33   A celiac angiogram is performed to evaluate suspected upper gastrointestinal bleeding. What artery is identified by the arrows in the images given below?

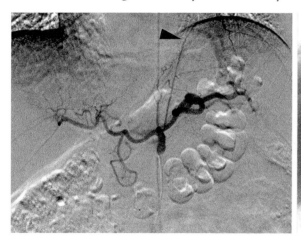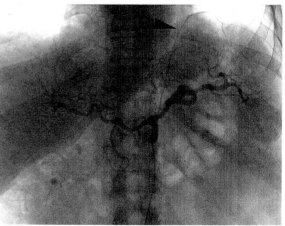

A. Celiac artery
B. Splenic artery
C. Left gastric artery
D. Common hepatic artery
E. Left inferior phrenic artery

34   A 56-year-old man with a history of bleeding duodenal ulcer and prior endoscopic treatment, presents urgently to interventional radiology with hypotension and bright red blood per rectum. A magnified DSA image demonstrates a pseudoaneurysm of the gastroduodenal artery (GDA) with brisk bleeding into the lumen of the duodenum. Where should microcoils be placed to effectively treat this bleed?

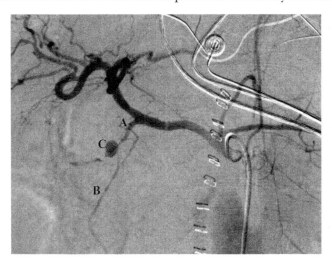

A. A (proximal GDA)
B. B (distal GDA)
C. C (within the pseudoaneurysm)
D. A and B (proximal and distal GDA)

35   A 10-year-old woman with fever and abdominal pain presents with perforated appendicitis. A CECT scan is performed demonstrating an 8 × 8 × 6 cm abscess (Ab) in the mid-pelvis. What is the best approach for image-guided drainage catheter placement?

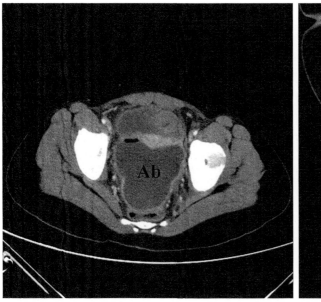
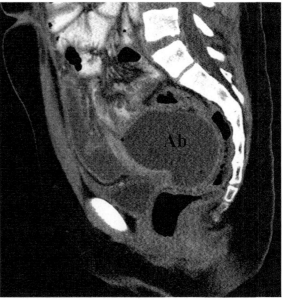

A. US-guided transabdominal
B. CT-guided transgluteal
C. US-guided transrectal
D. Catheter placement is not indicated

36   A 50-year-old woman with cirrhosis and a history of right iliac fossa kidney transplant presents for ultrasound-guided paracentesis. Eight liters of fluid are obtained from a left lower abdomen access site. What is the SAAG calculation performed for fluid analysis?

A. Serum total protein minus ascites albumin
B. Serum albumin plus ascites albumin
C. Serum albumin minus ascites albumin
D. Serum amylase minus ascites amylase

37   A 15-year-old girl presents with repeated episodes of hematemesis and a mesenteric angiogram is requested. During the procedure, the SMA is selected and angiography demonstrates what pathology?

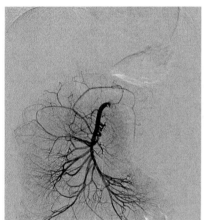 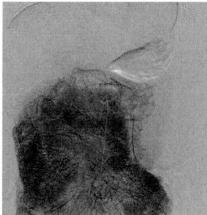 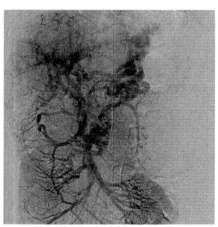

A. Arteriovenous malformation in the colon
B. Blunt trauma to the liver with pseudoaneurysm formation
C. Chronic portal vein thrombosis with cavernous transformation
D. Diffuse mucosal hemorrhage of the small and large bowel

38   The IR team receives a request from surgery for CT-guided placement of a percutaneous drainage catheter. The patient is a 53-year-old man with necrotizing pancreatitis for approximately 5 weeks, and CECT demonstrates pancreatic and peripancreatic walled-off necrosis. He is symptomatic with pain and fevers and cannot tolerate nasojejunal feeds. What is the best management strategy?

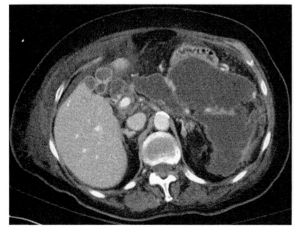 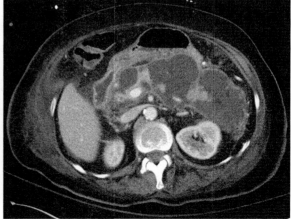

A. Place an 8-Fr pigtail drain using a midline transperitoneal approach
B. Place a 14-Fr pigtail drain using a left retroperitoneal approach
C. No indication for drainage catheter
D. Perform 20-gauge needle aspiration only

39   A CECT is performed to evaluate a patient with nausea and vomiting. What additional history is most likely present?

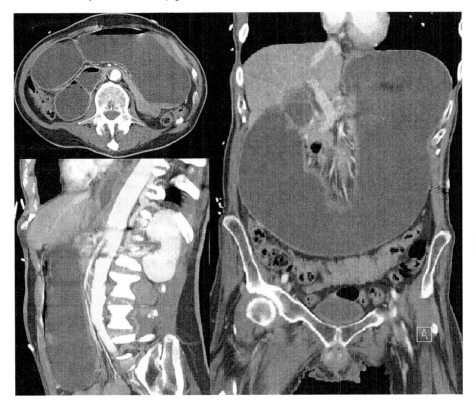

A. Remote abdominal trauma
B. Poorly controlled diabetes mellitus
C. Long history of smoking
D. Significant weight loss

40   A patient presents to the ER with hematochezia, jaundice, and feeling weak. She underwent percutaneous liver biopsy 2 days prior. A CECT is performed. Which is the correct conclusion?

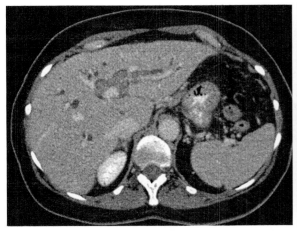
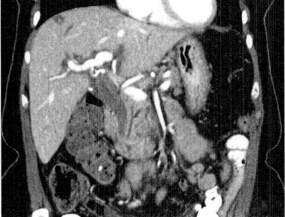

A. Complication of liver biopsy
B. Underlying pancreatic malignancy
C. Brisk small bowel bleed
D. Worsening cirrhosis

41   During workup for a transarterial chemoembolization (TACE) procedure to treat
intrahepatic metastases, the patient reports a history of prior surgery with choledo-
chojejunostomy. Which complication is the patient at increased risk for developing
after the embolization?

A. Portal vein thrombosis
B. Hepatic abscess formation
C. Hepatic infarct
D. Biliary stricture

42   Which of the following scenarios would be acceptable for liver transplantation
according to the Milan criteria for hepatocellular carcinoma?

A. 1 tumor 5.8 cm
B. 2 tumors 1.7 cm and 3.3 cm
C. 3 tumors 1.4 cm, 2.0 cm, 2.8 cm
D. 4 tumors 1.2 cm, 1.4 cm, 1.5 cm, 1.8 cm

43   A patient with known capsular HCC (arrow) presents to the ED with severe acute
abdominal pain. Given the findings on this CT scan, what is this patient at increased
risk for?

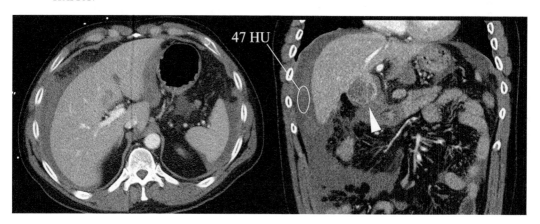

A. Spontaneous bacterial peritonitis (SBP)
B. Hepatic tumor thrombus
C. Future need of TIPS
D. Intraperitoneal metastasis

44   A patient status post remote cadaveric liver transplantation with hepaticojejunostomy presents with cholangitis. An MRCP is performed confirming central biliary
stones (arrows). What is the best initial approach to treat this condition?

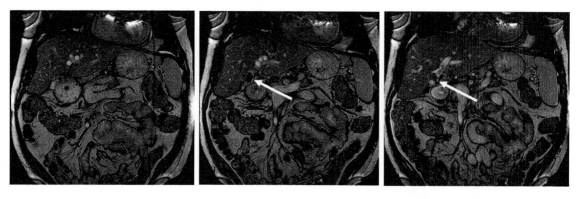

A. Percutaneous drainage followed by rendezvous with endoscopy for stone removal
B. Percutaneous drainage followed by surgical laparotomy for stone removal
C. Percutaneous drainage followed by percutaneous stone removal
D. Lifetime percutaneous biliary drainage

45 What is the management for the pathology demonstrated here?

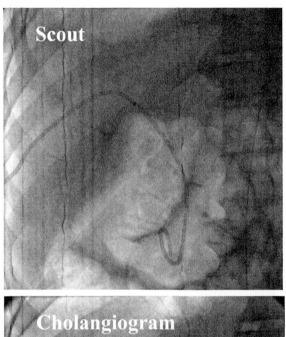

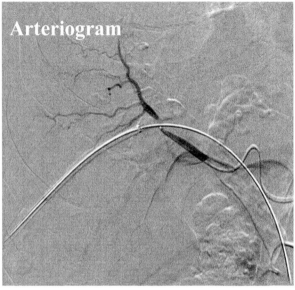

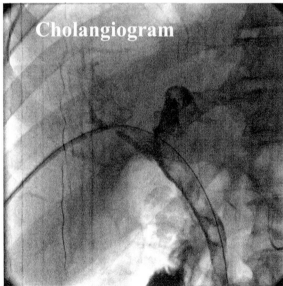

A. Biliary drain removal and "fresh stick" 1 week later
B. Anticoagulation for portal clot
C. Coil embolization of the hepatic artery
D. Exchange biliary drain and leave uncapped to bag drainage

ANSWERS AND EXPLANATIONS

1 **Answer A.** The standard of care for the treatment of HCC is to follow a liver cancer staging and treatment system such as the Barcelona Clinic Liver Cancer (BCLC) model for HCC.

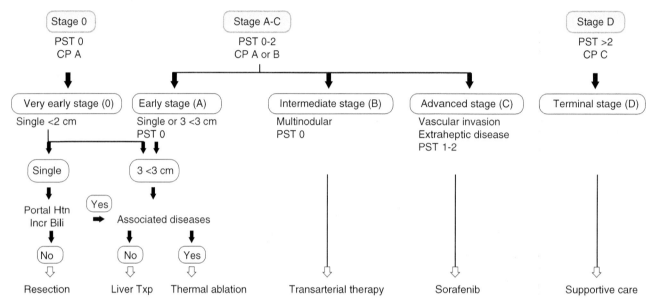

Figure 1-1   BCLC algorithm for the management of HCC. CP, Child-Pugh score; PST, ECOG performance status. Adapted from Forner A, Reig ME, De Lope CR, Bruix J. Current strategy for staging and treatment: the BCLC update and future prospects. *Semin Liver Dis.* 2010;30(1):61-74.

First-line treatments for very early and early stage HCC strive for a curative result, namely through surgical resection, liver transplantation, or ablation (choice A). The transarterial liver-directed therapies (choices B and C) are most commonly utilized in intermediate or even advanced-stage patients and generally are considered noncurative. There are exceptions, such as performance of a radiation segmentectomy with yttrium-90 to achieve results akin to ablation or surgery, but this is beyond the scope of this book. Importantly, the transarterial treatments can shrink or stabilize the tumor(s) in hopes of downstaging to a curative treatment, maintaining transplant candidacy, and/or providing palliation/extension of life.

References: Forner A, Reig ME, De Lope CR, Bruix J. Current strategy for staging and treatment: the BCLC update and future prospects. *Semin Liver Dis.* 2010;30(1):61-74.

Hickey R, Vouche M, Sze DY, et al. Cancer concepts and principles: primer for the interventional oncologist-part II. *J Vasc Interv Radiol.* 2013;24(8):1167-1188.

Kinoshita A, Onoda H, Fushiya N, Koike K, Nishino H, Tajiri H. Staging systems for hepatocellular carcinoma: current status and future perspectives. *World J Hepatol.* 2015;7(3):406-424.

Llovet JM, Brú C, Bruix J. Prognosis of hepatocellular carcinoma: the BCLC staging classification. *Semin Liver Dis.* 1999;19(3):329-338.

2 **Answer B.** The initial scout image on the left suggests incorrect gastrostomy tube positioning. For orientation, the gastric air bubble is fairly well seen, and the tube tip is right of midline in the region where the pylorus would be located. Contrast is injected through the tube, and the duodenum opacifies (choice A is incorrect) at the tube tip, confirming the internal fixation balloon is postpyloric. Postpyloric tube position can result in gastric outlet obstruction, leaking along the tube tract, and abdominal pain. Only intraluminal contrast is identified on the images, excluding choices C and D.

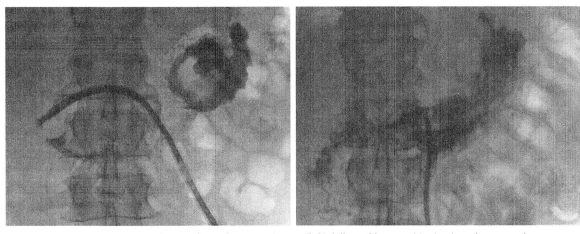

Figure 2-1 Initial postpyloric placement image (left) followed by repositioning into the stomach (right).

Reference: Lyon SM, Pascoe DM. Percutaneous gastrostomy and gastrojejunostomy. *Semin Intervent Radiol.* 2004;21(3):181-189.

3   **Answer C.**   Gastrostomy tube placement can be performed by surgeons, endoscopists, or interventional radiologists. Typical indications include dysphagia or swallowing disorders, unmet nutritional needs, and gastric outlet obstruction. The most widely held absolute contraindication is untreated hypocoagulable state. The presence of gastric varices, inability to insufflate the stomach, and inability to safely access the stomach are additional contraindications. Ascites, once considered a contraindication, can be handled by performing preprocedure paracentesis (choice C) decreasing the risk of peritonitis and delayed tract maturation. If there is significant preprocedure ascites or rapid reaccumulation, sonographic follow-up and repeat paracentesis can be performed while the tract matures over 7 to 10 days.

Reference: Lyon SM, Pascoe DM. Percutaneous gastrostomy and gastrojejunostomy. *Semin Intervent Radiol.* 2004;21(3):181-189.

4   **Answer C.**   The optimal tract for percutaneous cholecystostomy tube placement crosses a small amount of liver parenchyma in order to tamponade any possible bile leak (choice C). Peritoneal nontranshepatic approach (choice B) is suboptimal, but acceptable if it is the only option, such as with a markedly dilated gallbladder. The posterior approach (choice D) results in an inappropriately long trajectory and does not include a good tract of hepatic parenchyma. For all percutaneous procedures, vascularity in the projected path of the intervention must be considered. Choice A demonstrates potential crossing of the inferior epigastric artery, which could lead to a major bleeding complication.

Reference: Bakkaloglu H, Yanar H, Guloglu R, et al. Ultrasound guided percutaneous cholecystostomy in high-risk patients for surgical intervention. *World J Gastroenterol.* 2006;12(44):7179-7182.

5   **Answer A.**   The cholangiogram depicts a short-segment focal narrowing or stricture of the common hepatic duct. The nearby metallic clips and lack of cystic duct suggest previous surgery to the region. This is confirmed by the very short distance between the hepatic duct confluence and the bowel. Benign strictures occur in approximately 10% of patients who have undergone hepaticojejunostomy (choice A). If the cystic duct is absent, presumably the gallbladder is absent; therefore Mirizzi syndrome is not feasible. Choledochal cysts do not present as strictures. Primary sclerosing cholangitis is not typically found as a singular focal stricture, and given the postoperative appearance, benign stricture is the most likely option.

Reference: Abdelrafee A, El-Shobari M, Askar W, Sultan AM, El Nakeeb A. Long-term follow-up of 120 patients after hepaticojejunostomy for treatment of post-cholecystectomy bile duct injuries: a retrospective cohort study. *Int J Surg.* 2015;18:205-210.

6   Answer C.   The sheath commonly used to guide the biopsy needle for this procedure is curved and therefore can be directed anteriorly, posteriorly, etc. The standard technique is to catheterize the right hepatic vein and aim the biopsy sheath and needle anteriorly (choice C). As the right hepatic vein is normally positioned posteriorly in the liver, by directing the biopsy needle anteriorly, it is unlikely to transgress the liver capsule, thereby reducing the risk of a bleeding complication.

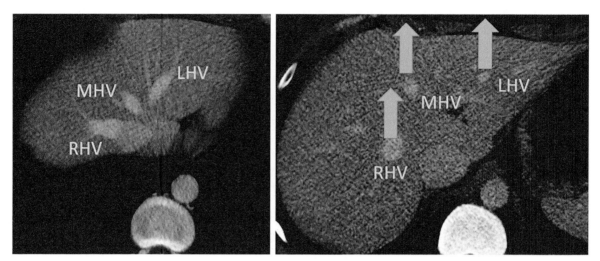

Figure 6-1   The blue arrows denote projected biopsy needle tract through the liver from the right (RHV), middle (MHV), and left (LHV) hepatic veins.

Reference: Dohan A, Guerrache Y, Boudiaf M, Gavini JP, Kaci R, Soyer P. Transjugular liver biopsy: indications, technique and results. *Diagn Interv Imaging.* 2014;95(1):11-15.

7   Answer A.   TIPS creation is a significant alteration in physiology. Even when performed pristinely, the physiologic changes can overwhelm an already abnormal liver. Model for end-stage liver disease (MELD) is a scoring system initially developed to estimate short-term survival after TIPS. Notably, a more recent version of the MELD score includes a correction for the sodium level; however, this has not yet been validated in studies for TIPS. We use the original MELD score in patient evaluation for TIPS. The MELD score was subsequently found to be useful in triaging patients for liver transplantation and is still used routinely in both applications.

$$MELD = 9.6 \times \log e \text{ (creatinine mg/dL)} + 3.8 \times \log e \text{ (bilirubin mg/dL)} + 11.2 \times \log e \text{ (INR)} + 6.4$$

While there is no absolute cutoff value for MELD score before TIPS, there are data to guide the patient and clinician in making an informed decision regarding the risks and benefits. For example, a MELD ≥18 has been shown to have 1- and 3-month mortality of 18% and 35%, respectively, after elective TIPS.

References: Ferral H, Gamboa P, Postoak DW, et al. Survival after elective transjugular intrahepatic portosystemic shunt creation: prediction with model for end-stage liver disease score. *Radiology.* 2004;231(1):231-236.

Kamath PS, Wiesner RH, Malinchoc M, et al. A model to predict survival in patients with end-stage liver disease. *Hepatology.* 2001;33(2):464-470.

Montgomery A, Ferral H, Vasan R, Postoak DW. MELD score as a predictor of early death in patients undergoing elective transjugular intrahepatic portosystemic shunt (TIPS) procedures. *Cardiovasc Intervent Radiol.* 2005;28(3):307-312.

8   Answer C. The case demonstrates a grossly abnormal hepatic venogram. There is a disorganized network of collateral hepatic veins, which are not draining the liver effectively. A normal right hepatic vein is not visualized peripherally or centrally. Reference a normal right hepatic venogram (Figure 8-1).

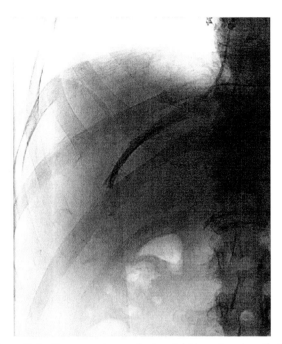

Figure 8-1   Venogram from selective right hepatic vein catheterization.

This is the angiographic picture of Budd-Chiari from hepatic vein thrombosis. The appearance of well-developed small-caliber tortuous collaterals is consistent with a chronic process; therefore choices A, B, or D would not likely be successful therapies. TIPS creation (choice C) and liver transplantation are the typical options for this presentation. In contradistinction, presented is an example of acute clot in the left axillary vein of a different patient (Figure 8-2).

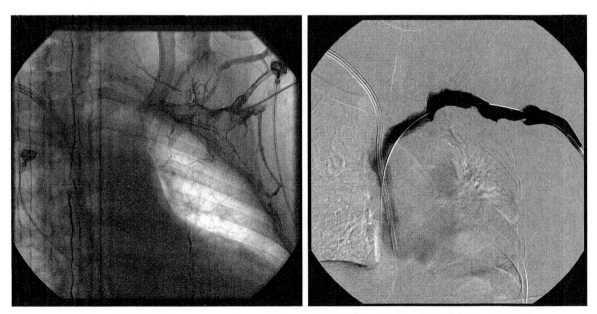

Figure 8-2   Catheter venogram demonstrating acute left axillary vein thrombosis (left image). Note the vein is expanded by a large filling defect, and the vessel maintains its expected anatomic course (not a collateral). This clot would be expected to respond to standard treatments for acute thrombus such as anticoagulation, tPA, or clot maceration/aspiration. Following overnight catheter-directed tPA fibrinolysis (right image), there is patency of the left axillary and central veins with no filling defects or stenosis.

References: Garcia-Pagán JC, Heydtmann M, Raffa S, et al. TIPS for Budd-Chiari syndrome: long-term results and prognostics factors in 124 patients. *Gastroenterology*. 2008;135(3):808815.

Han G, Qi X, Zhang W, et al. Percutaneous recanalization for Budd-Chiari syndrome: an 11-year retrospective study on patency and survival in 177 Chinese patients from a single center. *Radiology*. 2013;266(2):657-667.

Molmenti EP, Segev DL, Arepally A, et al. The utility of TIPS in the management of Budd-Chiari syndrome. *Ann Surg*. 2005;241(6):978-981.

Smith M, Durham J. Evolving indications for tips. *Tech Vasc Interv Radiol*. 2016;19(1):36-41.

9   **Answer E.**   When the TIPS procedure was initially investigated in animal studies, the shunt tract was created and dilated open with angioplasty alone. This technique was quickly discovered to have poor shunt patency. The next step in TIPS evolution was the placement of uncovered stents in the shunt tract. In-stent stenosis occurred (thought to be due to bile leak around the intraparenchymal portion of the uncovered stent), and ultimately a hybrid covered/uncovered stent was found to be superior. The intraparenchymal portion of the hybrid stent is covered, and the terminal 2 cm of the portal venous end is uncovered to ensure portal patency.

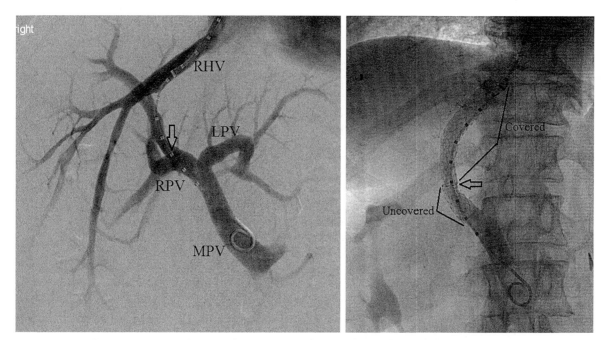

Figure 9-1   Hepatoportogram from TIPS procedure pre (left) and post (right) deployment of the hybrid covered/uncovered stent. Marker pigtail catheter is seen coming from the right hepatic vein, traversing through the liver parenchyma and entering the right portal vein at the level of the arrow (the traditional route for TIPS). Postdeployment image (right) demonstrating stent extending from the right portal to the right hepatic vein. Note the metallic ring (arrow) delineating the uncovered portion of the stent that lies within the right portal vein, from the covered portion of the stent that lies within the parenchymal tract and extends into the right hepatic vein. LPV, left portal vein; MPV, main portal vein; RHV, right hepatic vein; RPV, right portal vein.

References: Cejna M. Should stent-grafts replace bare stents for primary transjugular intrahepatic portosystemic shunts? *Semin Intervent Radiol*. 2005;22(4):287-299.

Clark TW. Stepwise placement of a transjugular intrahepatic portosystemic shunt endograft. *Tech Vasc Interv Radiol*. 2008;11(4):208-211.

10   **Answer D.** Two DSA images are presented with the end-hole catheter positioned in the proximal segment of the main splenic artery. The left image is in the arterial phase, and the right image is in the parenchymal phase (outflow veins not yet present). On the arterial phase image, near the splenic hilum, there is contrast exiting the normal pathway of the splenic artery. On the more delayed image, a well-defined spherical structure becomes opacified with contrast, consistent with a saccular aneurysm (choice D). Active arterial extravasation would show contrast dispersing in a random and uncontained manner; therefore choice B is incorrect. These images are earlier than the venous phase, excluding choice C (incidentally, seeing true venous extravasation from an arterial injection is rare). Choice A, arteriovenous fistula, would be represented as early opacification of an outflow vein, which is not seen here.

Reference: Lakin RO, Bena JF, Sarac TP, et al. The contemporary management of splenic artery aneurysms. *J Vasc Surg.* 2011;53(4):958-964.

11   **Answer C.** The commonly accepted minimum diameter for treating a true aneurysm of the splenic artery is 2.0 to 2.5 cm, assuming no complicating factors. Other indications for treatment include a rapidly enlarging aneurysm or one that has ruptured. For women who may become pregnant or patients undergoing liver transplantation, some suggest treating all true splenic artery aneurysms regardless of size because of an increased risk of rupture in those conditions. One additional category is that of a symptomatic (painful) aneurysm; this suggests the possibility of imminent rupture that could result in catastrophic bleeding. All symptomatic aneurysms should be fixed urgently.

Reference: Lakin RO, Bena JF, Sarac TP, et al. The contemporary management of splenic artery aneurysms. *J Vasc Surg.* 2011;53(4):958-964.

12   **Answer D.** There is robust collateral arterial supply to the visceral organs. Occluding the splenic artery proximally (not at the hilum) will virtually never cause end-organ ischemia. Collateral supply to the spleen includes pancreatic arterial branches, short gastric arteries, and the gastroepiploic artery as a continuation of the gastroduodenal artery. In this case, the embolization was intentionally performed with the coil pack extending from the distal segment of the main splenic artery into the upper and lower pole arteries. This "isolation" technique closed the front and back door to the aneurysm, resulting in immediate thrombosis. Following the embolization, the gastroepiploic artery nicely communicated with the residual patent lower pole splenic artery branch, allowing for continued perfusion of the splenic parenchyma.

Reference: Madoff DC, Denys A, Wallace MJ, et al. Splenic arterial interventions: anatomy, indications, technical considerations, and potential complications. *Radiographics.* 2005;25(suppl 1):S191-S211.

13   **Answer C.** On the AP and lateral view abdominal aortograms, neither the celiac artery nor the superior mesenteric artery (SMA) opacify, and a hypertrophied inferior mesenteric artery (IMA) is present giving rise to a large cephalad coursing collateral (Figure 13-1, small arrowheads). On the lateral view there is a bulky, eccentric atherosclerotic plaque where the celiac and SMA origins would normally be seen. This is the angiographic picture of chronic mesenteric ischemia, which is most often due to atherosclerotic disease. Slowly over time, the mesenteric arteries become narrowed and even occluded, with collateral pathways developing, which help prevent acute ischemia and bowel loss. Symptoms do not usually present until 2 of the 3 major mesenteric arteries become occluded. The classic triad is that of postprandial abdominal pain, food fear or avoidance, and subsequent weight loss. Both endovascular stenting and open surgical revascularization are acceptable treatments.

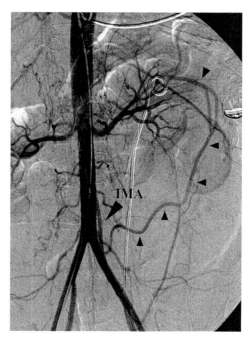

Figure 13-1   Abdominal aortogram.

When there is compromise of the SMA or IMA, arterial collaterals hypertrophy between the distributions, allowing for bowel perfusion and viability. The two named pathways often discussed are the arc of Riolan and the marginal artery of Drummond. The arc of Riolan refers to a pathway more centrally located in the root of the mesentery, often arising shortly after the middle colic artery and connecting to the proximal IMA. The marginal artery of Drummond refers to a pathway that develops more peripherally along the mesenteric border of the colon, connecting the distal middle colic branches (SMA origin) to the distal left colic branches (IMA origin).

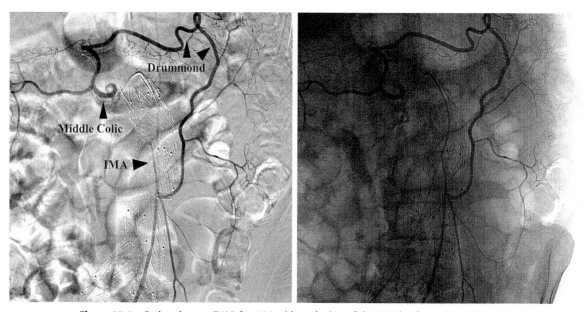

Figure 13-2   Patient is post-EVAR for AAA with exclusion of the IMA by the endograft. Angiography from the SMA shows filling of the middle colic artery, which demonstrates its characteristic "T" shape with right and left branches perfusing the transverse colon. A contiguous arterial collateral has hypertrophied connecting the SMA to IMA distributions (marginal artery of Drummond).

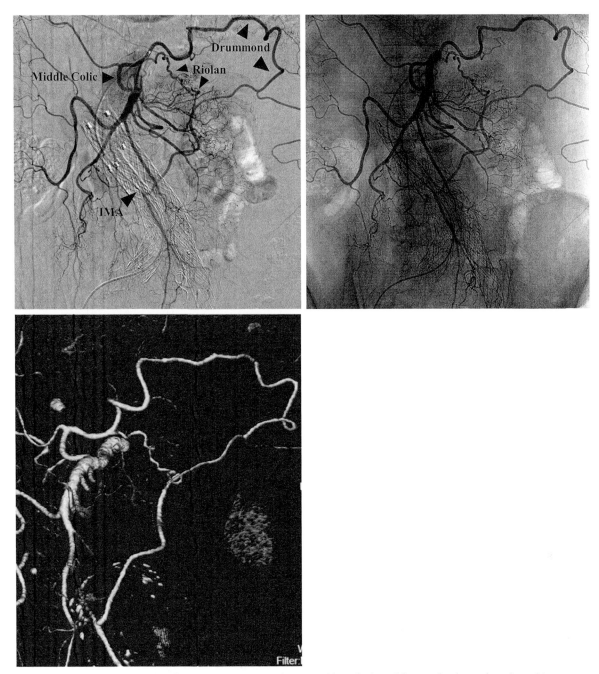

Figure 13-3   Another patient post-EVAR for AAA with exclusion of the IMA by the endograft. In this example, angiography from the SMA shows both central (arc of Riolan) and peripheral (marginal artery of Drummond) collateral arterial pathways connecting the SMA and IMA distributions. A 3D volume-rendered CTA image (bottom) highlights the pathways.

Reference: Hohenwalter EJ. Chronic mesenteric ischemia: diagnosis and treatment. *Semin Intervent Radiol.* 2009;26(4):345-351.

14   **Answer B.**   The case images depict the hepatic artery following liver transplantation. Understanding the orientation and anatomy is crucial to accurately interpret the images, and reviewing the operative report is often necessary. The following diagrams with corresponding angiography demonstrate the surgical anatomy and pathology present here.

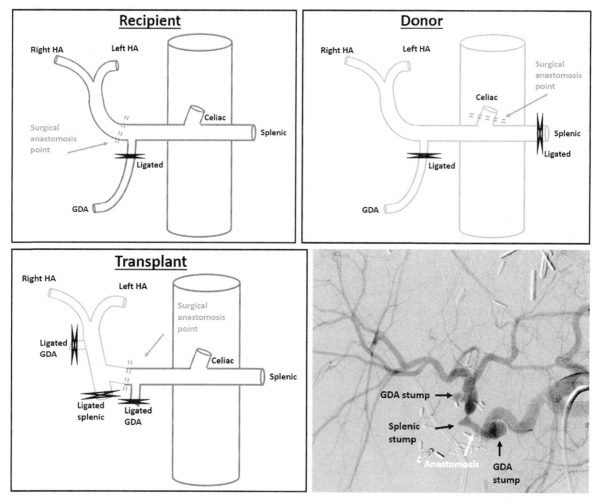

Figure 14-1   Posttransplant hepatic arterial anatomy. The irregular outpouchings must be recognized as surgically ligated vessel stumps, and not pseudoaneurysms, pathologically thrombosed vessels, or active extravasation. GDA, gastroduodenal artery; HA, hepatic artery.

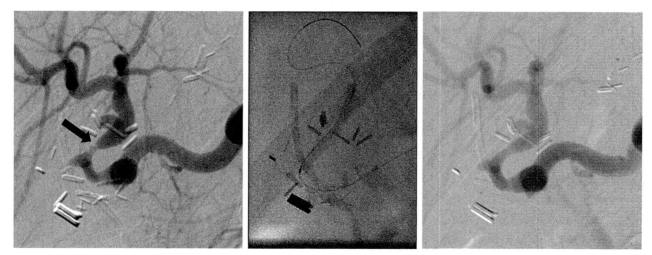

Figure 14-2   The true abnormality is the focal arterial narrowing (arrow) likely from clamp injury at the time of surgery. Balloon angioplasty (middle) is performed, and completion DSA (right) shows no residual stenosis.

Reference: Amesur NB, Zajko AB. Interventional radiology in liver transplantation. *Liver Transpl.* 2006;12(3):330-351.

15 **Answer B.** Portal hypertension can be classified into presinusoidal, sinusoidal, and postsinusoidal causes. Presinusoidal pathology is found upstream from the liver sinusoids. An example of this is portal vein thrombosis. Postsinusoidal pathology relates to the venous outflow of the liver, classically seen with Budd-Chiari or right heart failure. Sinusoidal portal hypertension is due to hepatic parenchymal diseases, most commonly cirrhosis. During endovascular evaluation, a catheter is positioned in the proximal right hepatic vein, and the measured pressure is the free hepatic vein pressure (FHVP). Subsequently, a surrogate for the portal venous pressure can be obtained by wedging an end-hole catheter into a hepatic venule or inflating a balloon occlusion catheter in the proximal hepatic vein. The measured pressure is the wedged hepatic vein pressure (WHVP). The hepatic venous pressure gradient (HVPG), or difference between wedged and free hepatic vein pressures, is a measure of how the liver sinusoids affect the portal pressure. Normal HVPG is <5 mmHg. An HVPG of >10 mmHg is the most commonly used criteria for clinically significant sinusoidal portal hypertension. These patients would potentially benefit from a TIPS (choice B). The pressures in choice A represent a patient with right heart failure and an HVPG <5 mmHg. The pressures in choice C represent a normal patient.

References: Fidelman N, Kwan SW, Laberge JM, Gordon RL, Ring EJ, Kerlan RK. The transjugular intrahepatic portosystemic shunt: an update. *AJR Am J Roentgenol.* 2012;199(4):746-755.

Silva-Junior G, Baiges A, Turon F, et al. The prognostic value of hepatic venous pressure gradient in patients with cirrhosis is highly dependent on the accuracy of the technique. *Hepatology.* 2015;62(5):1584-1592.

16 **Answer B.** The best medical evidence supports a post-TIPS goal portosystemic pressure gradient between 5 and 12 mmHg for the indication of variceal bleeding. Following TIPS, if the gradient between the portal and systemic veins remains high, the pressure within the varices will also be elevated, increasing the risk of rupture. If the gradient is too low, the detoxification function of the liver may be compromised as a significant amount of blood is shunted back to the right heart. This can lead to uncontrollable hepatic encephalopathy. For the indication of refractory ascites, the goal portosystemic pressure gradient is less well delineated, although many practitioners use the same criteria as for variceal bleeding.

Reference: Fidelman N, Kwan SW, Laberge JM, Gordon RL, Ring EJ, Kerlan RK. The transjugular intrahepatic portosystemic shunt: an update. *AJR Am J Roentgenol.* 2012;199(4):746-755.

17 **Answer C.** The portosystemic gradient across a TIPS is typically optimized at a value between 5 and 12 mmHg. If the gradient is too high (>12 mmHg), the TIPS can be dilated with balloon angioplasty to increase the shunt diameter. This decreases the resistance in the shunt, lowering the pressure gradient and increasing the blood flow back to the right heart. If the gradient is too low, the detoxification function of the liver may be compromised as a significant amount of blood is shunted back to the right heart. This can lead to refractory hepatic encephalopathy (choice C). In this situation the TIPS can be constrained, decreasing the luminal diameter, increasing the resistance and thereby reducing the amount of blood shunted away from the liver. There are several techniques to constrain a TIPS, discussed elsewhere in this book. Choices A and B relate to inadequate shunting and are therefore incorrect. HCC (choice D) should not factor into TIPS function.

Reference: Madoff DC, Wallace MJ. Reduced stents and stent-grafts for the management of hepatic encephalopathy after transjugular intrahepatic portosystemic shunt creation. *Semin Intervent Radiol.* 2005;22(4):316-328.

18 **Answer A.** The images depict the portal venous system of the liver, pre (left) and post (right) embolization. On the post image, contrast opacifies the main and left portal veins only. There is no further flow in the right portal vein and its branches following coil and particle embolization. Portal vein embolization (PVE) is a technique used to redirect portal blood flow before partial hepatectomy in patients with an inadequate future liver remnant (FLR). Inadequate FLR is commonly defined as <20% in patients with a normal liver and <40% in those with a compromised liver (FLR% = FLR volume/total healthy liver volume × 100). In the case example, a right PVE will cause hypertrophy of the tumor-free left hepatic lobe in preparation for a right hepatectomy. Growth of the FLR after PVE is time dependent, with most growth occurring between 2 and 6 weeks. We typically reimage at 4 weeks post-PVE to assess the results of the procedure. Portal hypertension and Budd-Chiari would not benefit from PVE (choices C and D). Identification that these images represent the portal venous system, not the biliary tree, excludes choice B.

References: Hemming AW, Reed AI, Howard RJ, et al. Preoperative portal vein embolization for extended hepatectomy. *Ann Surg.* 2003;237(5):686-691.

May BJ, Madoff DC. Portal vein embolization: rationale, technique, and current application. *Semin Intervent Radiol.* 2012;29(2):81-89.

Wajswol E, Jazmati T, Contractor S, Kumar A. Portal vein embolization utilizing N-butyl cyanoacrylate for contralateral lobe hypertrophy prior to liver resection: a systematic review and meta-analysis. *Cardiovasc Intervent Radiol.* 2018;41(9):1302-1312.

19   **Answer B.**   Cholecystostomy tube placement is typically done in patients with calculous or acalculous cholecystitis who cannot undergo immediate surgical cholecystectomy. Once the catheter is placed, the patient is followed clinically to ensure improvement. If the patient improves and has no further symptoms, drain removal can be considered. Algorithms for removal vary from practice to practice but most wait at least 3 weeks with the tube in place, which allows the percutaneous tract to epithelialize and reduces the risk of a bile leak upon tube removal. Before removal, the most important step is to confirm patency of the cystic and common bile duct to ensure adequate internal physiologic drainage will occur. This is easily done with contrast injection of the tube under fluoroscopy (choice B). If there is persistent duct obstruction, recurrent cholecystitis is more likely to occur. Although the presence or absence of gallstones should be noted on the cholecystogram, tube removal can be considered with or without stones. A low drain output (choice C) may indicate patency of the cystic duct, but can also be seen with cholecystostomy tube dysfunction because of malposition or obstruction. Although scintigraphy can help evaluate for a suspected bile leak, it is not the standard of care before removal.

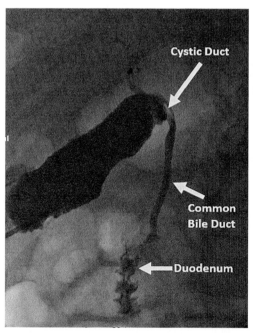

Figure 19-1 Fluoroscopic cholecystogram in a patient who recovered from acalculous cholecystitis. After 6 weeks of catheter drainage, contrast study showed no gallstones and widely patent cystic and common bile ducts. The tube was removed with no reported recurrence of cholecystitis.

Reference: Alvino DML, Fong ZV, Mccarthy CJ, et al. Long-term outcomes following percutaneous cholecystostomy tube placement for treatment of acute calculous cholecystitis. *J Gastrointest Surg.* 2017;21(5):761-769.

Gulaya K, Desai SS, Sato K. Percutaneous cholecystostomy: evidence-based current clinical practice. *Semin Intervent Radiol.* 2016;33(4):291-296.

Wise JN, Gervais DA, Akman A, Harisinghani M, Hahn PF, Mueller PR. Percutaneous cholecystostomy catheter removal and incidence of clinically significant bile leaks: a clinical approach to catheter management. *AJR Am J Roentgenol.* 2005;184(5):1647-1651.

20   **Answer B.**   The DSA image shows abrupt occlusion of the SMA approximately 4 cm beyond its origin and just beyond a large patent jejunal branch. The proximal arterial segment is healthy appearing, without underlying flow limiting stenosis. There is poor collateralization distally consistent with an acute presentation. In the distal segment of the jejunal branch, there is another segment of nonopacification with reconstitution distally. The constellation of findings point to an embolus as the underlying etiology. In situ thrombosis more commonly occurs in the first few centimeters of the SMA at a site of preexisting atherosclerotic narrowing; collaterals have often already formed secondary to the underlying arterial stenosis. The clinical presentation also may be less abrupt as a result of these developed collaterals. Choice C occurs in critically ill patients on vasoactive infusions. Angiography often demonstrates diffuse small caliber of the mesenteric artery branches with short and long segmental narrowings. Venous thrombosis is an important cause of mesenteric ischemia but would be best assessed in the venous phase of angiography, or with multiphase CECT. Once a patient is diagnosed with acute mesenteric ischemia, the treatment often depends on the etiology, duration of presentation, and whether or not there is evidence of devitalized bowel. Anticoagulation is the mainstay of initial medical management, followed by surgical or endovascular revascularization. Surgical intervention has the distinct advantage of offering both revascularization of the occluded artery, and visual inspection of the bowel and resection if needed.

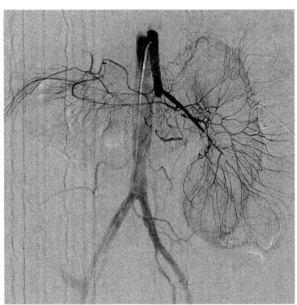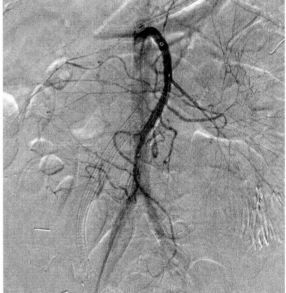

Figure 20-1 DSA images pre (left) and post (right) endovascular recanalization of an acute SMA embolus. The embolus was mostly removed with a suction catheter, and the artery was then ballooned and stented with excellent restoration of flow to the distal branches.

References: Clair DG, Beach JM. Mesenteric ischemia. *N Engl J Med.* 2016;374(10):959-968.

Stone JR, Wilkins LR. Acute mesenteric ischemia. *Tech Vasc Interv Radiol.* 2015;18(1):24-30.

Salsano G, Salsano A, Sportelli E, et al. What is the best revascularization strategy for acute occlusive arterial mesenteric ischemia: systematic review and meta-analysis. *Cardiovasc Intervent Radiol.* 2018;41(1):27-36.

21 **Answer C.** The accepted bilirubin cutoff for lobar yttrium-90 radioembolization is 2.0 mg/dL. The bilirubin level is one of several parameters interventionalists should assess when considering radioembolization to the liver. Choices A and B are within normal limits, and choice C is a significantly elevated bilirubin concerning for biliary obstruction or liver failure.

The practice guidelines on radioembolization adapted from the American College of Radiology-Society of Interventional Radiology:

Indications:

1. The presence of unresectable primary or secondary liver malignancies. The tumor burden should be liver dominant or liver only. Patients should have a performance status that will allow them to benefit from therapy (ECOG performance status of 0 or 1 or Karnofsky score of 70 or more)

2. Life expectancy >3 months

Relative contraindications:

1. Tumor burden >70% of the parenchyma

2. Total bilirubin greater than 2 mg/dL (in the absence of obstructive cause). Operators may choose to treat more selectively (sublobar or segmental) when the bilirubin is elevated beyond 2 mg/dL

3. Pretreatment technetium-99m macroaggregated albumin (MAA) study demonstrating unacceptable shunt fraction between the liver and the lung parenchyma

4. Prior radiation therapy that included a significant volume of the liver

5. Chemotherapy agents in the preceding 4 weeks known to be unsafe when used with radioembolization

6. Pregnancy

Absolute contraindications:

1. Inability to catheterize the hepatic artery to safely deliver microspheres

2. Fulminant liver failure

3. Pretreatment technetium-99m MAA study demonstrating significant reflux or nontarget deposition to the gastrointestinal organs that cannot be corrected

References: Coldwell D, Sangro B, Wasan H, Salem R, Kennedy A. General selection criteria of patients for radioembolization of liver tumors: an international working group report. *Am J Clin Oncol*. 2011;34(3):337-341.

Kennedy A, Nag S, Salem R, et al. Recommendations for radioembolization of hepatic malignancies using yttrium-90 microsphere brachytherapy: a consensus panel report from the radioembolization brachytherapy oncology consortium. *Int J Radiat Oncol Biol Phys*. 2007;68(1):13-23.

Padia SA, Lewandowski RJ, Johnson GE, et al. Radioembolization of hepatic malignancies: background, quality improvement guidelines, and future directions. *J Vasc Interv Radiol*. 2017;28(1):1-15.

Sangro B, Salem R, Kennedy A, Coldwell D, Wasan H. Radioembolization for hepatocellular carcinoma: a review of the evidence and treatment recommendations. *Am J Clin Oncol*. 2011;34(4):422-431.

22 **Answer B.** Side effects after transarterial radioembolization (TARE) are common, typically occurring in the first 3 weeks after treatment, and they last for a few to several days. Fatigue is most commonly reported along with nausea, vomiting, low-grade fever, and abdominal pain. Prolonged fatigue coupled with a marked increase in the bilirubin level is concerning for something more sinister. Generally speaking, the liver is somewhat radiation intolerant. Historically, with initial attempts at external beam radiation treatments to the liver, it was found that at doses needed to kill tumor, the risk of radiation-induced liver disease was fairly high. This in part led to the development of selective internal radiation therapy (SIRT) or TARE, whereby microscopic radioactive particles are delivered transarterial, disproportionately travelling to the hypervascular liver tumors and sparing as much healthy liver as possible. Unfortunately, even with transarterial technique, there are cases where the liver responds poorly to the radiation and radioembolization-induced liver disease (REILD) occurs. Careful preprocedural assessment helps to reduce this risk by screening out poor candidates for TARE. REILD typically presents 4 to 8 weeks after treatment with elevated levels of bilirubin, transaminitis, and worsening ascites. Ultimately, it can be a fatal process or the patient can recover over a period of months. If there is question as to the diagnosis, liver biopsy may be helpful. While it is an important consideration, bacterial cholangitis would present more acutely with high-grade fever, jaundice, and abdominal pain. Antibiotics and drainage of obstructed bile ducts are paramount to recovery. Hepatic artery thrombosis can occur anytime the artery is interrogated with a catheter. When it does occur in a native liver, the clinical consequence is usually negligible.

References: Gil-Alzugaray B, Chopitea A, Iñarrairaegui M, et al. Prognostic factors and prevention of radioembolization-induced liver disease. *Hepatology*. 2013;57(3):1078-1087.

Hamoui N, Ryu RK. Hepatic radioembolization complicated by fulminant hepatic failure. *Semin Intervent Radiol*. 2011;28(2):246-251.

Riaz A, Awais R, Salem R. Side effects of yttrium-90 radioembolization. *Front Oncol*. 2014;4:198.

23   Answer A.   Endoscopy is an endoluminal procedure that can be both diagnostic and therapeutic. Percutaneous cholangiogram with stent placement is by definition more invasive as you must transgress the liver, a well-vascularized organ, during the procedure. Current American College of Radiology recommendations are to perform endoscopy with stenting for most presentations of benign and malignant biliary obstruction. A notable exception is when the level of biliary obstruction is at or above the hepatic duct confluence (think Klatskin tumor), in which case percutaneous stenting is more likely to be successful. Additionally, if the patient has had surgery that precludes endoscopic access to the ampulla (such as a gastric bypass), a percutaneous procedure will be the preferred approach. Surgery is virtually never performed before endoscopic or percutaneous biliary decompression, and there is no role for arterial embolization in the hopes of shrinking an obstructing mass.

Reference: Ray CE, Lorenz JM, Burke CT, et al. ACR appropriateness criteria radiologic management of benign and malignant biliary obstruction. *J Am Coll Radiol*. 2013;10(8):567-574.

24   Answer C.   The images show a 2 cm arterially enhancing round mass in the right lobe of the liver with washout on the portal venous phase. Note the cirrhotic morphology of the liver with enlarged left lateral segment and nodular surface. Keeping in line with the BCLC staging and treatment model (discussed earlier in this chapter), this is the ideal patient for thermal ablation. He has early stage cirrhosis and early stage HCC. The available ablation technologies include chemical ablation (percutaneous ethanol injection) and energy-based ablation (microwave, radiofrequency, cryo, laser, ultrasound, and irreversible electroporation). Percutaneous ethanol injection has fallen out of favor given the major advancements made in the other ablation technologies, and relatively poorer performance in treating larger lesions. Choices A, B, and D are appropriate for intermediate to advanced stage disease and are mainly used for downstaging or palliation/extension of life.

References: Ahmed M, Solbiati L, Brace CL, et al. Image-guided tumor ablation: standardization of terminology and reporting criteria–a 10-year update. *Radiology*. 2014;273(1):241-260.

Foltz G. Image-guided percutaneous ablation of hepatic malignancies. *Semin Intervent Radiol*. 2014;31(2):180-186.

25   Answer B.   Current expert opinion is to ablate with a margin of 5 to 10 mm for primary and secondary liver malignancies. The intended margin is often defined by several factors including hepatic reserve and proximity to adjacent critical structures such as the gallbladder or bowel. An ablative margin is necessary to ensure complete coverage of the target tumor and address microscopic tumor or metastases in the immediate periphery that are not demonstrated with current imaging techniques. At our institution, we aim for a 10 mm ablative margin whenever feasible.

Reference: Foltz G. Image-guided percutaneous ablation of hepatic malignancies. *Semin Intervent Radiol*. 2014;31(2):180-186.

26 **Answer C.** After thermal ablation of liver tumors, an immediate CECT helps to assess for residual unablated tumor, to evaluate the zone of ablation (and associated ablative margin), and to detect immediate complications. Scanning protocols vary, but the authors typically perform CECT with arterial and portal venous phase imaging following every hepatic ablation. The arterial phase image demonstrates residual enhancing tumor (particularly for HCC and other arterial enhancing secondary malignancies), and the portal venous phase depicts the zone of ablation (nonenhancing hypoattenuating area adjacent to enhancing liver parenchyma). The field of view is increased to incorporate the entire liver and complete path of any instrument used in the procedure, in order to assess for complications such as bleeding or injury to adjacent structures. Local tumor progression, which is a new focus of tumor at the margin of the ablation (choice A), should be assessed on follow-up imaging. The presence of tumors outside the liver (choice B) should be known before performing tumor treatment. Immediately after a tumor treatment is not an appropriate time to stage the patient. Naturally, the development of new extrahepatic tumors will be assessed on longer-term follow-up imaging.

TABLE 26-1 Cross-sectional Imaging After Thermal Ablation for Hepatic Malignancy.

Immediate (technical success)	Assess for residual unablated tumor
	Determine the zone of ablation
	Determine the ablative margin
	Evaluate for immediate complications
One month (technique efficacy)	Assess for residual unablated tumor
	Evaluate for complications
Three months	Assess for local tumor progression
	Assess for distant tumor
	Evaluate for delayed complications

Adapted from Bouda D, Lagadec M, Alba CG, et al. Imaging review of hepatocellular carcinoma after thermal ablation: the good, the bad, and the ugly. *J Magn Reson Imaging*. 2016;44(5):1070-1090.

References: Ahmed M, Solbiati L, Brace CL, et al. Image-guided tumor ablation: standardization of terminology and reporting criteria – a 10-year update. *Radiology*. 2014;273(1):241-260.

Bouda D, Lagadec M, Alba CG, et al. Imaging review of hepatocellular carcinoma after thermal ablation: the good, the bad, and the ugly. *J Magn Reson Imaging*. 2016;44(5):1070-1090.

27 **Answer D.** On CECT immediately after thermal ablation, the zone of ablation is demonstrated by a round to oval, nonenhancing hypoattenuating area. It is less well seen on arterial phase when compared with portal venous phase images, as the surrounding parenchyma enhances relatively greater on the latter. Within the zone of ablation, there may be gas (round and linear) and heterogeneously attenuating debris. Ablation probe tracts are often seen as linear hypoattenuating structures extending to the liver capsule. As time progresses, a rim of enhancement/hyperemia may develop at the margin of the zone of ablation and last a period of 1 to 4 months. This is expected as long as it is thin and relatively uniform. Discontinuous irregular nodular enhancement that enlarges over time is highly concerning for unablated tumor or local tumor progression. Within the zone, the gas resolves (it can be present for weeks), and the internal contents become more homogenous and hypoattenuating. Months after the ablation, the zone shrinks progressively and can be associated with capsular retraction, calcifications, and small dilated biliary radicals.

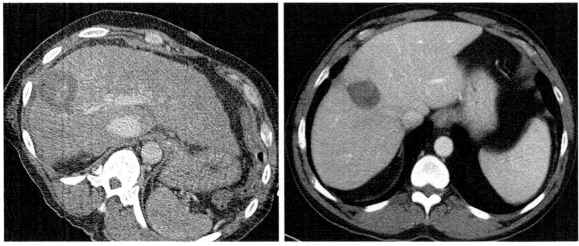

Figure 27-1 Immediate (left) and 9-month follow-up (right) CECT images following right lobe microwave thermal ablation of a solitary HCC. On the immediate postprocedure image, the zone of ablation is defined by the round nonenhancing hypoattenuating area in the right lobe. Note the internal higher attenuation debris, an expected finding and not indicative of unablated tumor or active hemorrhage. On the 9-month follow-up image, the zone of ablation is nonenhancing and uniformly hypoattenuating. The measured size is smaller, and there is associated retraction of the surrounding liver parenchyma.

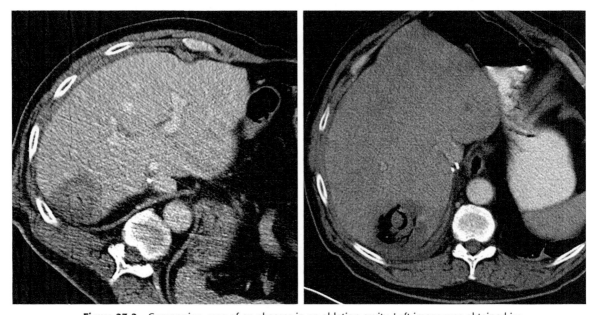

Figure 27-2 Companion case of an abscess in an ablation cavity. Left image was obtained immediately after thermal ablation of recurrent HCC in a transplanted liver. Note the minimal central linear gas present. Approximately 2 weeks later, the patient presented with pain and fever. CECT now demonstrated increasing gas throughout the ablation zone. This was successfully managed with antibiotics and percutaneous catheter drainage.

Reference: Bouda D, Lagadec M, Alba CG, et al. Imaging review of hepatocellular carcinoma after thermal ablation: the good, the bad, and the ugly. *J Magn Reson Imaging*. 2016;44(5):1070-1090.

Kim KR, Thomas S. Complications of image-guided thermal ablation of liver and kidney neoplasms. *Semin Intervent Radiol*. 2014;31(2):138-148.

28   Answer C.   In patients with cirrhosis and portal hypertension, hepatic encephalopathy (HE) is common, and often very treatable with medications such as lactulose and rifaximin. HE can be due to liver failure (synthetic dysfunction) and/or related to underlying portosystemic shunts. With shunt physiology, portal venous blood is diverted through collateral channels to the systemic venous blood, resulting in an increased exposure of the brain to certain metabolites such as ammonia and manganese. The most common example is encephalopathy that occurs after TIPS. When a TIPS is not present, an underlying spontaneous portosystemic shunt should be sought in patients who demonstrate recurrent encephalopathy despite maximal medical therapy and no other identifiable cause. Biliary obstruction will present with jaundice, and although hepatic hydrothorax is a manifestation of portal hypertension, it does not produce encephalopathy.

References: Philips CA, Kumar L, Augustine P. Shunt occlusion for portosystemic shunt syndrome related refractory hepatic encephalopathy-A single-center experience in 21 patients from Kerala. *Indian J Gastroenterol.* 2017;36(5):411-419.

Saad WE. Portosystemic shunt syndrome and endovascular management of hepatic encephalopathy. *Semin Intervent Radiol.* 2014;31(3):262-265.

29   Answer C.   A portosystemic shunt is a low resistance connection between the portal venous system (high pressure in the setting of cirrhosis) and the systemic venous system (low pressure). Even in the presence of a patent portal vein, the shunt may be diverting a significant amount of blood away from the liver and directly back to the systemic veins and ultimately the right heart. Closure of the shunt with embolization eliminates the low resistance pathway, causing an immediate increase in portal venous flow and pressure. If there are preexisting gastroesophageal varices, the increased pressure after embolization can result in acute variceal hemorrhage. Ascites may begin to accumulate as well.

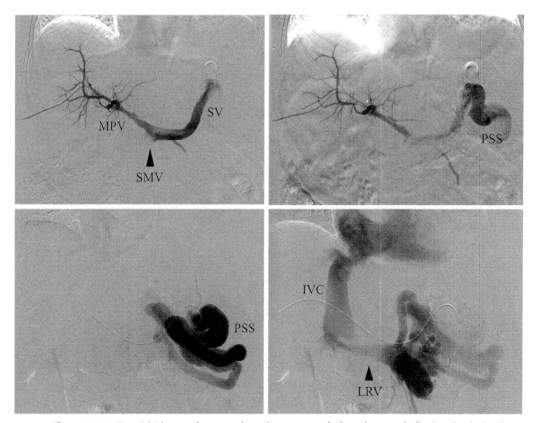

Figure 29-1   Four DSA images from transhepatic portogram before shunt embolization, beginning in the upper left image. There is contrast opacification of the intra- and extrahepatic portal veins, as well as a large, tortuous vessel (PSS) arising from the splenic vein that ultimately drains into the left renal vein (bottom right image). Note the diminutive appearance of the main portal vein and its intrahepatic branches due to chronic shunting away from the liver. IVC, inferior vena cava; LRV, left renal vein; MPV, main portal vein; PSS, portosystemic shunt; SMV, superior mesenteric vein; SV, splenic vein.

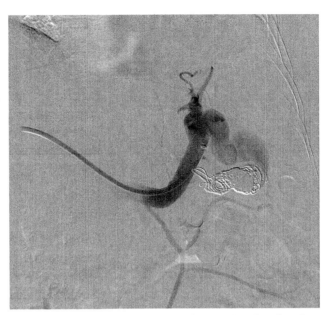

Figure 29-2 DSA image after embolization with a dense coil pack in the afferent segment of the portosystemic shunt. Both the splenic vein and inferior mesenteric vein are opacified. Preembolization main portal vein pressure measured 17 mmHg. Post embolization main portal vein pressure measured 32 mmHg. Upper endoscopy showed no varices before the embolization. Following the procedure, the patient's hepatic encephalopathy resolved with no recurrence 2 years later.

References: Philips CA, Kumar L, Augustine P. Shunt occlusion for portosystemic shunt syndrome related refractory hepatic encephalopathy-A single-center experience in 21 patients from Kerala. *Indian J Gastroenterol*. 2017;36(5):411-419.

Saad WE. Portosystemic shunt syndrome and endovascular management of hepatic encephalopathy. *Semin Intervent Radiol*. 2014;31(3):262-265.

30   **Answer A.**   The images depict a three-phase CECT examination with precontrast, arterial, and delayed phases. The imaged vasculature gives you the necessary information to delineate the phase of contrast enhancement. The finding of interest is a distended loop of colon in the right lower abdomen. Note on the precontrast image, there is no high attenuation material seen within the bowel lumen. On the arterial phase, there is new intraluminal high attenuation that matches that of the adjacent iliac arteries. On the delayed phase, the high attenuation collection has spread out and begins to layer against the right lateral wall. All of these findings indicate extravasating iodinated contrast from active colonic bleeding (choice A). Necrosis of the colon may show a spectrum of findings including bowel dilatation, wall thickening, absent wall enhancement, pneumatosis, and portal venous gas. An abscess would present as an extraluminal collection of fluid and/or air. Over time, a well-formed rim of enhancement will develop. Ectopic varices can form at many different locations in the abdomen or pelvis and certainly can cause bleeding; however, high-attenuation arterial phase intraluminal contrast extravasation should not occur from venous pathology.

References: Artigas JM, Martí M, Soto JA, Esteban H, Pinilla I, Guillén E. Multidetector CT angiography for acute gastrointestinal bleeding: technique and findings. *Radiographics*. 2013;33(5):1453-1470.

Feuerstein JD, Ketwaroo G, Tewani SK, et al. Localizing acute lower gastrointestinal hemorrhage: CT angiography versus tagged RBC scintigraphy. *AJR Am J Roentgenol*. 2016;207(3):578-584.

31   **Answer B.**   The celiac artery branches into the left gastric artery, splenic artery, and common hepatic artery supplying the distal esophagus through the duodenum. The SMA branches into jejunal branches, ileal branches, ileocolic artery, right colic artery, and middle colic artery supplying the jejunum through the transverse colon. The inferior mesenteric artery branches into the left colic artery, sigmoid branches, and superior rectal (hemorrhoidal) artery supplying the splenic flexure of the colon through the rectum. The internal iliac artery has anterior and posterior divisions and has collateral circulation to the rectum through the middle and inferior hemorrhoidal arteries.

Reference: Uflacker R. In: *Atlas of Vascular Anatomy, An Angiographic Approach.* LWW; 2007:457-654.

32   **Answer C.**   Endovascular treatment of lower gastrointestinal bleeding is most commonly performed by microcatheterization of arterial branches as close to the source as possible (choice C). Microcoils (other embolics can be used as well) are then deployed, occluding the extravasating branch. If limited superselective embolization is performed, ischemic complications are rare. In this case, a more proximal embolization at the level of the ileocolic artery (choice A) or cecal artery (choice B) would be ineffective, as robust collateral arcades exist closer to the bowel wall. The arcades anastomose along the inner margin of the colon forming the marginal artery of Drummond. If superselective embolization cannot be performed, vasoconstrictor infusion can be initiated with repeat angiographic assessments to assess for hemostasis, although this technique is not commonly used today.

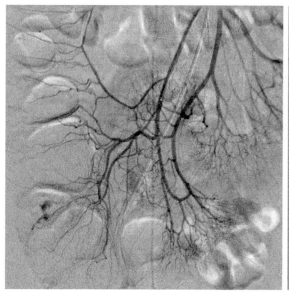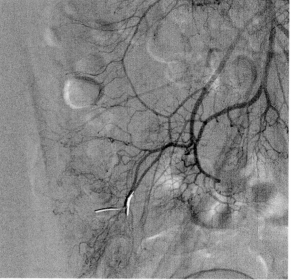

Figure 32-1 Pre-embolization DSA image (left) demonstrating a brisk bleed from the cecum. Note the long straight arteries extending out to the bowel wall termed vasa recta. Postembolization DSA image (right) after superselective embolization with straight coils into the extravasating vasa recta branch as well as slightly more proximal.

References: Bouhaidar DS, Strife BJ. Transcatheter intervention for non-variceal gastrointestinal bleeding: what have we learned in 45 years? *Dig Dis Sci.* 2013;58(7):1819-1821.

Frisoli JK, Sze DY, Kee S. Transcatheter embolization for the treatment of upper gastrointestinal bleeding. *Tech Vasc Interv Radiol.* 2004;7(3):136-142.

Kuo WT. Transcatheter treatment for lower gastrointestinal hemorrhage. *Tech Vasc Interv Radiol.* 2004;7(3):143-150.

Walker TG. Acute gastrointestinal hemorrhage. *Tech Vasc Interv Radiol.* 2009;12(2):80-91.

33 **Answer E.**   The celiac artery traditionally branches into the common hepatic artery, left gastric artery, and splenic artery although numerous variations are commonly found in practice (discussed elsewhere in this book in detail). The right and left inferior phrenic arteries have a variable origin, with the most common being the supraceliac abdominal aorta or the base of the celiac artery as seen here (left artery only; right inferior phrenic originated directly from the aorta). The inferior phrenic arteries demonstrate an initial steep course cephalad and curve laterally as they run along the right and left hemidiaphragm. The inferior phrenic arteries have significant clinical importance in conditions such as hepatocellular carcinoma and bronchial hemorrhage from chronic lung disease, as the artery can become parasitized causing treatment failure or recurrence. It is also prone to injury with diaphragmatic trauma.

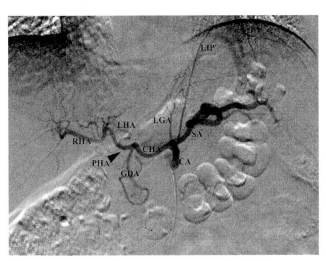

Figure 33-1   Catheter angiography after selection of the celiac artery. CA, celiac artery; CHA; common hepatic artery; GDA, gastroduodenal artery; LGA, left gastric artery; LHA; left hepatic artery; LIP, left inferior phrenic artery; PHA, proper hepatic artery; RHA, right hepatic artery; SA, splenic artery.

Reference: Uflacker R. In: *Atlas of Vascular Anatomy, An Angiographic Approach.* LWW; 2007:457-654.

34 **Answer D.**   This case illustrates the importance of understanding endovascular treatment options for aneurysms and pseudoaneurysms, as well as collateral arterial pathways that can result in treatment failure. The first question we ask before any embolization is whether or not the parent artery can be sacrificed. Each vascular territory is different, and some arteries are "end organ" and others can be occluded without risking organ ischemia/infarction. In the case example, there is a saccular pseudoaneurysm arising from the proximal GDA, with jet of extravasating contrast into the adjacent duodenal lumen. Collateral flow from both the SMA (through the pancreaticoduodenal arcade) and celiac artery (splenic artery to left gastroepiploic artery) will prevent distal stomach and duodenal ischemia after occlusion of the GDA.

Having decided that the parent artery can be sacrificed, the operator must then consider if there are collateral blood flow pathways that might cause a treatment failure. A coil occluding the proximal GDA (choice A) will certainly result in treatment failure as retrograde flow through the gastroepiploic artery will backfill the distal GDA and the pseudoaneurysm (see question 12 for example of GDA to gastroepiploic collateralization). Similarly, treatment at choice B will occlude the backdoor pathway, but allow the inflow to persist. Coils within the pseudoaneurysm can be effective, but a pseudoaneurysm is a contained arterial rupture by definition, and catheter, wire, or coil manipulation within the sac can take a nonbleeding pseudoaneurysm to a frank rupture. Ideally, treatment would consist of arterial occlusion distal and proximal to the pseudoaneurysm. This isolates the pseudoaneurysm from the circulation as seen in Figure 34-1. Notably, with true aneurysms, coiling of the aneurysm sac alone may be a good option as the aneurysm wall is otherwise intact and flow preservation through the parent artery is achieved.

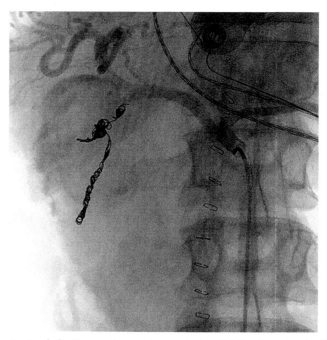

Figure 34-1 Postembolization angiogram demonstrating distal and proximal coil occlusion of the GDA (isolation technique). Coils unintentionally migrated into the pseudoaneurysm sac while forming the pack.

With parent arteries that cannot be sacrificed, flow preservation can also be achieved with covered stent grafts (think EVAR for AAA) and stent or balloon-assisted coiling. Percutaneous thrombin or glue injection into the pseudo-/aneurysm can also be considered in certain instances.

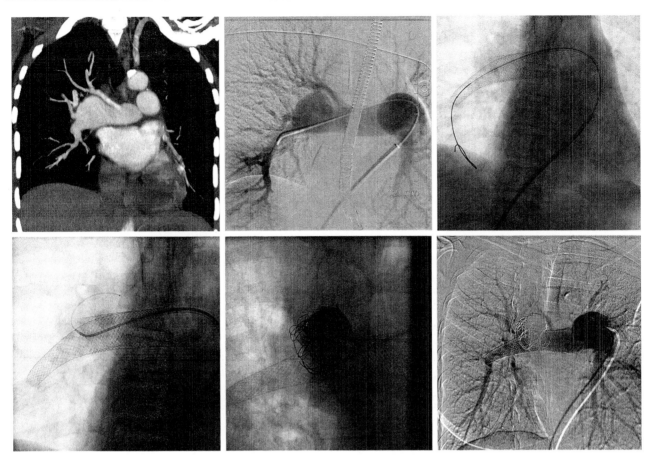

Figure 34-2 Companion case of a broad necked pseudoaneurysm arising from the right pulmonary artery, which developed after a surgical lymph node biopsy. Coronal CECT image (top left) demonstrates the pseudoaneurysm. Endovascular embolization was planned for flow preservation to the right lung using a stent-assisted coiling technique. Uncovered stents were deployed in the right pulmonary artery across the pseudoaneurysm, providing a scaffold to then pack the sac with coils (top right). A microcatheter was advanced through the interstices of the stents into the pseudoaneurysm sac (bottom left), and several meters of coil were deployed (middle bottom). Completion angiogram showed no further filling of the pseudoaneurysm with preserved flow to right pulmonary artery branches.

References: Belli AM, Markose G, Morgan R. The role of interventional radiology in the management of abdominal visceral artery aneurysms. *Cardiovasc Intervent Radiol*. 2012;35(2):234-243.

Hemp JH, Sabri SS. Endovascular management of visceral arterial aneurysms. *Tech Vasc Interv Radiol*. 2015;18(1):14-23.

35   **Answer C.**   In this case, the best approach for abscess drainage catheter placement is US-guided transrectal. We use transabdominal (using the bladder as an acoustic window) or transrectal ultrasound to visualize the abscess cavity. A barium enema catheter or dilator is used as a needle sheath and introduced transrectally. The needle is then advanced into the fluid collection, a wire is coiled, serial dilation is performed, and a locking pigtail drainage catheter is advanced over the wire into position. The pigtail is formed and locked in the collection, and the cavity is drained of all infected fluid. The catheter is then secured to the thigh and is well tolerated in terms of comfort. Patients can then undergo interval appendectomy at a later date, once the abscess has been completely eradicated and inflammation has subsided. Transabdominal access, whether with CT or US, would not be safe in this case as the needle and subsequent drainage catheter would traverse adjacent blood vessels, bladder, or uninvolved bowel. Transgluteal catheter placement is usually a good option for mid-pelvic abscess, but the ideal needle tract is medial, close to the sacrum, and through the sacrospinous ligament in order to avoid nerves and blood vessels. Based on the images presented, there was perhaps a small window on the right, but the level is significantly cranial to the sacrospinous ligament, increasing the risk of traversing important neurovascular structures. Another drawback of CT guidance is the radiation exposure to the child. Choice D is incorrect as catheter drainage of the pelvic abscess is arguably the most important step in treatment when dealing with a pelvic abscess. If the abscess measures less than 3 cm, needle aspiration (no catheter) of the abscess can be considered.

References: Brown C, Kang L, Kim ST. Percutaneous drainage of abdominal and pelvic abscesses in children. *Semin Intervent Radiol.* 2012;29(4):286-294.

Mcdaniel JD, Warren MT, Pence JC, Ey EH. Ultrasound-guided transrectal drainage of deep pelvic abscesses in children: a modified and simplified technique. *Pediatr Radiol.* 2015;45(3):435-438.

36   **Answer C.**   Ascites fluid analysis is critical for the determination of underlying etiology. The SAAG or serum ascites albumin gradient is calculated by subtracting the ascites albumin level from the serum albumin level (choice C). Ideally these levels are measured simultaneously. When the SAAG is >1.1 g/dL, the ascites is most commonly due to hepatic causes such as cirrhosis with portal hypertension, and less commonly congestive heart failure. When the SAAG is <1.1 g/dL, the ascites may be due to malignancy, infection such tuberculosis, or spontaneous bacterial peritonitis.

TABLE 36-1   Ascitic Fluid Analysis Based on Etiology

	Cirrhosis	CHF	Malignancy	Infection
Total protein	<25 g/L	<25 g/L	>25 g/L	>25 g/L
SAAG	>1.1 g/dL	>1.1 g/dL	<1.1 g/dL	<1.1 g/dL
Glucose	Normal	Normal	Decreased	Decreased
Lactate dehydrogenase	Decreased	Normal to decreased	Increased	Normal to increased
Cell count	>250/μL or normal			>250/μL or normal
Culture	Occasionally positive			Positive or false negative

Adapted from Huang LL, Xia HH, Zhu SL. Ascitic fluid analysis in the differential diagnosis of ascites: focus on cirrhotic ascites. *J Clin Transl Hepatol.* 2014;2(1):58-64.
CHF, Congestive heart failure.

Reference: Huang LL, Xia HH, Zhu SL. Ascitic fluid analysis in the differential diagnosis of ascites: focus on cirrhotic ascites. *J Clin Transl Hepatol.* 2014;2(1):58-64.

37   **Answer C.**   Three sequential DSA images depict the arterial phase, parenchymal phase, and finally the portal venous phase from a power injection of the SMA. On the arterial phase image, the SMA and its branches perfusing the bowel from the duodenum through transverse colon appear normal. Note the absence of an early draining vein that would indicate an arteriovenous malformation or fistula. On the

parenchymal phase, contrast has filled the wall of the bowel appropriately. There is no extravasation. On the portal venous phase, contrast has filled peripheral mesenteric veins, which coalesce into the superior mesenteric vein centrally. Normally, the SMV joins the splenic vein in the upper abdomen with a single main portal vein coursing towards the liver and ultimately branching into the right and left portal veins. Instead, there is a tangle of dilated and tortuous collaterals that have formed to circumvent a chronic main portal vein occlusion. Additionally, several dilated and tortuous veins have formed coursing towards the gastroesophageal junction. These are gastroesophageal varices. In summary, this is a classic angiographic picture of presinusoidal portal hypertension due to chronic portal vein occlusion with cavernous transformation.

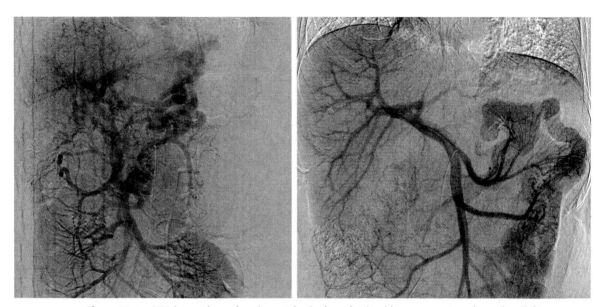

Figure 37-1 DSA image from chronic portal vein thrombosis with cavernous transformation (left) compared with a normal portal venogram (right). Both were performed by injecting the superior mesenteric artery and holding out for the portal venous phase.

References: Arora A, Sarin SK. Multimodality imaging of primary extrahepatic portal vein obstruction (EHPVO): what every radiologist should know. *Br J Radiol.* 2015;88(1052):20150008.

Gallego C, Velasco M, Marcuello P, Tejedor D, De Campo L, Friera A. Congenital and acquired anomalies of the portal venous system. *Radiographics.* 2002;22(1):141-159.

Uflacker R. In: *Atlas of Vascular Anatomy, An Angiographic Approach.* LWW; 2007:699-802.

38 **Answer B.** The management of necrotizing pancreatitis has evolved in the last few years with increased utilization of minimally invasive surgical, endoscopic, and percutaneous techniques. In this case, the patient has necrotizing pancreatitis on CECT with development of walled-off necrosis (WON), which is a persistent fluid collection (>4 wk from onset of necrotizing pancreatitis) with defined walls. Note the foci of fat within the peripancreatic collection and irregular contour of the wall, which helps delineate it as WON. These collections can be sterile or become superinfected. Indications for drainage catheter placement include sepsis from superinfection of necrotic tissue, and control of symptoms from the collection due to mass effect such as pain, obstruction, and inability to tolerate feeds. The favored percutaneous approach is left retroperitoneal when possible, to avoid peritoneal transgression. Also, as part of a step-up approach, future minimally invasive necrosectomy can utilize the left retroperitoneal approach catheter tract to assist with that operation. In general, drains for necrotizing pancreatitis should be large (>10 Fr) to assist with removal of fluid and/or debris. Fine needle aspiration is useful for diagnostic purposes only, in cases where these is a question of an infected fluid collection.

References: Shyu JY, Sainani NI, Sahni VA, et al. Necrotizing pancreatitis: diagnosis, imaging, and intervention. *Radiographics*. 2014;34(5):1218-1239.

Van Santvoort HC, Besselink MG, Bakker OJ, et al. A step-up approach or open necrosectomy for necrotizing pancreatitis. *N Engl J Med*. 2010;362(16):1491-1502.

39 **Answer D.**   The CECT images depict marked distention of the stomach, and first and second portions of the duodenum with collapse of the third portion of the duodenum. These findings point to the level of obstruction in the midduodenum. The axial and sagittal-oblique reconstructions show that the SMA tightly opposed the adjacent abdominal aorta. Note the transition point in the bowel from obstructed to unobstructed specifically at the level of the SMA crossing the duodenum. The constellation of findings are consistent with SMA syndrome, a vascular phenomenon of complete or partial duodenal obstruction due to vascular compression. Patients frequently present with a history of significant weight loss, often due to an underlying condition (medical, surgical, and/or psychiatric). As the obstruction evolves, progressive fullness, nausea, vomiting, and malnutrition can occur. Treatment is aimed at the underlying condition, and weight gain can be curative. Surgical treatment may be necessary to reposition the bowel or circumvent the obstruction.

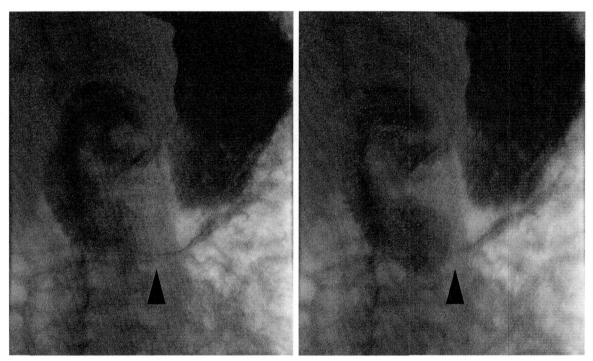

Figure 39-1   A young female with history of marked weight loss due to an anxiety disorder. Fluoroscopic examination with oral barium demonstrates dilation of the stomach, and first and second portions of the duodenum with transition point (arrowhead) in the mid transverse segment. Note the decompressed appearance of distal duodenum.

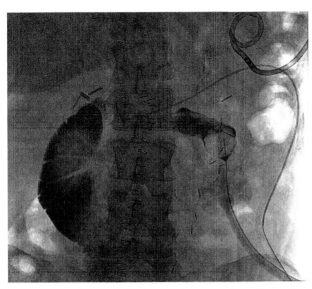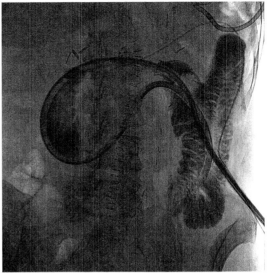

Figure 39-2 Companion case of a patient with excessive weight loss following gastric bypass surgery. A feeding tube for nutrition is placed into the excluded stomach. When used, the tube continually leaks along the percutaneous tract concerning for a downstream bowel obstruction. Tube contrast study shows a distended first and second portions of the duodenum with no passage of contrast left of midline (left image). A CTA showed SMA compression of the duodenum. A gastro-jejunostomy tube is subsequently placed beyond the midduodenal obstruction for distal feeding (right image). Note the decompressed bowel left of midline.

Reference: Lamba R, Tanner DT, Sekhon S, Mcgahan JP, Corwin MT, Lall CG. Multidetector CT of vascular compression syndromes in the abdomen and pelvis. *Radiographics*. 2014;34(1):93-115.

40   **Answer A.**   In patients with gastrointestinal bleeding, diagnostic investigation aims to localize the source to the upper or lower tract. An uncommon but important etiology for upper tract bleeding is transpapillary hemorrhage from the liver or pancreas via their respective ducts into the duodenum. If brisk, there can be hematochezia rather than melena. As in this case, a history of trauma or instrumentation is often elicited, which produces a communication between the parenchymal vasculature and ductal system. For the pancreas, pancreatitis and pseudocyst formation are common precursors. The images presented depict diffuse biliary dilatation with internal high-attenuation fluid consistent with blood products. Angiography should be performed to identify and embolize the vascular injury (an arterial pseudoaneurysm with fistula to the bile duct in this case), while endoscopic retrograde cannulation of the common bile duct with balloon sweep and sphincterotomy can treat symptomatic and/or unresolved biliary obstruction from blood clots.

Reference: Behrens G, Ferral H. Transjugular liver biopsy. *Semin Intervent Radiol*. 2012;29(2):111-117.

41   **Answer B.**   TACE is typically performed using (1) an emulsion of chemotherapeutic agent with lipiodol aka conventional (cTACE) or (2) chemotherapeutic agent loaded onto embolic beads aka drug-eluting bead chemoembolization (DEBTACE). TACE has been used extensively for the treatment of primary and secondary malignancies in the liver. Ideally, catheter position will be as selective as possible, although depending on the tumor type and distribution of disease, the treatment can be delivered in lobar fashion. The embolization is often repeated depending on the tumor response and goals of care. Patient selection is important to avoid complications from the procedure, considering that the treatment is embolic with some degree of ischemia caused. Adequate hepatic reserve and absence of portal vein thrombosis are two important inclusion criteria. An additional important

consideration is whether the patient has biliary incompetence from prior surgery such as hepaticojejunostomy or prior manipulation such as sphincterotomy or biliary stenting. Several studies have identified biliary incompetence as a significant risk factor for the development of hepatic abscess after TACE procedures. Antibiotic protocols have been studied and perhaps the most promising approach is an extended course of moxifloxacin given before and after the procedure.

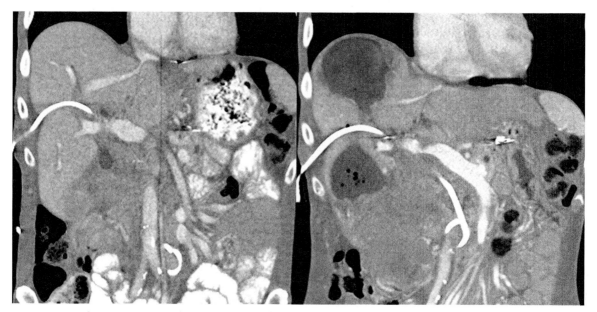

Figure 41-1   Coronal CECT images pre (left) and post (right) right lobar TACE in a patient with metastatic gastric cancer. Note the indwelling internal-external biliary drainage catheter. Despite periprocedural antibiotics, the patient developed large hepatic abscesses after the embolization, treated with prolonged antibiotics and catheter drainage.

References: Brown DB, Nikolic B, Covey AM, et al. Quality improvement guidelines for transhepatic arterial chemoembolization, embolization, and chemotherapeutic infusion for hepatic malignancy. *J Vasc Interv Radiol*. 2012;23(3):287-294.

Khan W, Sullivan KL, Mccann JW, et al. Moxifloxacin prophylaxis for chemoembolization or embolization in patients with previous biliary interventions: a pilot study. *AJR Am J Roentgenol*. 2011;197(2):W343-W345.

Kim W, Clark TW, Baum RA, Soulen MC. Risk factors for liver abscess formation after hepatic chemoembolization. *J Vasc Interv Radiol*. 2001;12(8):965-968.

Woo S, Chung JW, Hur S, et al. Liver abscess after transarterial chemoembolization in patients with bilioenteric anastomosis: frequency and risk factors. *AJR Am J Roentgenol*. 2013;200(6):1370-1377.

42   **Answer C.**   A significant arm of interventional radiology is oncologic work centered on the treatment of cirrhosis and HCC. Ideally, these patients are reviewed and discussed among a multidisciplinary team as their care is often complex and affected by a myriad of different issues ranging from psychosocial to physical. As liver transplantation is one of the most important treatment options for patients with cirrhosis and HCC, team members should be familiar with the Milan criteria. There can be 1 tumor ≤5.0 cm in diameter or up to 3 tumors, each of which is ≤3.0 cm in diameter. Patients cannot have hepatic vascular invasion or extrahepatic malignancy. Keeping a patient within these criteria is often a task for the interventional radiologist through the use of downstaging procedures such as transarterial embolization. It is worth noting that there are variations or extensions of Milan criteria, which may be used at some institutions.

References: Clavien PA, Lesurtel M, Bossuyt PM, et al. Recommendations for liver transplantation for hepatocellular carcinoma: an international consensus conference report. *Lancet Oncol.* 2012;13(1):e11-e22.

Mazzaferro V, Regalia E, Doci R, et al. Liver transplantation for the treatment of small hepatocellular carcinomas in patients with cirrhosis. *N Engl J Med.* 1996;334(11):693-699.

43   **Answer D.**   The CECT images demonstrate a shrunken cirrhotic liver and a round tumor with central necrosis extending off the surface of the liver exophytically. There is complex fluid around the liver and spleen consistent with hemorrhage. With the history of acute abdominal pain, the constellation of findings point to a ruptured HCC. Unfortunately, studies have shown HCC rupture is a risk factor for peritoneal seeding. The patient in the case example was treated in the acute setting for continued hemorrhage with transarterial particle embolization (see Figure 43-1). In the short term, he had excision of the tumor with a central hepatectomy. Years later an enlarging peritoneal nodule distant to the liver was identified and biopsy proven to be metastatic HCC (see Figure 43-2).

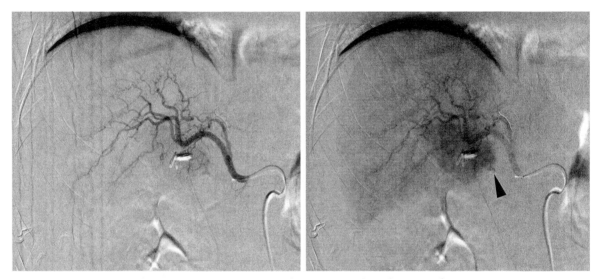

Figure 43-1   Angiography from the proper hepatic artery shows hypervascular segment 4 HCC with jet of contrast extravasation (arrowhead) from ongoing hemorrhage. Notice the right lateral border of the liver is displaced from the abdominal wall from known perihepatic hematoma.

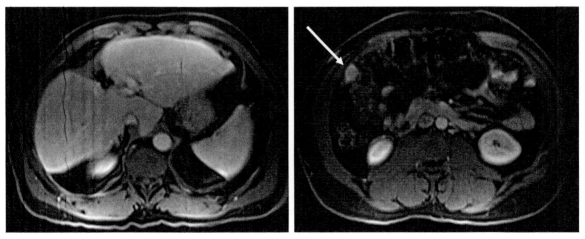

Figure 43-2   Axial T1 fat sat + gad MRI images 3 years after embolization and resection of ruptured segment 4 HCC. Right image shows surgical scar with no recurrence. Unfortunately, a new peritoneal nodule (arrow) is discovered, biopsy proven to be HCC.

References: Matsukuma S, Sato K. Peritoneal seeding of hepatocellular carcinoma: clinicopathological characteristics of 17 autopsy cases. *Pathol Int.* 2011;61(6):356-362.

Sonoda T, Kanematsu T, Takenaka K, Sugimachi K. Ruptured hepatocellular carcinoma evokes risk of implanted metastases. *J Surg Oncol.* 1989;41(3):183-186.

44   Answer C. Percutaneous treatment of biliary stones is in the purview of the interventional radiologist. This mostly comes into play if the patient has anatomy preclusive to endoscopy (such as hepaticojejunostomy or Roux-en-Y gastric bypass) or has failed endoscopic intervention. As this minimally invasive percutaneous option exists, this would be a more reasonable treatment compared with laparotomy. Once percutaneous access is made into the biliary system, several tools can be employed to facilitate clearing the stone(s). We commonly start with cholangioplasty to dilate any preexisting stenosis and then follow with antegrade balloon sweeps into the bowel. This often works well for small stones. With large stones, they can be broken down using specially made baskets or even standard vascular loop snares (see Figure 44-1). Once fragmented, the stone debris can be aspirated or swept antegrade into the bowel. Multiple procedures may be needed with serial upsizing of the biliary drainage catheter to help treat any underlying stenosis and allow for stones and debris to pass on their own. Finally, percutaneous choledocoscopy with lithotripsy may be available at certain centers.

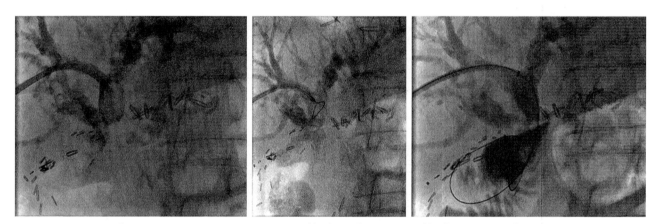

Figure 44-1   Percutaneous stone removal in the patient presented in the case example. Large central stone is seen as a filling defect on antegrade cholangiogram (left). A combination of loop snare fragmentation (middle) and balloon sweep successfully removes the stone with completion cholangiogram (right) showing a patent central bile duct with flow into the bowel.

Reference: García-García L, Lanciego C. Percutaneous treatment of biliary stones: sphincteroplasty and occlusion balloon for the clearance of bile duct calculi. *AJR Am J Roentgenol.* 2004;182(3):663-670.

45   Answer C. The case images demonstrate a complication from a right flank approach internal-external biliary drainage catheter. On the image labeled "hepatic arteriogram," the drainage catheter has been removed over a wire and an arteriogram performed from a catheter in a branch of the right hepatic artery. There is obvious deformity to the artery where the biliary catheter crosses the vessel but no frank extravasation. On the unsubtracted image labeled "cholangiogram," contrast has been injected into the biliary tree, demonstrating diffuse biliary dilatation with extensive intraluminal filling defects that represent blood clots in obstructed bile ducts. In addition, the right hepatic artery is opacified on the cholangiogram, confirming an arteriobiliary fistula.

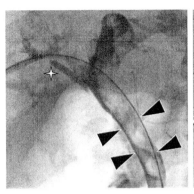
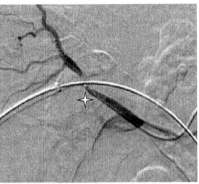
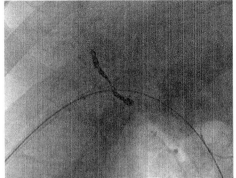

Figure 45-1 Hepatic artery injury (star) from percutaneous biliary catheter on cholangiogram and arteriogram. The common bile duct is obstructed by extensive blood clots (arrowheads). This is treated with coil embolization of the artery, proximal and distal to the injury to prevent backbleeding (right).

Of note, the biliary drainage catheter can tamponade the bleeding intermittently, making evaluation challenging. When a blood vessel to bile duct connection is suspected in the setting of an indwelling catheter, angiography with and without (removed over a wire) the tube in place should be performed to thoroughly evaluate for a connection.

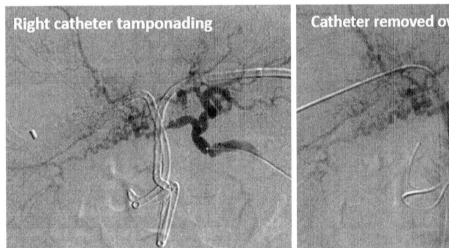
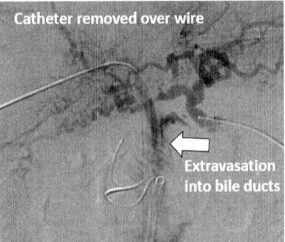

Figure 45-2 Companion case demonstrating arteriobiliary fistula, which is only identified when the biliary drainage catheter is removed over a wire. The patient presented with multiple episodes of intermittent gastrointestinal bleeding.

Percutaneous biliary drainage is a vital procedure for the treatment of acute and chronic biliary pathology. Although it can be a life-saving intervention, it is not without risk. In general, when creating the percutaneous tract to the bile ducts, the more central the access is relative to the liver hilum, the more likely the operator will transgress a large blood vessel. Additionally, one must take into account possible pleural transgression. For fluoroscopic-guided right-sided biliary access, classic teaching is to start with the needle entry at or below the 10th intercostal space just anterior to the midaxillary line. The needle should be parallel to the table, and aimed 20° to 30° cranial.

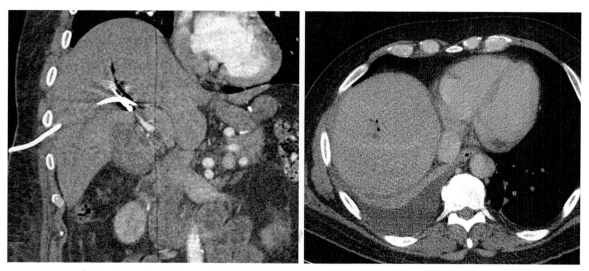

Figure 45-3   The patient in the case example with the arteriobiliary fistula also had the drain placed at the eighth intercostal space with resultant bile leak into the pleural space. Fortunately, this was managed with pleural catheter drainage alone; the biliary-pleural communication closed in a matter of weeks and both tubes were removed uneventfully.

Reference: Covey AM, Brown KT. Percutaneous transhepatic biliary drainage. *Tech Vasc Interv Radiol*. 2008;11(1):14-20.

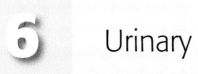

Urinary

QUESTIONS

1 An 8-year-old male undergoes a percutaneous native kidney core needle biopsy. In the recovery area, he is tachycardic and hypotensive. A noncontrast computed tomography (CT) demonstrates a massive left perirenal hematoma and he is taken emergently to the interventional radiology (IR) suite. What is the best treatment option after these images are obtained?

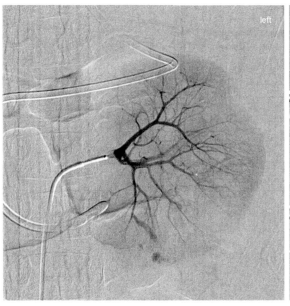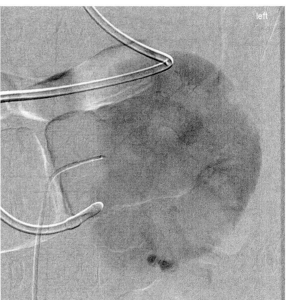

    A. Watchful waiting, no safe position to perform embolization
    B. Superselective coil embolization
    C. Embolize with particles
    D. Surgical partial nephrectomy

2 Which of the following is an indication for a renal arteriogram in a pediatric patient?

    A. Hydronephrosis
    B. Recurrent urinary tract infection
    C. Hypertension
    D. Nephrolithiasis

3   Which of the following is the most common cause of pediatric renal arterial stenosis?

   A. Fibromuscular dysplasia
   B. Atherosclerosis
   C. Neurofibromatosis 1
   D. Polyarteritis nodosa

4   An adult female with cervical cancer and known vesicovaginal fistula presents for urinary diversion. Which is the most appropriate initial procedure?

   A. Bilateral PCN (percutaneous nephrostomy) catheter placement
   B. Bilateral NUS (nephroureteral stent) placement
   C. Bilateral double-J ureteral stent placement
   D. Bilateral ureteral embolization with plugs

5   PCN catheter placement carries which risk of bleeding?

   A. Category I low risk of bleeding, easy to detect or control
   B. Category II moderate risk of bleeding
   C. Category III significant risk of bleeding, difficult to detect or control

6   A 75-year-old female presents to the emergency room (ER) with left flank pain and weakness. She is febrile and hypotensive, which quickly escalates to the need for pressors. She has normal coagulation laboratory test results but does have a history of vascular disease with bilateral renal artery stents, and she takes clopidogrel (Plavix) 75 mg daily. What is the most appropriate treatment plan?

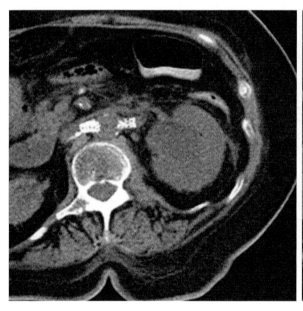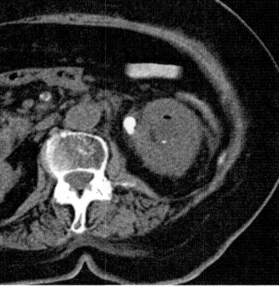

   A. Give intravenous (IV) antibiotics, hold clopidogrel for 5 days, and then place a left PCN catheter
   B. Give IV antibiotics and place a left PCN catheter emergently
   C. Give IV antibiotics and percutaneous placement of a left internal double-J ureteral stent emergently
   D. Give IV antibiotics and reimage in 48 hours; if there is persistent obstruction, place a left PCN catheter and internal double-J ureteral stent

7   A 35-year-old female with malignant distal right ureteral obstruction presents for PCN catheter placement. Which would be the preferred access path (arrows) for tube placement?

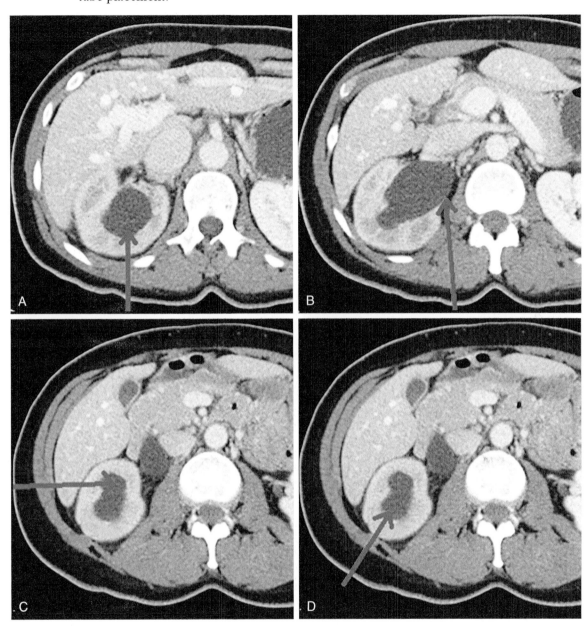

A. A
B. B
C. C
D. D

8   A 63-year-old male undergoes renal transplantation in the right iliac fossa. The
     patient does not make urine in the immediate post-op period. Based on the follow-
     ing images, what is the best explanation for the transplant kidney dysfunction?

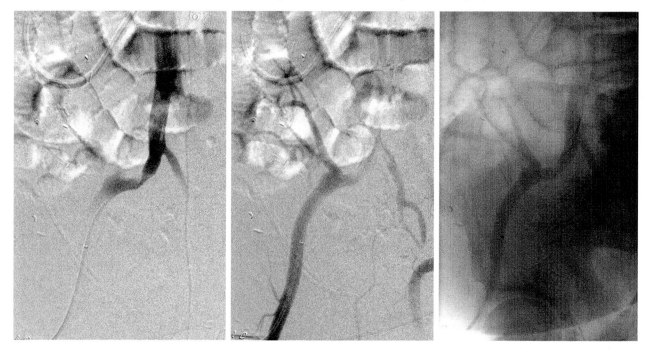

    A. Transplant renal artery thrombosis
    B. External iliac artery stenosis
    C. Transplant renal vein thrombosis
    D. Transplant kidney urinary obstruction

9   Which of the following interventions is most appropriate in this patient with right
     flank pain?

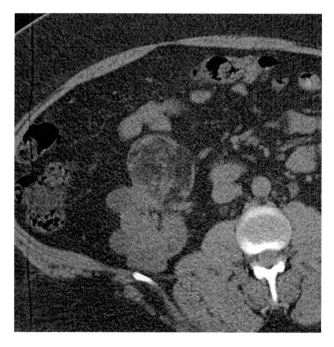

    A. PCN catheter placement
    B. Percutaneous cyst sclerosis
    C. Percutaneous double-J stent placement
    D. Transarterial embolization

10   What is the most commonly used tumor diameter for considering prophylactic embolization of a renal angiomyolipoma (AML)?

A. >2 cm
B. >3 cm
C. >4 cm
D. >5 cm

11   Which of the following scenarios is best suited for percutaneous thermal ablation of a renal cell carcinoma (RCC)?

A. 6 cm solitary tumor
B. Life expectancy of 9 months
C. Underlying von Hippel-Lindau
D. Metastasis confined to the lungs

12   Which of the following is most likely to be found in this kidney transplant recipient?

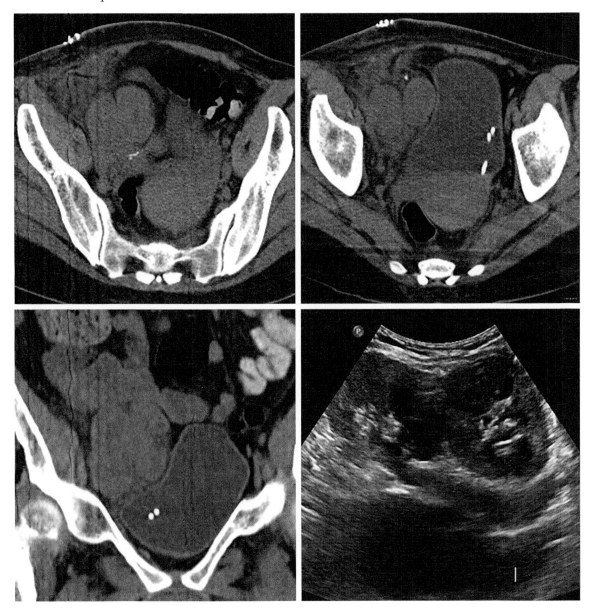

A. Two ureteral stents
B. Transplant renal artery stent
C. PCN catheter
D. Bladder outlet obstruction

13   Which of the following should be avoided if possible when performing PCN access for the purpose of nephrolithotomy?

    A. Access above the 12th rib
    B. Access to a peripheral calyx
    C. Prone positioning of the patient
    D. Upper pole calyceal access

14   This pyelogram is obtained the day following percutaneous nephrolithotomy (PCNL) for a large central stone. Which of the following should be performed next?

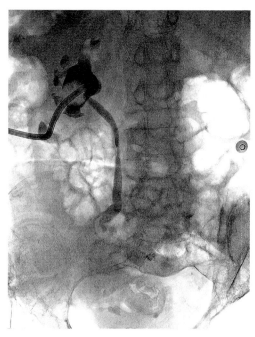

    A. Remove the balloon nephrostomy catheter
    B. Obtain additional fluoroscopic images
    C. Take patient emergently to the operating room (OR)
    D. Renal angiogram with embolization

15   What is the best interpretation of the following computed tomography angiography (CTA) images with respect to the changes in the right kidney?

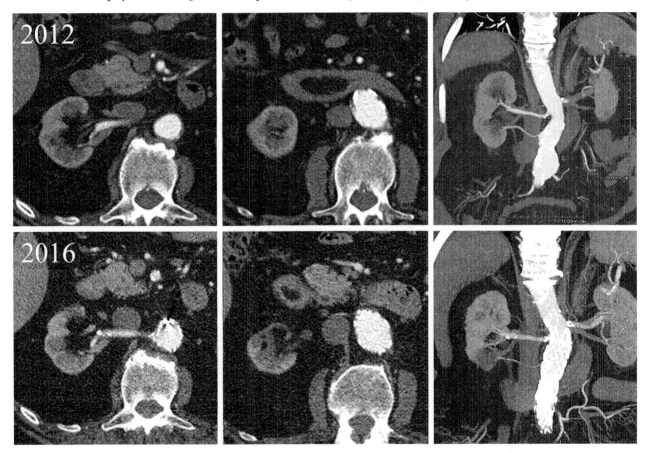

A. Postablation changes
B. Interval growth of angiomyolipoma
C. Traumatic injury
D. Expected changes

16   What is the most likely cause of this transplant kidney ureteral stricture?

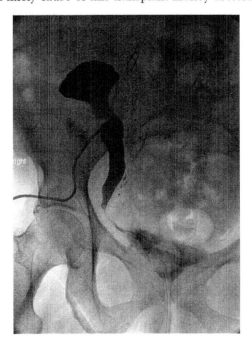

A. Ischemic
B. Infectious
C. Rejection
D. Kinking

17   Which intervention could you offer to this patient with kidney pathology who is a
     surgical candidate?

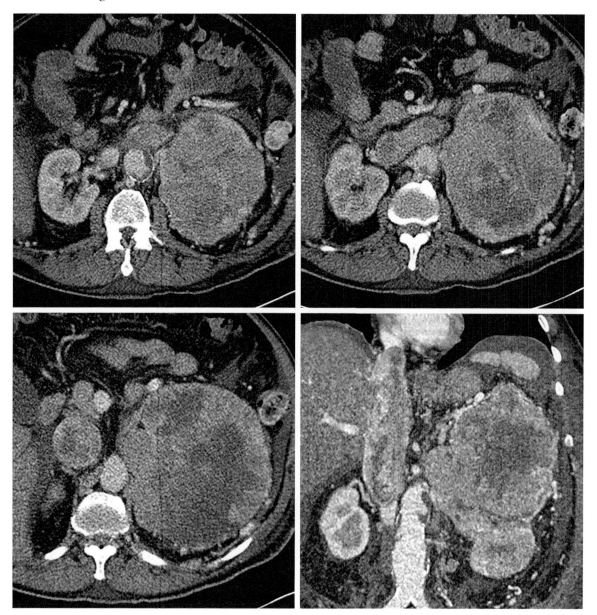

A. Transarterial radioembolization
B. Percutaneous thermal ablation
C. Transarterial alcohol embolization
D. Prophylactic nephrostomy catheter placement

18   Based on these images, what is the most likely underlying pathology?

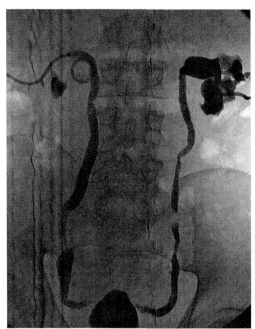 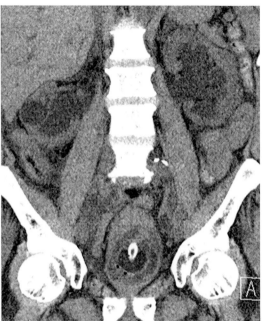

A. Nephrolithiasis
B. Bladder cancer
C. Iatrogenic injury
D. Ureterocolic fistula

19   What is the diameter size threshold for treating this asymptomatic pathology?

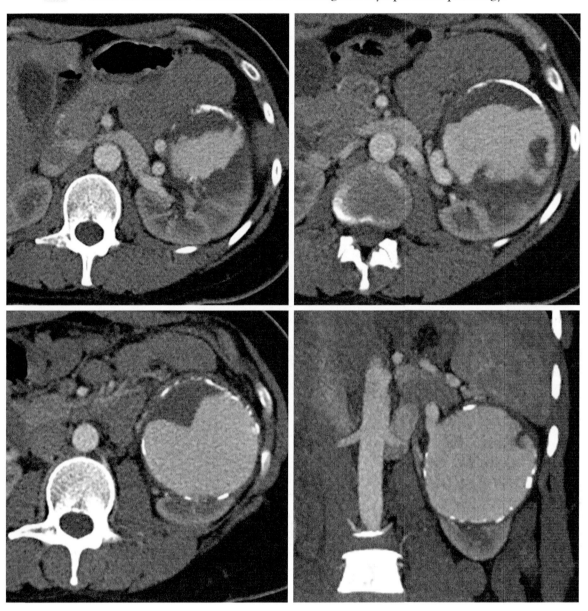

A. >2 cm
B. >3 cm
C. >4 cm
D. No size threshold, only treat if symptomatic

20   An unstable blunt trauma patient is transported directly to the OR for laparotomy. In the OR, there is suspected bleeding from the right kidney and the trauma team requests emergent angiography. Based on the angiographic image, what is the best course of action?

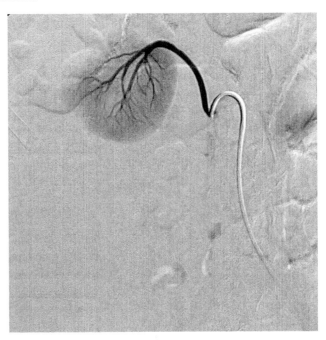

A. Coil embolize the right renal artery
B. No intervention indicated
C. Additional angiography required
D. Return to the OR

21   Which is the most common major complication with percutaneous thermal ablation for RCC?

A. Ureteral injury
B. Nerve damage
C. Hemorrhage
D. Bowel injury
E. Tumor tract seeding

ANSWERS AND EXPLANATIONS

1   **Answer B.**   Embolization of a renal artery or one of its branches is not without consequence as it is an end-organ vessel and some degree of renal parenchyma, and therefore kidney function, will be sacrificed. If there is active bleeding from an intrarenal branch, as this case demonstrates, a microcatheter can be guided as close to the injury as possible, and superselective embolization can be performed such that it infarcts a relatively small amount of kidney parenchyma. Watchful waiting is not appropriate, as there is clearly active bleeding, the patient is hemodynamically unstable, and embolization should at least be attempted. Particles work well in the kidney for tumor embolization, but when there is a focal arterial injury, they offer less control than a coil and risk nontarget embolization through reflux. Surgery should only be entertained if minimally invasive techniques fail.

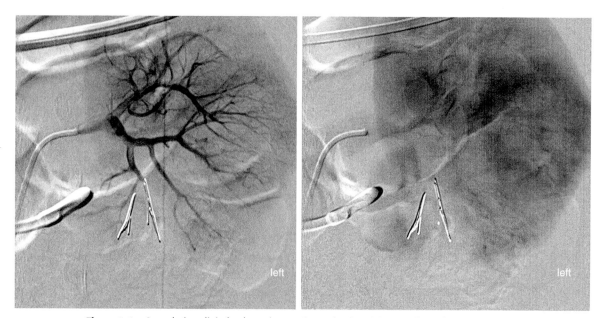

Figure 1-1   Completion digital subtraction angiography (DSA) images from the case example after superselective coil embolization of 2 lower pole renal artery branches that demonstrated active bleeding. Straight, fibered coils were used in this instance, as the injured arteries were quite small in caliber. Note the lack of parenchymal filling corresponding to the embolization territory on the parenchymal phase (right image). This will become a small renal infarct.

References: Schwartz MJ, Smith EB, Trost DW, Vaughan ED. Renal artery embolization: clinical indications and experience from over 100 cases. *BJU Int.* 2007;99(4):881-886.

Tøndel C, Vikse BE, Bostad L, Svarstad E. Safety and complications of percutaneous kidney biopsies in 715 children and 8573 adults in Norway 1988–2010. *Clin J Am Soc Nephrol.* 2012;7(10):1591-1597.

2   **Answer C.**   Hypertension affects 1% to 2% of the pediatric population, with renal artery stenosis as the cause 5% to 25% of the time. The following (Figure 2-1) is an example of a 14-year-old presenting with systolic blood pressure in the 180s for several months despite multiple medications. The lesion was treated with angioplasty alone, and the patient subsequently experienced normalization of the blood pressure. Hydronephrosis, recurrent urinary tract infection, and nephrolithiasis often warrant radiologic workup; however, they are not indications for a catheter arteriogram.

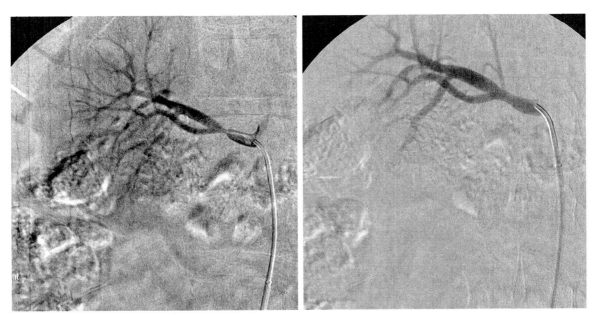

Figure 2-1   Pre (left) and post (right) images from renal artery angioplasty to treat pediatric reno-vascular hypertension. Both main renal artery and branch artery stenoses benefit from angioplasty. Operators have published clinical response treating lesions with as little as 30% luminal narrowing.

References: Srinivasan A, Krishnamurthy G, Fontalvo-herazo L, et al. Angioplasty for renal artery stenosis in pediatric patients: an 11-year retrospective experience. *J Vasc Interv Radiol.* 2010;21(11):1672-1680.

Zhu G, He F, Gu Y, et al. Angioplasty for pediatric renovascular hypertension: a 13-year experience. *Diagn Interv Radiol.* 2014;20(3):285-292.

3   **Answer A.**   In the Western literature, fibromuscular dysplasia is the leading cause of pediatric renal artery stenosis. In the East, Takayasu arteritis is often listed as the most common cause. Neurofibromatosis, midaortic syndrome, and polyarteritis nodosa are less likely causes. Atherosclerosis is virtually absent in the pediatric population.

References: Srinivasan A, Krishnamurthy G, Fontalvo-Herazo L, et al. Angioplasty for renal artery stenosis in pediatric patients: an 11-year retrospective experience. *J Vasc Interv Radiol.* 2010;21(11):1672-1680.

Zhu G, He F, Gu Y, et al. Angioplasty for pediatric renovascular hypertension: a 13-year experience. *Diagn Interv Radiol.* 2014;20(3):285-292.

4   **Answer A.**   This question addresses the basics of urologic intervention. A PCN catheter is a drainage catheter with a distal pigtail that is positioned in the collecting system of the kidney, often the renal pelvis. It functions primarily as an external drainage catheter. When attached to a bag, it relieves distal urinary obstruction but also provides urinary diversion in the setting of a distal leak (as in the case example). An NUS is like a PCN catheter, except that it extends all the way to the bladder. It has proximal (renal pelvis) and distal (bladder) pigtails. It can be attached to a bag for external drainage or capped for internal drainage. It maintains percutaneous access to the kidney, ureter, and bladder. It is often used for stone intervention, in the setting of ureteral injuries or fistulas (to maintain contiguity), or when internal drainage is desired but the patient cannot undergo retrograde procedures. In the case example, an NUS does not offer benefit beyond a PCN and, because of the catheter extending into the bladder, is likely to cause some continued leakage of urine and possibly unnecessary irritation to the underlying vesico-vaginal fistula. A double-J ureteral stent can be placed percutaneously (antegrade approach) or cystoscopically (retrograde approach). It primarily serves to keep

the urine flowing from the kidney to the bladder, and often used in the setting of ureteral obstruction (stone, stenosis) or ureteral leak. As the urine will drain to the bladder, patients should have normal bladder function. In the case example, it provides no benefit to the patient. Ureteral embolization is a procedure that can be performed when permanent ureteral occlusion is desired. Plugs, coils, glue, and other embolics can be deployed in the ureters to completely block urine flow to the distal ureter and/or bladder. A PCN is required to drain the kidney. This is often a procedure of last resort and not appropriate as an initial urinary diversion tactic.

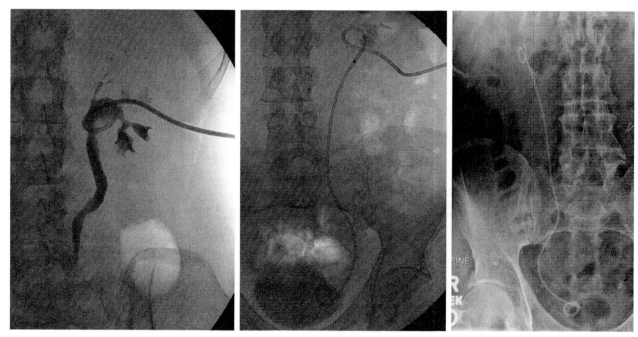

Figure 4-1 Example of a percutaneous nephrostomy (PCN) catheter (left), nephroureteral stent (NUS) (middle), and double-J stent (right).

References: Dagli M, Ramchandani P. Percutaneous nephrostomy: technical aspects and indications. *Semin Intervent Radiol.* 2011;28(4):424-437.

Makramalla A, Zuckerman DA. Nephroureteral stents: principles and techniques. *Semin Intervent Radiol.* 2011;28(4):367-379.

5   **Answer C.** There are guidelines from the Society of Interventional Radiology, which categorize common procedures into 1 of 3 levels of bleeding risk. Based on the assessed risk of bleeding that a procedure carries, operators can then appropriately manage coagulation parameters, antiplatelet and anticoagulation medications in the periprocedural period.

TABLE 5-1   Bleeding Risk for IR Procedures

Category I: *Low-Risk of Bleeding, Easy to Detect or Control*

• Venous access	• Thoracentesis
• Superficial biopsy or drainage	• Routine drain exchange
• Paracentesis	• IVC filter placement

Category II: *Moderate Risk of Bleeding*

• Arterial intervention	• Spine intervention
• Venous intervention	• Transjugular liver biopsy

Category III: *Significant Risk of Bleeding, Difficult to Detect or Control*

• TIPS	• Kidney biopsy
• PTC with drain placement	• PCN catheter placement

Adapted from Patel IJ, Davidson JC, Nikolic B, et al. Consensus guidelines for periprocedural management of coagulation status and hemostasis risk in percutaneous image-guided interventions. *J Vasc Interv Radiol*. 2012;23(6):727-736.
IR, interventional radiology; *IVC*, inferior vena cava; *PCN*, percutaneous nephrostomy; *PTC*, percutaneous transhepatic cholangiography; *TIPS*, transjugular intrahepatic portosystemic shunt.

Memorizing the guideline is not recommended, but a basic concept of level of risk should be known and the guideline frequently referenced when triaging procedures. For the highest risk procedures (Category III), all mitigable risk factors should be addressed; platelets should be greater than 50,000/μL, international normalized ratio (INR) should be <1.5, and all anticoagulation/antiplatelet medications should be held if possible.

Reference: Patel IJ, Davidson JC, Nikolic B, et al. Consensus guidelines for periprocedural management of coagulation status and hemostasis risk in percutaneous image-guided interventions. *J Vasc Interv Radiol*. 2012;23(6):727-736.

6   **Answer B.**   This question is a bit of a reality check to the preceding question. Periprocedural coagulation guidelines are extremely important. Decades of research and numerous consensus meetings have tried to establish best practice. However, guidelines will always be guidelines and must be used in the context of each individual patient. In this example, there is an unstable patient with presumed sepsis, and imaging showing an obstructed left ureter due to a large calcific stone, left hydronephrosis with collecting system, and/or parenchymal gas locules. The patient needs source control. Although the risk of bleeding is higher in the setting of Plavix, the lifesaving benefit to immediate left renal decompression outweighs the risk. A sidenote about Plavix worth knowing: although the binding and disabling of platelets by the drug is irreversible, the half-life is about 6 hours. Therefore, if the drug is held for 24 to 48 hours, the medication will mostly be eliminated and a transfusion of fresh platelets can be expected to function appropriately.

References: Patel IJ, Davidson JC, Nikolic B, et al. Consensus guidelines for periprocedural management of coagulation status and hemostasis risk in percutaneous image-guided interventions. *J Vasc Interv Radiol*. 2012;23(6):727-736.

Thiele T, Sümnig A, Hron G, et al. Platelet transfusion for reversal of dual antiplatelet therapy in patients requiring urgent surgery: a pilot study. *J Thromb Haemost*. 2012;10(5):968-971.

7   **Answer D.**   PCN catheter placement can be performed with a few different techniques, but there are some basic principles regarding the access path to be aware of. As discussed elsewhere, the kidney is a very vascular organ, earning a category III risk for periprocedural risk of bleeding. Best practice is to avoid passing through and subsequently dilating a tract across a large vessel. This can be accomplished by accessing a peripheral calyx, which avoids the large hilar vessels, and targeting the posterolateral kidney where there is a relative avascular zone in the parenchyma (the avascular plane of Brodel). On the patient, the skin entry translates to roughly a full hand breadth lateral from the midline spinous process in the subcostal space. Among the choices, D fits all the criteria for safe percutaneous access. Choice A is medial and intercostal, increasing the risk of pleural transgression. Choice B is medial and direct access to the central renal pelvis without intervening parenchyma. This type of access increases the risk of central vascular injury, collecting system injury, and urinary extravasation. Choice C is anterior and transhepatic, which is unnecessary.

References: Dagli M, Ramchandani P. Percutaneous nephrostomy: technical aspects and indications. *Semin Intervent Radiol.* 2011;28(4):424-437.

Dyer RB, Regan JD, Kavanagh PV, Khatod EG, Chen MY, Zagoria RJ. Percutaneous nephrostomy with extensions of the technique: step by step. *Radiographics.* 2002;22(3):503-525.

8   **Answer B.**   The images show pelvic arteriography, not venography or urography (excluding choices C and D). There is a moderate to severe focal stenosis of the external iliac artery, just proximal to the arterial anastomosis of the transplant kidney. The transplant renal artery appears widely patent. The etiology of the inflow stenosis is not always clear, with a differential including preexisting atherosclerosis or iatrogenic injury during transplantation. In this patient, the inflow lesion was treated with a self-expanding bare-metal stent with good angiographic result and subsequent improvement in kidney function.

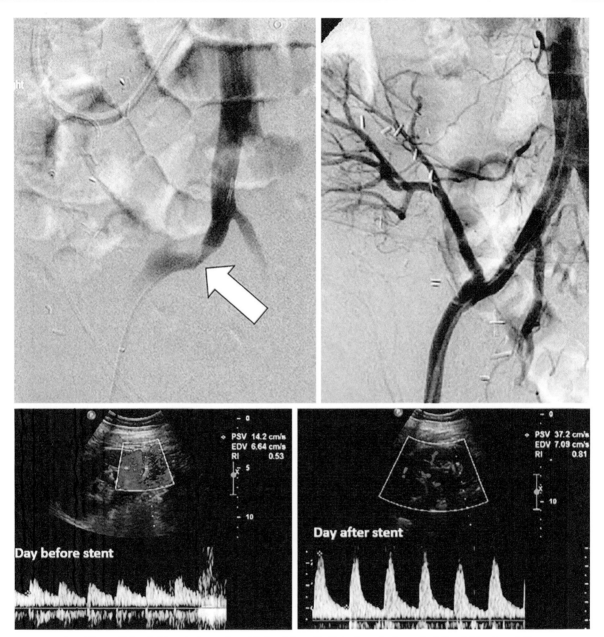

Figure 8-1 Pelvic arteriography with focal flow-limiting stenosis (arrow) of the right external iliac artery as the source of transplant kidney dysfunction. Preprocedural ultrasound shows evolving parvus et tardus waveform, which normalizes after stent placement (right images).

References: Kolli KP, Laberge JM. Interventional management of vascular renal transplant complications. *Tech Vasc Interv Radiol*. 2016;19(3):228-236.

Rajan DK, Stavropoulos SW, Shlansky-Goldberg RD. Management of transplant renal artery stenosis. *Semin Intervent Radiol*. 2004;21(4):259-269.

9   **Answer D.**   There is an exophytic mass arising from the right kidney with macroscopic fat, which is the hallmark of an AML. AML often occurs sporadically (approximately 80% of cases) or may be associated with the phakomatoses, such as tuberous sclerosis (seen here), von Hippel-Lindau, or neurofibromatosis 1. It can also be seen with lymphangioleiomyomatosis (LAM). When these lesions grow to a large size, they can be symptomatic and also carry a risk for significant spontaneous bleeding. Transarterial embolization can be performed to shrink the tumor, which can palliate the symptoms and/or alleviate the risk of bleeding. There is no evidence for obstructive urinary pathology; therefore, choices A and C are incorrect. Although renal cyst sclerosis can be performed, the cysts present are quite small and the dominant pathology is clearly the AML.

References: Kiefer RM, Stavropoulos SW. The role of interventional radiology techniques in the management of renal angiomyolipomas. *Curr Urol Rep.* 2017;18(5):36.

Li D, Pua BB, Madoff DC. Role of embolization in the treatment of renal masses. *Semin Intervent Radiol.* 2014;31(1):70-81.

10   **Answer C.**   As discussed previously, larger renal AMLs carry a risk for spontaneous hemorrhage. In the literature, >4 cm is most commonly used as the threshold for treatment in an asymptomatic patient. Other factors that may be considered are overall degree of vascularity and size of aneurysms within the tumor. Regarding embolization technique, permanent particles or alcohol are the most commonly used agents. At angiography, the appearance can be quite variable, largely depending on the proportion of lipomatous to vascular components. Classically, the tumor will be hypervascular, composed of abnormal tortuous arteries with variably sized aneurysms. Arteriovenous shunting is usually absent.

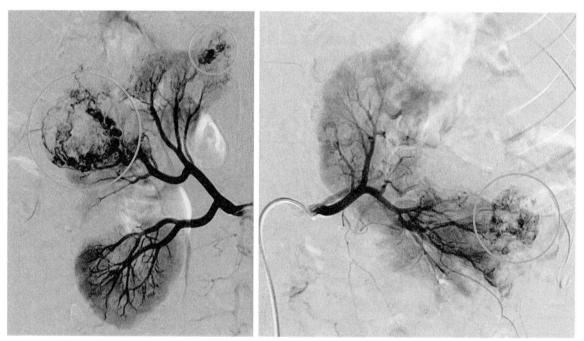

Figure 10-1   Bilateral renal arteriography in a patient with tuberous sclerosis and multiple angiomyolipomas (AMLs) (orange circles).

References: Kiefer RM, Stavropoulos SW. The role of interventional radiology techniques in the management of renal angiomyolipomas. *Curr Urol Rep.* 2017;18(5):36.

Li D, Pua BB, Madoff DC. Role of embolization in the treatment of renal masses. *Semin Intervent Radiol.* 2014;31(1):70-81.

11 **Answer C.**   If a patient has a predisposition to RCC, such as with von Hippel-Lindau, one should strongly consider percutaneous thermal ablation. Partial nephrectomy is a good surgery, but if the patient is expected to have recurrent tumors, the most minimally invasive nephron-sparing technique is ideal. Accepted indications for renal ablation include T1a (≤4 cm) tumors, increased risk of multiple tumors, solitary kidney, or poor surgical candidate. If the life expectancy is poor, the risk of the procedure outweighs the benefit. Metastatic disease is considered a contraindication to local treatment.

References: Higgins IJ, Hong K. Renal ablation techniques: state of the art. *AJR Am J Roentgenol.* 2015;205(4):735-741.

Krokidis ME, Orsi F, Katsanos K, Helmberger T, Adam A. CIRSE guidelines on percutaneous ablation of small renal cell carcinoma. *Cardiovasc Intervent Radiol.* 2017;40(2):177-191.

12 **Answer A.**   The case images demonstrate an en bloc double pediatric kidney transplant. This is not a common procedure and needs to be recognized. Typically, portions of the donor aorta and vena cava are transplanted along with the kidneys and anastomosed to the recipient iliac vessels, leaving the donor renal vessels untouched. As there are 2 separate collecting systems, there will be 2 ureteral stents (choice A) placed at transplantation.

Reference: Brunner MC, Matalon TA, Patel SK, Siliunas DA, Mcdonald V, Merkel FK. Percutaneous interventions in adults receiving pediatric "en bloc" double renal grafts. *Cardiovasc Intervent Radiol.* 1995;18(5):291-295.

13 **Answer A.**   The most commonly injured juxtarenal structures when accessing the collecting system of the kidney are the diaphragm and the pleura. Studies have shown rates of pleural transgression at the 11th intercostal space of 29% on the right and 14% on the left. This becomes even more important for PCNL access as the tract may subsequently be dilated up to 30 Fr (1 cm). Reported rates of pleural complications from nephrostomy access alone range from 0.1% to 0.6%, whereas in the setting of PCNL, it can be as high as 12%. During PCNL, intercostal approach transpleural access can result in irrigant pleural fluid accumulation, pneumothorax, hemothorax, pulmonary infection, and nephropleural fistula. It should be noted that the intercostal approach is not contraindicated; in fact, it is frequently used. However, operators should not necessarily choose this access path unless necessary for the stone intervention.

The remaining choices are all appropriate for PCN access for the purpose of PCNL. Peripheral calyceal access is desired, as less kidney parenchyma is transgressed and the operator can have greater instrument flexibility during stone removal. Prone or semiprone positioning is required to perform PCNL access, given the anatomic location of the kidneys. Lateral decubitus position can also be used; however, hyperinflation of the nondependent lung will occur, increasing the risk of pneumothorax. Upper pole calyceal access may be desired depending on the orientation of the kidney, collecting system, and/or position of the target stones. Both rigid and flexible instruments are used during PCNL, and the ideal access facilitates their use.

References: Dagli M, Ramchandani P. Percutaneous nephrostomy: technical aspects and indications. *Semin Intervent Radiol.* 2011;28(4):424-437.

Lee WJ, Smith AD, Cubelli V, et al. Complications of percutaneous nephrolithotomy. *AJR Am J Roentgenol.* 1987;148(1):177-180.

Pabon-ramos WM, Dariushnia SR, Walker TG, et al. Quality improvement guidelines for percutaneous nephrostomy. *J Vasc Interv Radiol.* 2016;27(3):410-414.

Springer RM. Planning and execution of access for percutaneous renal stone removal in a community hospital setting. *Semin Intervent Radiol.* 2015;32(3):311-322.

14   **Answer B.**   After PCNL, a common practice is to leave a PCN catheter in place, which tamponades the PCNL tract, drains the kidney, and maintains access to the kidney for subsequent urography and intervention if needed. When performing post-PCNL urography, interpreting physicians should identify residual stones, urinary obstruction, and urinary extravasation. Complete evaluation of the collecting system down to the bladder is performed. One must ensure that contrast progresses fully into the bladder, a concept sometimes missed by trainees focused on the intrarenal portion of the collection system. For the patient in the case example, additional imaging identified a complete distal ureteral obstruction from residual stones or clot. Either a PCN catheter should remain in place or double-J ureteral stent should be placed to ensure adequate drainage.

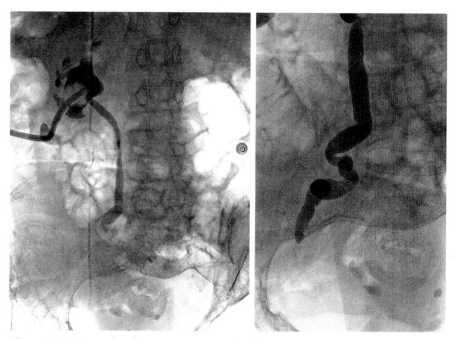

Figure 14-1   Urography after percutaneous nephrolithotomy (PCNL) with distal ureteral obstruction due to residual stones. Had the nephrostomy access been removed based on the initial image, the patient would have been left with untreated urinary obstruction.

References: Michel MS, Trojan L, Rassweiler JJ. Complications in percutaneous nephrolithotomy. *Eur Urol.* 2007;51(4):899-906.

Springer RM. Planning and execution of access for percutaneous renal stone removal in a community hospital setting. *Semin Intervent Radiol.* 2015;32(3):311-322.

15   **Answer D.**   To understand the change in appearance of the right kidney, one must recognize the patient has undergone interval endovascular aneurysm repair (EVAR) in the setting of 2 right renal arteries. After EVAR, the smaller and more caudally positioned accessory renal artery is clearly covered by the stent graft and demonstrates a diminutive appearance. As expected, the lower pole of the right kidney became ischemic resulting in corticomedullary atrophy and increased prominence of the renal sinus fat. Postablation changes, remote traumatic injury, or an underlying AML may appear similar; however, the constellation of findings best supports choice D.

Reference: Picel AC, Kansal N. Essentials of endovascular abdominal aortic aneurysm repair imaging: postprocedure surveillance and complications. *AJR Am J Roentgenol.* 2014;203(4):W358-W372.

16 **Answer A.**   PCN catheter placement in a transplant kidney is often performed for obstruction due to a ureteral stenosis. Published rates of transplant kidney ureteral stenosis formation range between 2% and 10%. Ischemia accounts for 90% of cases and is typically found at the ureterovesicular end. This is due to the vulnerable blood supply of the ureter the further from the renal artery. Other causes such as rejection, kinking, and extrinsic compression are less common. Treatment options include surgical revision, stenting, and/or ureteroplasty.

References: Dagli M, Ramchandani P. Percutaneous nephrostomy: technical aspects and indications. *Semin Intervent Radiol*. 2011;28(4):424-437.

Sandhu C, Patel U. Renal transplantation dysfunction: the role of interventional radiology. *Clin Radiol*. 2002;57(9):772-783.

17 **Answer C.**   Demonstrated on the images is a large hypervascular tumor arising from the left kidney consistent with primary renal malignancy. Currently, radio-embolization has an extremely limited role in the treatment of renal cancer and is mainly palliative in intent. Percutaneous thermal ablation is recommended for T1a lesions (≤4 cm) and, at some centers, is performed on larger lesions. This tumor is clearly >4 cm in size and at least T3 in staging, as this tumor grows into the left renal vein and IVC and ablation is not appropriate. Surgical resection is the treatment of choice. There is no role for prophylactic PCN catheter placement in an unobstructed kidney, and the procedure would incur additional risk of bleeding from the tumor replaced kidney. For surgical candidates, preoperative embolization, often performed with alcohol and/or embolic particles, can be performed to devascularize the tumor and kidney, aiding in resection and reducing operative blood loss. Some research has also shown improved long-term survival with prenephrectomy embolization when compared with resection alone.

References: Bakal CW, Cynamon J, Lakritz PS, Sprayregen S. Value of preoperative renal artery embolization in reducing blood transfusion requirements during nephrectomy for renal cell carcinoma. *J Vasc Interv Radiol*. 1993;4(6):727-731.

Sauk S, Zuckerman DA. Renal artery embolization. *Semin Intervent Radiol*. 2011;28(4):396-406.

Zielinski H, Szmigielski S, Petrovich Z. Comparison of preoperative embolization followed by radical nephrectomy with radical nephrectomy alone for renal cell carcinoma. *Am J Clin Oncol*. 2000;23(1):6-12.

18 **Answer B.**   When performing nephrostograms, it is important to not only evaluate tube positioning but study the entire urinary pathway. The urogram shows bilateral ureteral obstruction. The points of obstruction demonstrate cupped margins with dilation of the ureter above and below. This appearance is characteristic of chronic obstruction due to underlying intraluminal mass, most commonly transitional cell carcinoma. The patient also has a Foley catheter to treat bladder outlet obstruction (note the thickened bladder wall). The constellation of findings supports a diagnosis of underlying transitional cell cancer of the bladder with synchronous ureteral involvement. Transitional cell carcinoma arises from the bladder 90% of the time, and synchronous and/or metachronous upper tract lesions are found in up to 6% of patients.

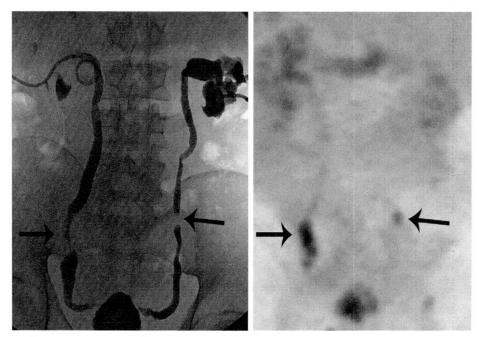

Figure 18-1   Corresponding maximum intensity projection (MIP) image from F-18 fludeoxyglucose positron emission tomography (FDG PET) shows focal tracer activity in the ureters corresponding to the strictures seen on urography (arrows).

References: Wong-you-Cheong JJ, Wagner BJ, Davis CJ. Transitional cell carcinoma of the urinary tract: radiologic-pathologic correlation. *Radiographics*. 1998;18(1):123-142.

Yousem DM, Gatewood OM, Goldman SM, Marshall FF. Synchronous and metachronous transitional cell carcinoma of the urinary tract: prevalence, incidence, and radiographic detection. *Radiology*. 1988;167(3):613-618.

19   **Answer A.**   The images demonstrate an avidly enhancing round lesion arising from the left kidney with peripherally calcified walls and mural thrombus. There is an enlarged feeding artery. This is a renal artery aneurysm. This particular lesion is atypical because of its large size (>8 cm in diameter); renal aneurysms are often <2 cm and discovered incidentally on imaging for some other reason. The most often quoted guideline for treatment in an asymptomatic patient is >2 cm in diameter (choice A). There admittedly is some degree of controversy here, as the natural course of these lesions is unclear; therefore, the risk of rupture is not fully known. Treatment options are surgical or endovascular. Renal artery aneurysms should also be treated when symptomatic or when they occur in women who are pregnant or of childbearing age.

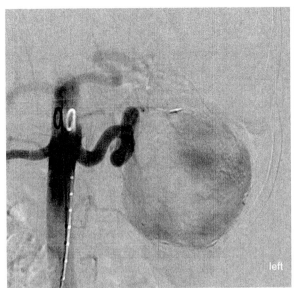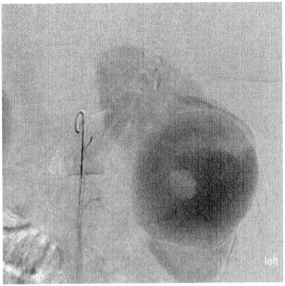

Figure 19-1 Aortography shows left renal artery aneurysm measuring >8 cm. The feeding artery was selected and occluded with a vascular plug. The aneurysm arose from a branch of the main renal artery, and virtually all of the kidney parenchyma was spared during the embolization.

References: Henke PK, Cardneau JD, Welling TH, et al. Renal artery aneurysms: a 35-year clinical experience with 252 aneurysms in 168 patients. *Ann Surg.* 2001;234(4):454-462.

Klausner JQ, Harlander-locke MP, Plotnik AN, Lehrman E, Derubertis BG, Lawrence PF. Current treatment of renal artery aneurysms may be too aggressive. *J Vasc Surg.* 2014;59(5):1356-1361.

20 **Answer C.** The images demonstrate selective catheterization of the right renal artery with angiography. What must be recognized is that only ⅓ of the expected kidney parenchyma is opacified with contrast. With or without prior cross-sectional imaging, one must be on guard for variant vascular anatomy. Duplicated/multiple renal arteries are fairly common, with reported incidence as high as 30%. If there is any doubt, a flush catheter aortogram can be performed to reveal additional arteries. In the case example, the upper pole artery was interrogated and angiography identified brisk active extravasation.

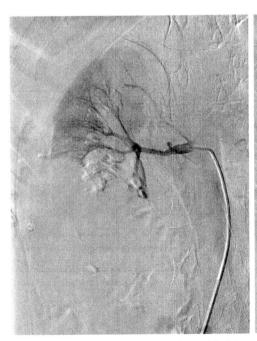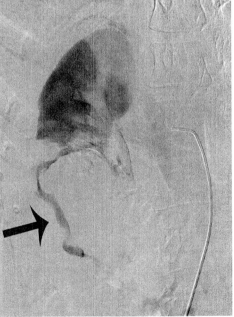

Figure 20-1 Blunt trauma patient with right renal angiogram demonstrating perfusion to the upper ⅔ of the right kidney and large laceration and active bleeding (arrow). A superselective coil embolization was performed.

References: Al-katib S, Shetty M, Jafri SM, Jafri SZ. Radiologic assessment of native renal vasculature: a multimodality review. *Radiographics*. 2017;37(1):136-156.

Ramaswamy RS, Darcy MD. Arterial embolization for the treatment of renal masses and traumatic renal injuries. *Tech Vasc Interv Radiol*. 2016;19(3):203-210.

21   **Answer C.**   The major complication rate for percutaneous thermal ablation of renal malignancies is between 3% and 7%. All of the provided answer choices have been reported, and a critical look at a sample case image reveals why.

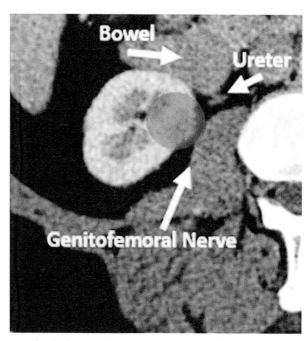

Figure 21-1   Example of a lower pole renal cell carcinoma (red shade) with location of adjacent bowel, ureter, and nerve identified by the arrows.

Renal tumors (especially those located in the medial lower pole) can be in close proximity to the ureter, bowel, and major nerves that travel along the periphery of the psoas muscle. When faced with potential nontarget thermal injury, adjunctive techniques such as hydrodissection can be used to displace adjacent structures away from the ablation zone. For protection of the collecting system and ureter, a stent can be placed preprocedurally and pyeloperfusion can be performed during the ablation (cool saline for heat ablation and warm saline for cryoablation). Although any of these complications can occur, major bleeding is the most common. Bleeding may be less common when using radiofrequency ablation (RFA) compared with cryoablation, which is attributed to coagulative effects. Tumor tract seeding, although reported and feared, is very uncommon and described in fewer than 1% of cases.

References: Atwell TD, Schmit GD, Boorjian SA, et al. Percutaneous ablation of renal masses measuring 3.0 cm and smaller: comparative local control and complications after radiofrequency ablation and cryoablation. *AJR Am J Roentgenol*. 2013;200(2):461-466.

Kim KR, Thomas S. Complications of image-guided thermal ablation of liver and kidney neoplasms. *Semin Intervent Radiol*. 2014;31(2):138-148.

Kurup AN. Percutaneous ablation for small renal masses-complications. *Semin Intervent Radiol*. 2014;31(1):42-49.

7

Reproductive Endocrine

1   A 20-year-old male with a varicocele detected on physical examination presents for evaluation. What side is most likely affected?

   A. Right
   B. Left
   C. Bilateral

2   Which is an indication for varicocele embolization?

   A. Priapism
   B. Testicular enlargement
   C. Pain
   D. Erectile dysfunction

3   As part of an embolization procedure to treat a symptomatic left varicocele, the left renal vein is catheterized. Which provocative maneuver during venography will help identify the pathologic gonadal vein?

   A. Valsalva
   B. Trendelenburg
   C. Deep inspiration
   D. Vasopressin infusion

4   At what level should the catheter be positioned to begin gonadal vein coil embolization to treat a left varicocele?

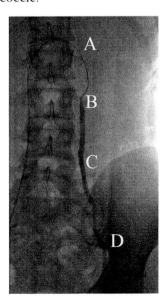

A. A
B. B
C. C
D. D

5   Which is an appropriate indication to sample this vein?

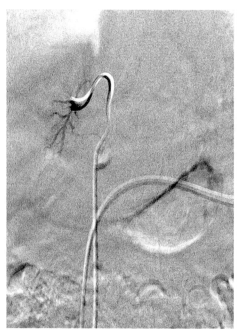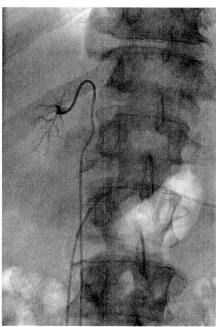

A. Chronic kidney disease
B. Hyperaldosteronism
C. Hypoglycemia
D. Transaminitis

6   Which clinical history most supports a diagnosis of high-flow priapism?

A. Overdose of phosphodiesterase type 5 (PDE5) inhibitor such as Viagra
B. Underlying sickle cell disease
C. Traumatic injury to the pelvis
D. Long-standing tobacco use

7   What is the role of interventional radiology (IR) for patients with priapism?

A. Diagnostic angiography only; embolization is contraindicated
B. Can therapeutically embolize high-flow pathology
C. No longer necessary with high-quality diagnostic ultrasound

8   Which of the following is an appropriate indication for embolization of the selected vessel?

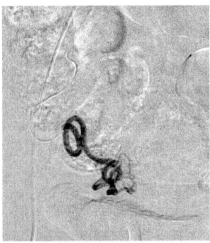
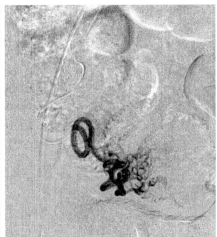
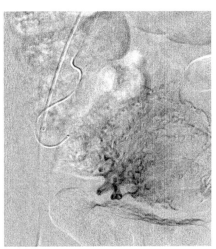
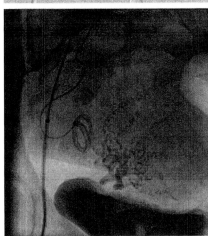

    A. Prolonged menstrual bleeding
    B. Refractory hemorrhoidal bleeding
    C. Benign prostatic hypertrophy
    D. Hemorrhagic cystitis

9   What is the most common method of embolization for symptomatic uterine fibroids?

    A. Bilateral uterine artery with particles
    B. Unilateral dominant uterine artery with particles
    C. Bilateral uterine artery with coils
    D. Unilateral dominant uterine artery with coils

10   Which of the following is the most likely reason for treatment failure after bilateral uterine artery embolization (UAE) for symptomatic fibroids?

    A. Embolization with permanent particles
    B. Misidentification of the uterine artery during the embolization
    C. Submucosal location of the fibroid
    D. Gonadal (ovarian) artery supply to the fibroids

11   Which of the following is an absolute contraindication for UAE for symptomatic fibroids?

    A. Infectious endometritis
    B. 10 cm pedunculated subserosal fibroid
    C. 3 cm intracavitary fibroid
    D. Desire for future pregnancies

12   A 46-year-old female is treated with bilateral UAE for symptomatic fibroids. Which of the following is the most likely complication after the procedure?

    A. Vesicouterine fistula
    B. Nontarget embolization with tissue ischemia
    C. Septicemia
    D. Permanent amenorrhea

13   A 43-year-old female reports years of pelvic fullness and heaviness, worse at the end of the day. To evaluate for pelvic venous congestion, which of the following is considered the gold standard for diagnosis?

    A. Magnetic resonance (MR) venogram
    B. Computed tomographic (CT) venogram
    C. Tagged red blood cell (RBC) scintigraphy
    D. Catheter venogram

14   Which of the following is a possible sequela of pelvic congestion syndrome?

    A. Development of lower extremity varicose veins
    B. Increased risk of deep vein thrombosis (DVT)
    C. Increased risk of colonic diverticular bleeding
    D. Development of portal hypertension

15   In which obstetric situation would predelivery placement of internal iliac artery (IIA) balloon occlusion catheters be indicated?

    A. Placental abruption
    B. Placenta percreta
    C. Vaginal birth after cesarean section (VBAC)
    D. Oligohydramnios

16   A 47-year-old patient presents for thyroid ultrasound to evaluate a left lobe nodule incidentally detected on a chest CT. Which is the appropriate next step?

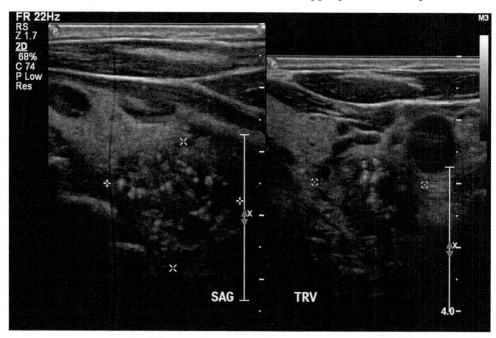

A. Follow-up ultrasound
B. Fine needle aspiration (FNA) biopsy if ≥1.0 cm
C. FNA biopsy if ≥1.5 cm
D. Benign nodule, no further follow-up

17   How should this image be interpreted?

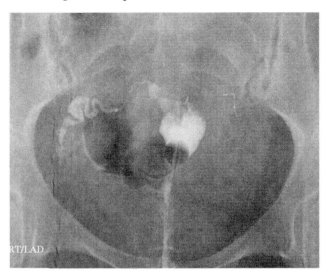

A. Complete sterility confirmed
B. Incomplete sterility confirmed
C. Variant anatomy
D. Inadequate study

ANSWERS AND EXPLANATIONS

1 **Answer B.**   Varicoceles are dilated veins of the pampiniform plexus and arise secondary to dysfunction of the renospermatic venous system. They can be primary (valvular incompetence or absence) or secondary (tumor compression, inferior vena cava [IVC] obstruction). Left-sided varicocele is most commonly found on physical examination. Bilateral and right-sided varicoceles are much less common on physical examination; however, when patients are evaluated with venography and/or duplex ultrasound, the incidence of bilateral pathology increases. Rapid development of large bilateral varicoceles and isolated right varicocele should prompt evaluation for secondary causes such as retroperitoneal tumor.

References: Baigorri BF, Dixon RG. Varicocele: a review. *Semin Intervent Radiol*. 2016;33(3):170-176.

Iaccarino V, Venetucci P. Interventional radiology of male varicocele: current status. *Cardiovasc Intervent Radiol*. 2012;35(6):1263-1280.

2 **Answer C.**   Accepted indications for varicocele embolization are symptomatic (painful) varicocele, massive varicoceles that impair quality of life, and varicocele in the setting of sub-/infertility. Testicular atrophy can occur with varicocele in adolescent males, representing another indication for treatment. Priapism is a painful erection unrelated to gonadal vein pathology. Erectile dysfunction often arises from penile arterial insufficiency, particularly in elderly males.

References: Baigorri BF, Dixon RG. Varicocele: a review. *Semin Intervent Radiol*. 2016;33(3):170-176.

Iaccarino V, Venetucci P. Interventional radiology of male varicocele: current status. *Cardiovasc Intervent Radiol*. 2012;35(6):1263-1280.

3 **Answer A.**   Valsalva maneuver raises intrathoracic pressure, impeding venous return to the right-sided heart. This transmits increased venous pressure upstream to the IVC and subsequently the left renal vein, eliciting reflux of contrast in the pathologic gonadal vein and improving visualization. Once the gonadal vein is selected with a catheter, additional venograms with Valsalva are performed to evaluate the anatomy and entire course of the vein. Trendelenburg or head-down position improves right-sided heart return by raising the abdomen, pelvis, and lower extremities above the level of the right atrium. Similarly, deep inspiration lowers intrathoracic pressure improving right-sided heart venous return. Both maneuvers are not likely to improve visualization of the gonadal vein.

References: Baigorri BF, Dixon RG. Varicocele: a review. *Semin Intervent Radiol*. 2016;33(3):170-176.

Iaccarino V, Venetucci P. Interventional radiology of male varicocele: current status. *Cardiovasc Intervent Radiol*. 2012;35(6):1263-1280.

4 **Answer D.**   Gonadal vein embolization should begin at or just above the level of the inguinal ligament to occlude the anterior pampiniform plexus and/or draining gonadal vein. Interventionalists commonly use agents such as coils, plugs, glue, and chemical sclerosants to occlude the target vein(s). Care must be taken not to embolize much below the inguinal ligament, as a painful thrombophlebitis can occur within the scrotum. Embolization too proximal (choices A, B, and C) can lead to recurrence, as parallel and collateral venous pathways can refill the varicocele through the patent lower segment of the gonadal vein.

References: Bittles MA, Hoffer EK. Gonadal vein embolization: treatment of varicocele and pelvic congestion syndrome. *Semin Intervent Radiol*. 2008;25(3):261-270.

Iaccarino V, Venetucci P. Interventional radiology of male varicocele: current status. *Cardiovasc Intervent Radiol*. 2012;35(6):1263-1280.

5 **Answer B.**   The vein selected and sampled must be identified to answer this question. The location is subphrenic, just right of midline, at the thoracolumbar junction. The size of the opacified venous bed is fairly small. The location is cranial

to that expected for the right renal vein. This is an example of right adrenal venography. There is variable appearance of the venous bed, and it can at times be quite challenging to select the vein ostium with a catheter. The procedure is performed to investigate the cause of primary hyperaldosteronism. In the setting of primary hyperaldosteronism, up to 62.5% of patients have a potentially resectable adrenal adenoma as the etiology. Others will have bilateral hyperplasia which is managed medically. Adrenal venous sampling is the gold standard to distinguish these 2 etiologies. Once the right and left adrenal veins are successfully sampled, the aldosterone and cortisol levels are measured. The aldosterone:cortisol ratio (AC ratio) for each kidney is calculated and then compared, known as the lateralization index. An abnormal lateralization index is >2, although some use >4.

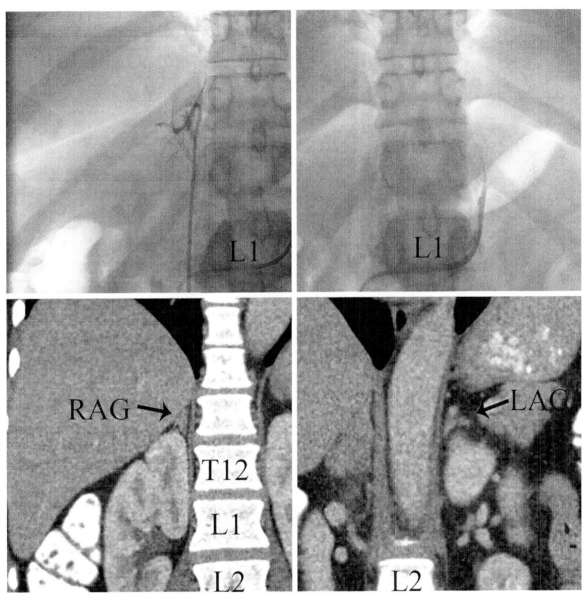

Figure 5-1 Adrenal venous sampling with computed tomography (CT) correlation. The right adrenal gland (RAG) most often drains directly to the inferior vena cava (IVC), with the vein ostium laterally or posterolaterally. The vein can sometimes be identified on CT. Note the RAG on coronal CT image corresponds in position and appearance to the selective venogram. The left adrenal gland (LAG) most often drains via the vertically oriented phrenicoadrenal venous trunk, which empties in the left renal vein. The phrenicoadrenal trunk is easily selected with a reverse curve catheter for sampling. Anatomic variants do exist, and those who perform this procedure need to be familiar with them to ensure successful sampling. T12, L1, L2; vertebral body levels.

A companion case demonstrates the evaluation of a female with hirsutism and amenorrhea, elevated peripheral venous testosterone level, and no evidence of pathology on imaging. Potential sites of abnormal androgen production include the adrenal glands and the ovaries. Therefore, a total of 4 veins were sampled for her, to include the bilateral gonadal and adrenal veins. Venous sampling revealed markedly elevated testosterone level from the left gonadal vein. After laparoscopic left oophorectomy, a Leydig cell tumor was found on pathology. Testosterone levels normalized, and her regular menses returned soon after.

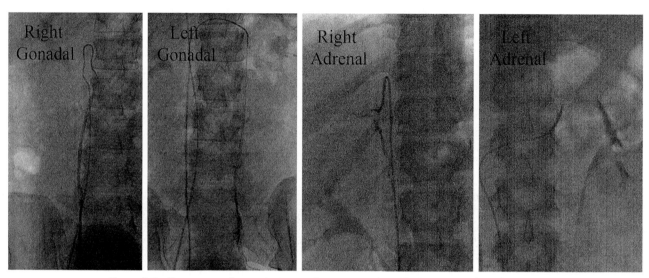

Figure 5-2 Venous sampling to detect occult testosterone-producing tumor. The right gonadal vein drains directly into the inferior vena cava (IVC) and uncommonly (~10%) into the right renal vein. The left gonadal vein drains into the left renal vein.

References: Barber B, Horton A, Patel U. Anatomy of the origin of the gonadal veins on CT. *J Vasc Interv Radiol*. 2012;23(2):211-215.

Kahn SL, Angle JF. Adrenal vein sampling. *Tech Vasc Interv Radiol*. 2010;13(2):110-125

Levens ED, Whitcomb BW, Csokmay JM, Nieman LK. Selective venous sampling for androgen-producing ovarian pathology. *Clin Endocrinol (Oxf)*. 2009;70(4):606-614.

Rossi GP. Update in adrenal venous sampling for primary aldosteronism. *Curr Opin Endocrinol Diabetes Obes*. 2018;25(3):160-171.

6   Answer C.   Priapism is categorized as low flow or high flow. Low-flow priapism, also termed ischemic, is typically painful and due to inadequate outflow of blood from the corpora cavernosa. Causes of low-flow priapism include blood dyscrasias such as sickle cell disease or medication toxicity but often are found to be idiopathic. High-flow priapism occurs when there is an acquired arteriovenous fistula between the cavernosal artery and adjacent venous sinusoids. This causes an erection; however, as blood outflow is not impaired, it is typically painless and strictly speaking is not an emergency. The most common cause of high-flow priapism is prior trauma. Choice B, sickle cell disease, is associated with low-flow priapism. Overdose of PDE5 inhibitor typically presents as hypotension and would not cause high-flow priapism. Interestingly, PDE5 inhibitors may actually help in some types of low-flow priapism.

References: Kim KR. Embolization treatment of high-flow priapism. *Semin Intervent Radiol*. 2016;33(3):177-181.

Montague DK, Jarow J, Broderick GA, et al. American Urological Association guideline on the management of priapism. *J Urol*. 2003;170(4 Pt 1):1318-1324.

7   Answer B.   As discussed previously, priapism is often grouped into low-flow and high-flow types. Differentiation is accomplished by evaluating the history, symptoms, duplex ultrasound, and/or gas analysis of penile blood aspirate. IR can play an important role in the treatment of high-flow priapism. Although not a common procedure, embolization of the offending arteriovenous fistula can be performed as a therapeutic intervention. Temporary agents such as Gelfoam or autologous blood clot are preferred for embolization. Permanent agents have also been used, but may increase the long term risk of erectile dysfunction.

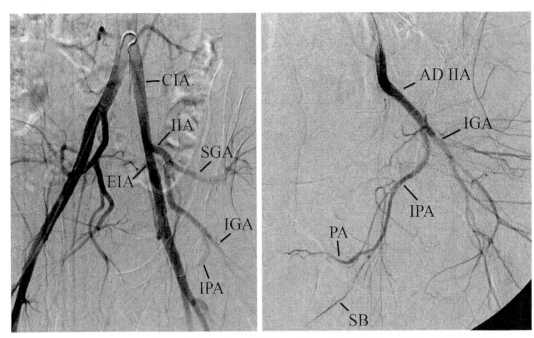

Figure 7-1   Images from pelvic arteriography in a patient with high-flow priapism. Digital subtraction angiography (DSA) images in left anterior oblique (LAO) projection demonstrate the branching of the internal iliac artery (IIA) into anterior and posterior divisions. The main posterior division branch is the superior gluteal artery (SGA). The anterior division gives off several branches, with the internal pudendal artery (IPA) of primary interest in this case. *AD IIA*, anterior division internal iliac artery; *CIA*, common iliac artery; *EIA*, external iliac artery; *IGA*, inferior gluteal artery; *PA*, penile artery; *SB*, scrotal branch.

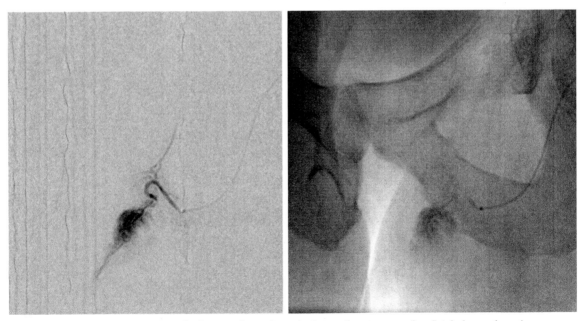

Figure 7-2   Angiography from a microcatheter in the penile artery reveals a fistula from a branch artery to the adjacent corpora sinusoids as the source of high-flow priapism. The fistula was closed with Gel-Bead embolization.

References: Kim KR. Embolization treatment of high-flow priapism. *Semin Intervent Radiol.* 2016;33(3):177-181.

Montague DK, Jarow J, Broderick GA, et al. American Urological Association guideline on the management of priapism. *J Urol.* 2003;170(4 Pt 1):1318-1324.

8 **Answer A.**   The vessel selected and opacified is the right uterine artery. UAE is most commonly performed for symptomatic uterine fibroids, which classically present with menorrhagia (choice A), metrorrhagia, pelvic pressure, pelvic pain, constipation, and/or difficulty with urination. The procedure enjoys high clinical success, with roughly 90% of patients experiencing reduction in bulk symptoms, and >90% experiencing elimination of abnormal uterine bleeding. UAE can also be used to treat symptomatic adenomyosis, vascular lesions of the uterus, postpartum hemorrhage, and bleeding uterine/cervical tumors. Regarding the other choices, hemorrhoidal bleeding can be treated with embolization, but this is done via the superior hemorrhoidal artery (branch of the inferior mesenteric artery) and/or from the middle/inferior hemorrhoidal arteries (branches of the anterior division of the IIA). The contrast-filled bladder caudal to the opacified arterial bed confirms that the vascular structure is not bladder or prostate.

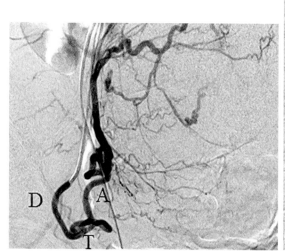
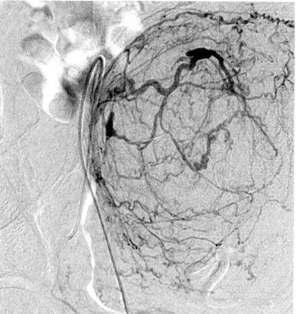

Figure 8-1 Digital subtraction angiography (DSA) images from right uterine artery embolization (UAE) for symptomatic fibroids showing classic uterine artery anatomy on the right with descending (D), transverse (T), and ascending (A) arterial segments. Typically, embolization is performed from the transverse segment, beyond the cervicovaginal branch. Late arterial phase image on the right shows extensive arterial network of the uterus with round mass becoming apparent because of underlying fibroid.

References: Dariushnia SR, Nikolic B, Stokes LS, Spies JB. Quality improvement guidelines for uterine artery embolization for symptomatic leiomyomata. *J Vasc Interv Radiol.* 2014;25(11):1737-1747.

Keung JJ, Spies JB, Caridi TM. Uterine artery embolization: a review of current concepts. *Best Pract Res Clin Obstet Gynaecol.* 2018;46:66-73.

Kohi MP, Spies JB. Updates on uterine artery embolization. *Semin Intervent Radiol.* 2018;35(1):48-55.

9   **Answer A.**   There is significant "cross talk" or collateralization between the right and left uterine arteries. This necessitates that both arteries are embolized; otherwise, the remaining patent uterine artery will continue to perfuse the fibroid(s) resulting in treatment failure. Rarely, the sole blood supply to a fibroid is a single uterine artery, in which case, unilateral embolization is appropriate. Regarding the best embolic agent, permanent particles are most commonly used, with trisacryl gelatin microspheres (TAGM) and polyvinyl alcohol (PVA) being well studied and demonstrating good efficacy. These embolics allow for distal penetration and optimal end-organ ischemia when sized appropriately. If coils are used, the site of arterial occlusion would be in the proximal portion of the uterine artery, effectively allowing for continued blood supply to the fibroid(s) via collaterals. Additionally, proximal occlusion with coils would eliminate the pathway for repeat embolization if needed.

References: Dariushnia SR, Nikolic B, Stokes LS, Spies JB. Quality improvement guidelines for uterine artery embolization for symptomatic leiomyomata. *J Vasc Interv Radiol.* 2014;25(11):1737-1747.

Keung JJ, Spies JB, Caridi TM. Uterine artery embolization: a review of current concepts. *Best Pract Res Clin Obstet Gynaecol.* 2018;46:66-73.

Kohi MP, Spies JB. Updates on uterine artery embolization. *Semin Intervent Radiol.* 2018;35(1):48-55.

10   **Answer D.**   In the setting of fibroids, the uterine artery is usually easy to identify based on its anatomical origin, typical course, tortuosity, and hypertrophy. Misidentification is virtually unseen (choice B incorrect). Technical success of uterine artery identification, selection, and embolization is >95%, and permanent particles are the embolic of choice (choice A incorrect). Virtually all submucosal, intramural, and subserosal fibroids can be successfully treated with UAE (choice C incorrect). Fibroid anatomy remains an important consideration in patient evaluation, however, as location should correlate with the patient's presenting symptoms. Although uncommon, a known mode of failure for UAE is the presence of partial or complete fibroid collateralization from the gonadal (ovarian) artery. After UAE, an untreated gonadal artery can provide blood supply and viability to the fibroid(s). As embolization of the gonadal artery may carry some risk of premature ovarian failure, it is not routinely embolized with the initial procedure unless it is the sole blood supply to the target fibroids. If there is clinical failure after initial bilateral UAE, embolization of the gonadal artery is then considered after the appropriate discussion of risks and benefits with the patient. The following is an example of an enlarged tortuous gonadal artery perfusing fibroids, which was identified after initial bilateral UAE.

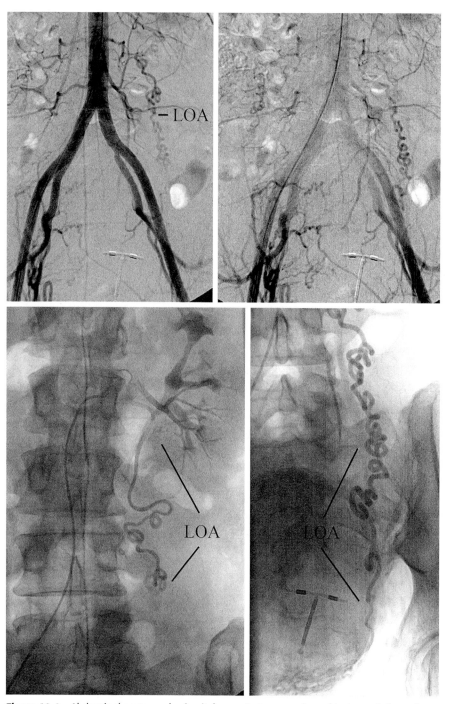

Figure 10-1   Abdominal aortography (top) demonstrates an enlarged tortuous left ovarian artery (LOA) descending into the pelvis. The ovarian arteries commonly originate directly from the infra-renal abdominal aorta. In this case, selective left renal arteriography (bottom) identifies a variant ovarian artery origin off the proximal segment of the main renal artery. The artery is traced into the pelvis where it perfuses multiple uterine fibroids.

References: Dariushnia SR, Nikolic B, Stokes LS, Spies JB. Quality improvement guidelines for uterine artery embolization for symptomatic leiomyomata. *J Vasc Interv Radiol*. 2014;25(11):1737-1747.

Kohi MP, Spies JB. Updates on uterine artery embolization. *Semin Intervent Radiol*. 2018;35(1):48-55.

Razavi MK, Wolanske KA, Hwang GL, Sze DY, Kee ST, Dake MD. Angiographic classification of ovarian artery-to-uterine artery anastomoses: initial observations in uterine fibroid embolization. *Radiology*. 2002;224(3):707-712.

11 **Answer A.**   Current Society of Interventional Radiology quality improvement guidelines define absolute contraindications for UAE to include viable pregnancy, active untreated infections, and suspected uterine/cervical/adnexal cancer (unless embolization is for palliation or as adjunct to surgery). Neither size nor location of a fibroid(s) is considered a contraindication (choices B and C). There had been long-standing caution with embolization of a narrow stalk pedunculated fibroid for fear of necrosis and detachment requiring surgical removal. This has been addressed in several recent studies, which showed safe treatment of these lesions. However, operators should know that the chance of successful treatment may be less when compared with other fibroid types. Intracavitary fibroids can also be treated successfully with UAE but with an increased risk of detachment and fibroid expulsion. Regarding fertility after UAE, there is a paucity of high-level evidence to support a contraindication or indication. Patients certainly can and do get pregnant after UAE, and recent data indicate post-UAE fertility may be similar to that of surgical myomectomy. In women desiring future fertility, an individualized fibroid treatment plan should be crafted in concert with the patient's Ob-Gyn provider.

References: Dariushnia SR, Nikolic B, Stokes LS, Spies JB. Quality improvement guidelines for uterine artery embolization for symptomatic leiomyomata. *J Vasc Interv Radiol.* 2014;25(11):1737-1747.

Keung JJ, Spies JB, Caridi TM. Uterine artery embolization: a review of current concepts. *Best Pract Res Clin Obstet Gynaecol.* 2018;46:66-73.

Pisco JM, Duarte M, Bilhim T, Cirurgião F, Oliveira AG. Pregnancy after uterine fibroid embolization. *Fertil Steril.* 2011;95(3):1121.e5-1121.e8.

12 **Answer D.**   The 3 most commonly reported complications after UAE for symptomatic fibroids are permanent amenorrhea (occurring in 20%-40% of patients >45 y of age), prolonged vaginal discharge (occurring in 2%-17%), and delayed fibroid expulsion. Less commonly encountered complications include septicemia, development of venous thromboembolic disease, and nontarget embolization with tissue ischemia. Vesicouterine fistula has been described but is quite rare.

References: Dariushnia SR, Nikolic B, Stokes LS, Spies JB. Quality improvement guidelines for uterine artery embolization for symptomatic leiomyomata. *J Vasc Interv Radiol.* 2014;25(11):1737-1747.

Kohi MP, Spies JB. Updates on uterine artery embolization. *Semin Intervent Radiol.* 2018;35(1):48-55.

13 **Answer D.**   Pelvic congestion syndrome (PCS) is a difficult diagnosis to make and often one of exclusion. Patients commonly present with noncyclical pelvic pain or fullness lasting >6 months. The symptoms are typically worse at the end of the day, exacerbated by prolonged standing, and can be associated with dyspareunia. A host of nonspecific symptoms are often reported as well. Magnetic resonance venography (MRV) and computed tomography venography (CTV) can help identify dilated veins and pelvic varicosities but are somewhat limited for dynamic vascular evaluation. Some advocate ultrasound, either transabdominal or transvaginal, as the best noninvasive study; however, the field of visualization can be significantly limited by adjacent organs. Classically, the gold standard for evaluation is catheter venography. With catheter venography, individual veins can be directly interrogated and size, flow direction, and valvular reflux can be quantified. Provocative maneuvers such as Valsalva or table tilt can also be performed to augment the study. PCS most commonly is a result of left gonadal vein reflux; however, the right gonadal vein and internal iliac veins can also be involved. When a dilated refluxing vein feeding pelvic varices is identified, endovascular embolization with coils, plugs, and/or sclerosants can be performed. Depending on the presenting symptom, clinical success of embolization ranges from 75% to 99% of treated patients.

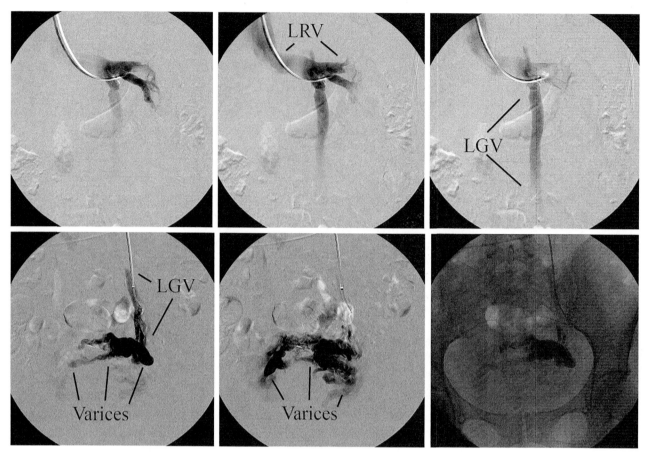

Figure 13-1 Catheter venography in a young female with debilitating chronic pelvic pain. The left renal vein (LRV) is catheterized, and venography with Valsalva (top images) shows reflux of contrast into a dilated left gonadal vein (LGV), which descends into the pelvis. The catheter is advanced further into the LGV and additional venography shows opacification of a large complex of pelvic varices (bottom images) with cross-pelvic filling.

References: Ignacio EA, Dua R, Sarin S, et al. Pelvic congestion syndrome: diagnosis and treatment. *Semin Intervent Radiol.* 2008;25(4):361-368.

Kim HS, Malhotra AD, Rowe PC, Lee JM, Venbrux AC. Embolotherapy for pelvic congestion syndrome: long-term results. *J Vasc Interv Radiol.* 2006;17(2 Pt 1):289-297.

14 **Answer A.** In PCS, dilated refluxing gonadal and/or internal iliac veins ineffectively drain blood from the pelvis. As the venous blood overwhelms the dysfunctional pelvic veins, preexisting communications with the pelvis become overflow collateral pathways and can result in vaginal, vulvar, and thigh varicosities (choice A). There is no known connection between pelvic venous congestion and the subsequent development of DVT. Diverticular bleeding (an arterial source) is unaffected; however, hemorrhoids can appear with PCS. Portal hypertension does not result from pelvic venous insufficiency; however, it may be a secondary cause of the condition. Other secondary causes of PCS include May-Thurner syndrome, nutcracker syndrome, and IVC obstruction.

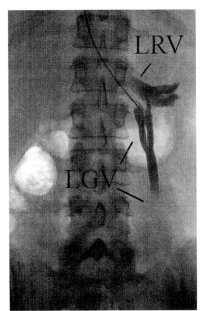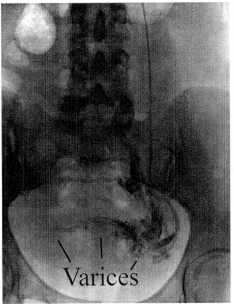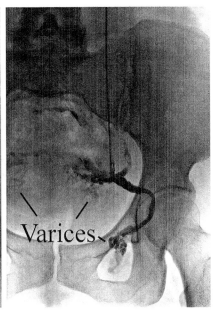

Figure 14-1 Unsubtracted venogram images in a young female with chronic pelvic pain and left lower extremity varicose veins. After catheterization of the left renal vein (LRV) (left), there is free reflux of contrast down a dilated left gonadal vein (LGV). Interrogation of the LGV (middle and right) shows filling of a large complex of pelvic varices as well as outflow pathway into the left inguinal region. On physical examination, there were large upper thigh varicosities. The pelvic and thigh varices were obliterated with sclerosant, and the LGV was closed with multiple coils and plugs.

References: Durham JD, Machan L. Pelvic congestion syndrome. *Semin Intervent Radiol.* 2013;30(4):372-380.

Ignacio EA, Dua R, Sarin S, et al. Pelvic congestion syndrome: diagnosis and treatment. *Semin Intervent Radiol.* 2008;25(4):361-368.

15 **Answer B.**   An invasive placenta increases the risk of maternal hemorrhage with childbirth. There are 3 types depending on the depth of placental invasion into the uterine wall with placenta accreta being the most common and least severe. This is followed by placenta increta and finally placenta percreta, where the placenta has grown through the uterine wall and outer lining into the adjacent tissues. With modern prenatal ultrasound, the diagnosis is often known or suspected. Before delivery, the IR physician can position a balloon occlusion catheter in the abdominal aorta, bilateral common or IIAs, with balloon inflation occurring immediately after delivery of the baby. In addition to causing cessation of flow to the pelvis, if postpartum hemorrhage cannot be controlled, subsequent catheter-directed arterial embolization of the uterine arteries can be performed expeditiously. There are overall promising data for this procedure, and it is routine in some centers. However, high-quality studies are scarce, and the US obstetric guidelines have not made a firm recommendation as to its implementation. Placental abruption (choice B) is a threat to the fetus and does not cause uncontrollable maternal bleeding. Although prior cesarean section is a risk factor for placental invasion, VBAC is not an indication on its own to place balloon occlusion catheters.

References: Knuttinen MG, Jani A, Gaba RC, Bui JT, Carrillo TC. Balloon occlusion of the hypogastric arteries in the management of placenta accreta: a case report and review of the literature. *Semin Intervent Radiol.* 2012;29(3):161-168.

Newsome J, Martin JG, Bercu Z, Shah J, Shekhani H, Peters G. Postpartum hemorrhage. *Tech Vasc Interv Radiol.* 2017;20(4):266-273.

Wu Q, Liu Z, Zhao X, et al. Outcome of pregnancies after balloon occlusion of the infrarenal abdominal aorta during caesarean in 230 patients with placenta praevia accreta. *Cardiovasc Intervent Radiol.* 2016;39(11):1573-1579.

16   **Answer B.**   Thyroid nodule biopsy is a difficult topic for board examination, as there are a wide variety of institution- and operator-dependent algorithms, all of which may be acceptable. Both the American Thyroid Association (ATA) and American College of Radiology (ACR) have published guidelines on thyroid nodule management, and operators should be familiar with these recommendations. Although differences exist, some similarities and common themes prevail regardless of which guideline is used. For example, both include 5 lesion categories ranging from benign to high suspicion of malignancy, using a combination of size and sonographic appearance, to stratify nodules and make a recommendation for biopsy. For testing purposes, clearly benign and malignant nodules should be recognized. A completely anechoic cyst with smooth regular walls is benign and requires no further follow-up. Solid nodules that are ≥1.0 cm, are hypoechoic, have irregular margins, and demonstrate microcalcifications (all present in the case example) will require biopsy no matter which algorithm is used.

TABLE 16-1   Summary Comparison of American Thyroid Association (ATA) and American College of Radiology (ACR) Thyroid Nodule Biopsy Guidelines

ATA			ACR TI-RADS		
Pattern	Example	Recommendation	Feature	Points	Recommendation
High suspicion	Hypoechoic nodule, irregular margin, microcalcs	Fine needle aspiration (FNA) if ≥1.0 cm	Composition	Cystic (0) Spongiform (0) Mixed cyst/solid (1) Solid (2)	Category 5 Points ≥7 FNA if ≥1.0 cm
Intermediate suspicion	Hypoechoic nodule, regular margin	FNA if ≥1.0 cm	Echogenicity	Anechoic (0) Hyper/Isoechoic (1) Hypoechoic (2) Very hypo (3)	Category 4 Points 4-6 FNA if ≥1.5 cm
Low suspicion	Partially cystic with eccentric solid area	FNA if ≥1.5 cm	Margin	Smooth (0) Ill defined (0) Lobulated (2) Irregular (2) Extrathyroidal extension (3)	Category 3 Points 3 FNA if ≥2.5 cm
Very low suspicion	Spongiform	FNA if ≥2.0 cm	Echogenic foci (calcifications)	Large comet tail (0) Macrocalc (1) Rim calc (2) Punctate/Micro (3)	Category 2 Points 2 No FNA
Benign	Cyst	No FNA	Shape	Wide (0) Tall (3)	Category 1 Points 0 No FNA

The ATA uses a pattern-based classification, whereas the ACR uses a scoring system based on sonographic features, with the sum total placing each nodule into 1 of 5 categories. See references Haugen et al and Middleton et al for further review of the ATA and ACR guidelines.

References: Haugen BR, Alexander EK, Bible KC, et al. 2015 American Thyroid Association Management Guidelines for adult patients with thyroid nodules and differentiated thyroid cancer: The American Thyroid Association Guidelines Task Force on thyroid nodules and differentiated thyroid cancer. *Thyroid.* 2016;26(1):1-133.

Middleton WD, Teefey SA, Reading CC, et al. Comparison of performance characteristics of American College of Radiology TI-RADS, Korean Society of Thyroid Radiology TIRADS, and American Thyroid Association Guidelines. *AJR Am J Roentgenol.* 2018;210(5):1148-1154.

Nachiappan AC, Metwalli ZA, Hailey BS, Patel RA, Ostrowski ML, Wynne DM. The thyroid: review of imaging features and biopsy techniques with radiologic-pathologic correlation. *Radiographics.* 2014;34(2):276-293.

17 **Answer B.** Hysterosalpingography (HSG) is covered for completeness. The study may be performed as part of an infertility workup, to evaluate tubal closure, and to assess for uterine and fallopian tube pathology. It should not be performed with active pelvic infection or during pregnancy. Ideally, the study is conducted in the first half of the menstrual cycle. A balloon catheter is passed into the cervical canal, gently inflated, and the uterine cavity is then filled with water-soluble contrast. There is opacification of the uterine cavity, followed by the fallopian tubes. If the fallopian tubes are patent, contrast will spill freely into the peritoneum (see Figure 17-1). In the case example, the left fallopian tube does not fill and an Essure coil is present in its expected location. The right fallopian tube fills with free peritoneal spillage of contrast indicating patency. This represents a failure of right tubal closure (choice B correct). With successful closure, the fallopian tubes will not fill (see Figure 17-2).

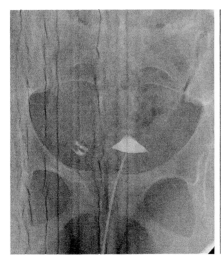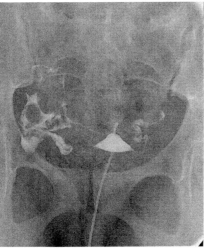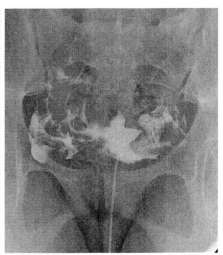

Figure 17-1 Sequential images from a normal hysterosalpingography (HSG) with patent right and left fallopian tubes and free spillage of contrast into the peritoneum.

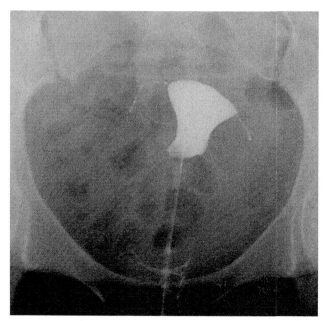

Figure 17-2   Hysterosalpingography (HSG) following successful bilateral fallopian tube closure with Essure-implanted contraceptive device.

In addition to uterine and fallopian tube pathology, it is worth knowing the imaging appearance of contrast intravasation. This occurs when contrast extends from the uterine cavity into the myometrium and draining pelvic veins. This can be subtle (see Figure 17-3) or more extensive (see Figure 17-4).

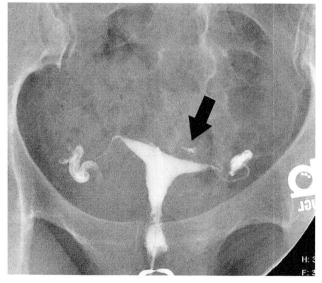

Figure 17-3   Contrast intravasation (arrow) during hysterosalpingography (HSG).

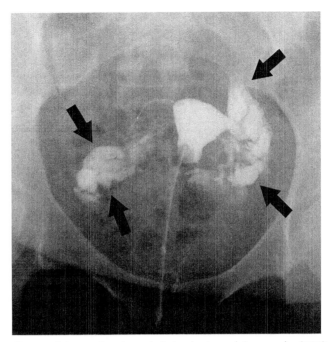

Figure 17-4   Contrast intravasation (arrow) during hysterosalpingography (HSG). Patient has indwelling Essure coils, and initial images (not shown) demonstrate no filling of the fallopian tubes consistent with tubal closure. Later image shows new tubular and curvilinear contrast bilaterally (arrows) from extensive intravasation with filling of periuterine venous and lymphatic channels.

References: Mcswain H, Shaw C, Hall LD. Placement of the Essure permanent birth control device with fluoroscopic guidance: a novel method for tubal sterilization. *J Vasc Interv Radiol.* 2005;16(7):1007-1012.

Thurmond AS. Fallopian tube catheterization. *Semin Intervent Radiol.* 2008;25(4):425-431.

Simpson WL, Beitia LG, Mester J. Hysterosalpingography: a reemerging study. *Radiographics.* 2006;26(2):419-431.

8

Noninvasive Imaging

1   On this CTA (computed tomography angiography) image obtained to evaluate a patient for suspected pulmonary embolism (PE), which of the following structures has abnormal contrast opacification?

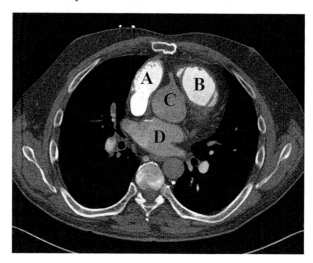

A. A
B. B
C. C
D. D

Hint:

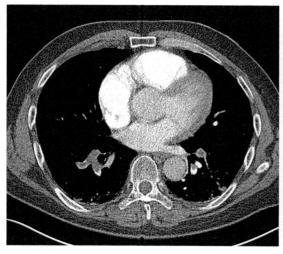
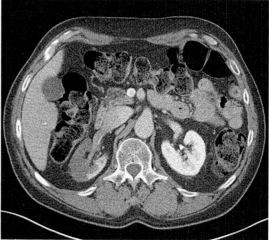

2   A 20-year-old male sustains a gunshot to the right thigh. A CTA is obtained and read out as complete transection of the right superficial femoral artery (SFA). The patient has palpable right pedal pulses. What is the explanation for the physical examination finding?

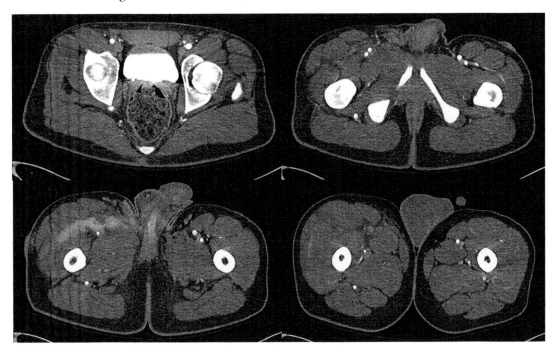

A. Variant anatomy
B. Misinterpretation of the CTA
C. Distal perfusion maintained by the profunda femoris artery

3   On the CTA images, how do you explain the findings in right hemiscrotum?

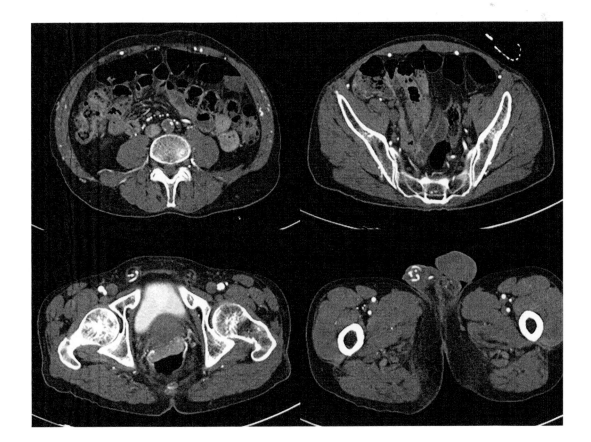

A. Varicocele
B. Arteriovenous malformation
C. Arterial collateral pathway
D. Normal anatomic variant

4   What pathology (arrows) is demonstrated on these contrast-enhanced computed tomography (CECT) images?

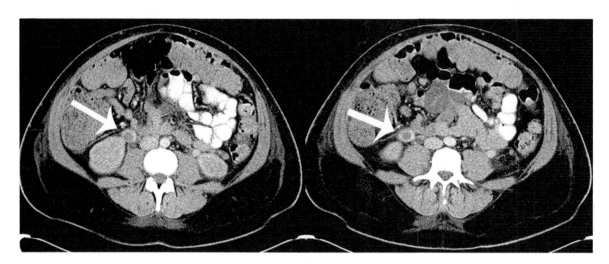

A. Clot in a duplicated inferior vena cava (IVC)
B. Clot in the gonadal vein
C. Clot in a circumaortic renal vein
D. Clot in the superior mesenteric vein (SMV)

5   Given the CECT images below, what is the most likely presenting symptom in this patient?

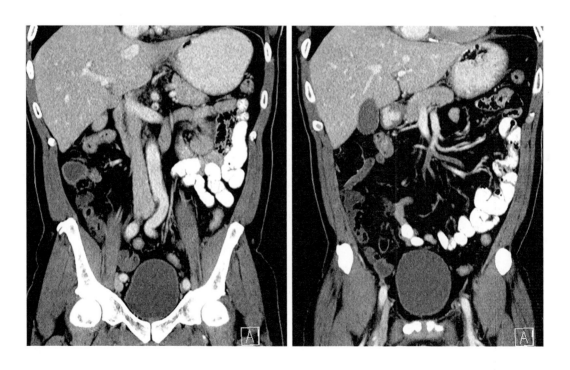

A. Lower extremity swelling
B. Bright red blood per rectum
C. Elevated liver function tests
D. Abdominal pain

6   What is the most likely etiology of the pathology (arrows) demonstrated?

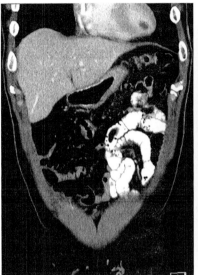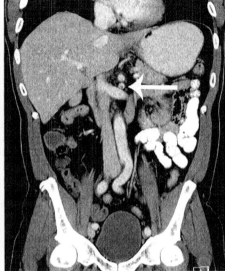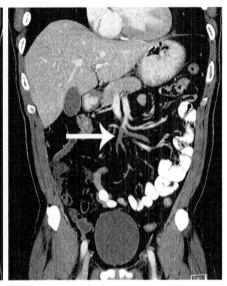

A. Embolus
B. Atherosclerosis
C. Vasculitis
D. Vasospasm

7   The medial aspect of the upper arm is evaluated for peripherally inserted central catheter (PICC) placement. What does the marked structure (arrows) represent?

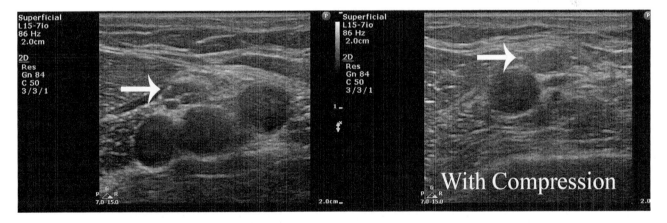

A. Thrombosed brachial vein
B. Radial artery
C. Median nerve
D. Biceps tendon

8   Which of the following is true regarding popliteal artery aneurysms (PAAs)?

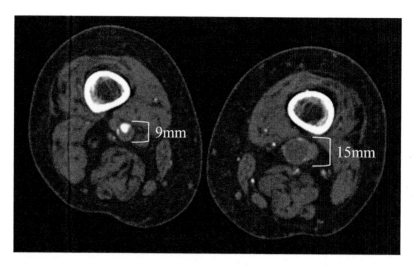

A. 30% to50% of patients with PAA have an abdominal aortic aneurysm
B. Patients typically present with PAA rupture
C. Diameter threshold to declare a PAA is 20 mm
D. Treatment is deferred if the PAA(s) remains asymptomatic

9   Based on the CTA images, which is the correct interpretation?

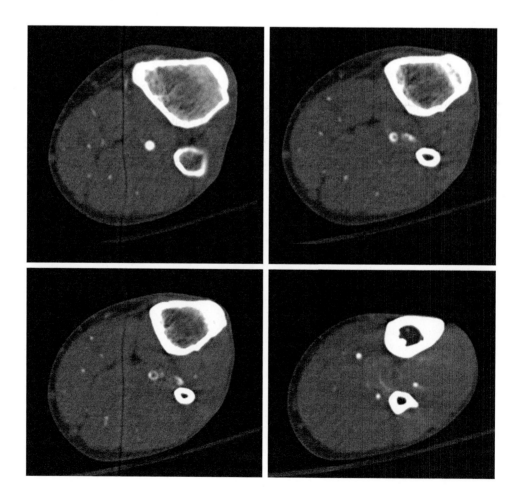

A. Normal arterial perfusion with computed tomography (CT) artifact
B. Chronic arterial occlusion
C. Acute arterial thromboembolus
D. Deep venous thrombosis

10 A 53-year-old male with a history of chronic pancreatitis presents with hematemesis. Given the findings on the CECT images, which of the following initial interventions is the most appropriate?

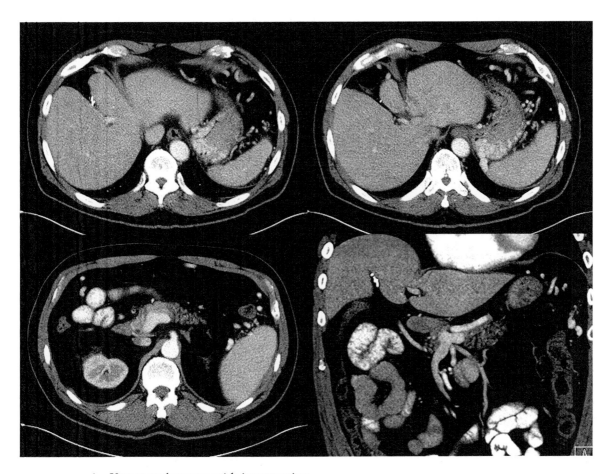

A. Upper endoscopy with intervention
B. Transjugular intrahepatic portosystemic shunt (TIPS) creation
C. Left gastric artery embolization
D. Surgical gastrectomy

11   A patient presents from an outside hospital with a right chest tunneled catheter, but nothing present on the left. An unenhanced CT chest is performed to evaluate shortness of breath, and an abnormality is identified in the upper mediastinum. What is the best management for the finding (arrows)?

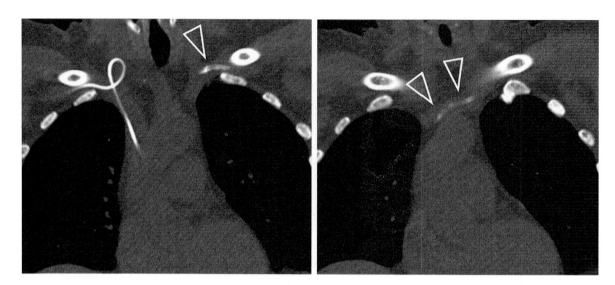

A. Interventional radiology (IR) suite for catheter fragment retrieval
B. Anticoagulation
C. No change in management

12   A 33-year-old female presents to the emergency department (ED) with abdominal bloating and pain. A CECT is performed. What is the diagnosis?

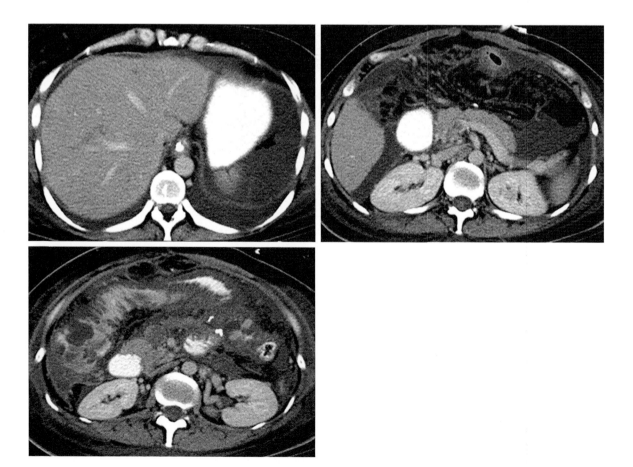

A. Acute liver failure from hepatic venous thrombosis
B. Acute mesenteric ischemia from superior mesentric artery (SMA) thrombosis
C. Acute mesenteric ischemia from SMV thrombosis
D. *Clostridium difficile* colitis

13 A 59-year-old male with Child-Pugh A cirrhosis presents for evaluation of a solitary lesion in segment 4 of the liver. He is completely asymptomatic. What is the most likely diagnosis based on these contrast-enhanced T1 FS MRI images?

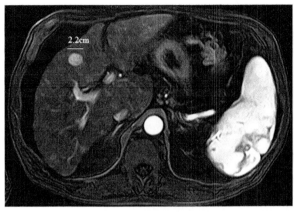 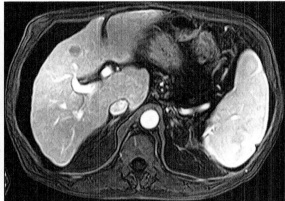

A. Hypervascular metastasis
B. Intrahepatic cholangiocarcinoma
C. Hepatocellular carcinoma (HCC)
D. Hemangioma

14   A 40-year-old male with alcoholic cirrhosis and a solitary 2.5 cm HCC in the right
lobe of the liver undergoes treatment with thermal ablation. CT scans are obtained
immediately following the ablation and at 3 months and 12 months after ablation.
Arrange the selected images from the follow-up CT scans in the order they were
acquired (immediate, 3, 12 mo).

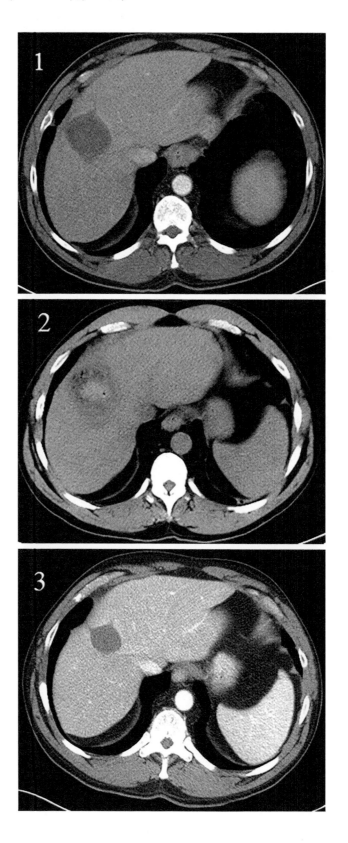

A. 1, 2, 3
B. 2, 1, 3
C. 3, 1, 2
D. 2, 3, 1

15   An adult patient with no history of trauma or surgery undergoes CECT evaluation to reassess a known aortic dissection. Based on the images presented, which of the following is the most likely clinical presentation for the additional pathology demonstrated (ignore the abdominal aortic dissection)?

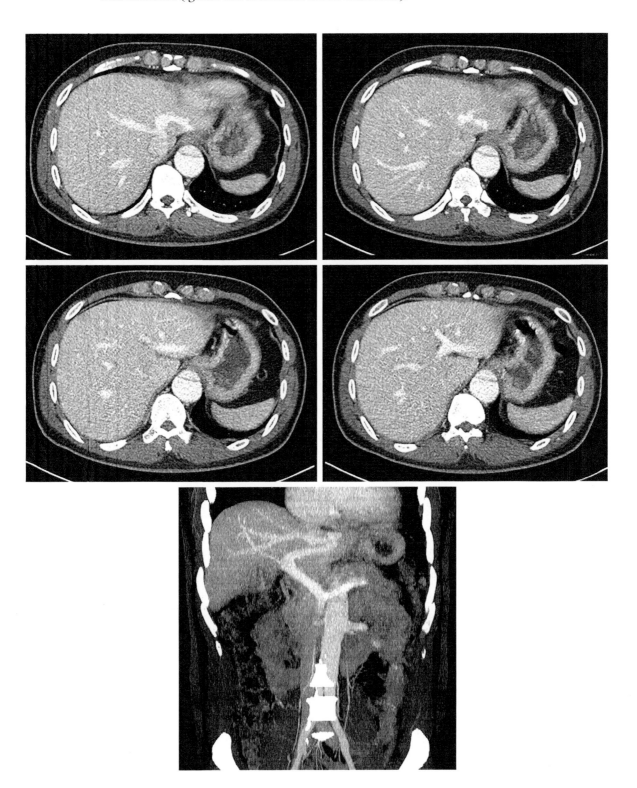

A. Encephalopathy
B. Weight loss
C. Abdominal pain
D. Hematochezia

16   Following a motor vehicle accident with blunt chest trauma, a patient is evaluated
with CECT. What finding is delineated by the arrows?

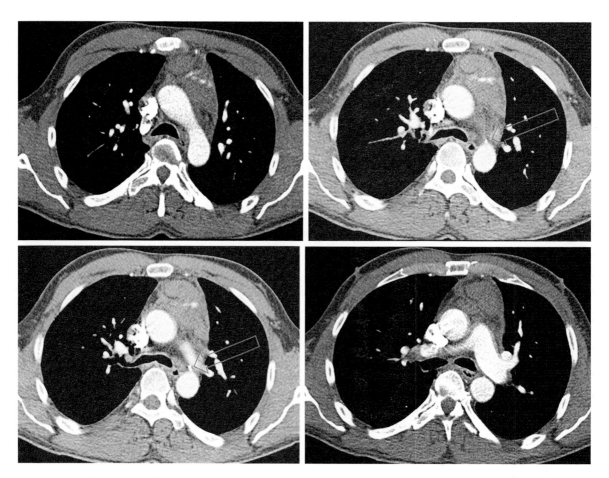

A. Aortic dissection flap
B. Aortic pseudoaneurysm
C. Active extravasation
D. Normal variant

17   What variant anatomy is demonstrated in this image?

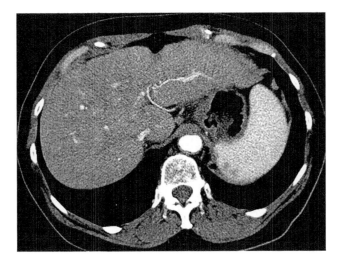

A. Hepatic artery
B. Portal Vein
C. Hepatic Vein
D. Aorta

18   What pathology explains the CECT findings in the liver?

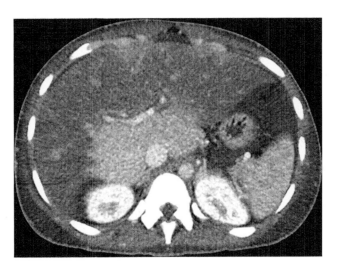

A. Hepatic artery occlusion
B. Portal vein occlusion
C. Hepatic vein occlusion
D. Biliary obstruction

19   Which of the following is most concerning for TIPS dysfunction?

A. Recurrent ascites
B. Hepatofugal flow in the parenchymal portal vein
C. Peak systolic velocity of 150 cm/s in the midportion of the stent

20 What is the best description for the appearance of this TIPS?

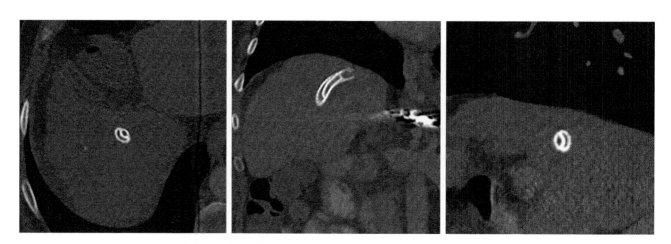

A. Stent maldeployment
B. Embolized foreign body
C. Expected postrevision appearance
D. CT artifact

21 There is a telephone consultation regarding an 82-year-old patient in the ED with back pain. The ED physician wants an opinion on the uploaded images whether vertebroplasty might be an option, as they decide whether to admit the patient. Without the benefit of a good physical examination, what is the best initial treatment plan? Left image is unenhanced CT. Right image is MRI T2 short TI inversion recovery (STIR).

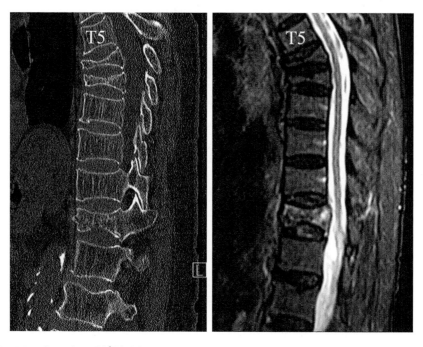

A. Vertebroplasty T6, T7, T11
B. Vertebroplasty T6, T7 only
C. Vertebroplasty T11 only
D. Conservative treatment, no indication for vertebroplasty

22   Where is the stent (arrow) located on these axial CTA images?

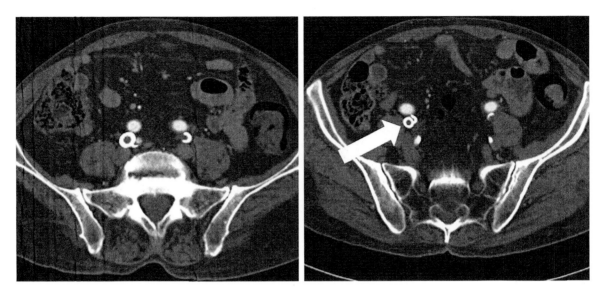

    A. Right external iliac vein
    B. Right external iliac artery
    C. Right iliac artery bypass graft
    D. Right internal iliac artery

23   Which treatment explains the change in appearance of this right hepatic dome lesion?

Pretreatment CECT:

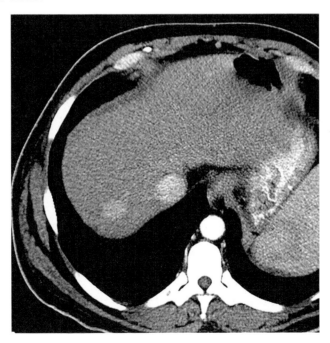

4 month posttreatment CECT (left) and CE T1 FS MRI (right):

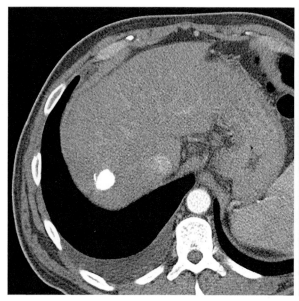
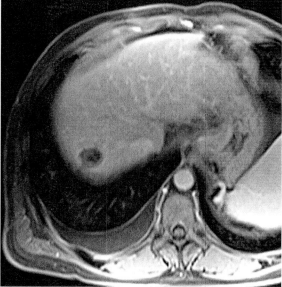

A. Conventional transarterial chemoembolization
B. Yttrium-90 radioembolization
C. Thermal ablation
D. Transarterial glue embolization

24   A new patient presents to Oncology clinic for follow-up of a right hepatic dome metastatic lesion from gastric cancer. He reports treatment a few years back at an outside hospital but is unsure what was done. Based on the provided pre- and post-treatment CECT images, what therapy did the patient receive?

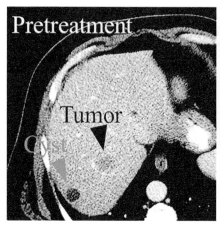
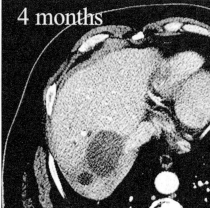
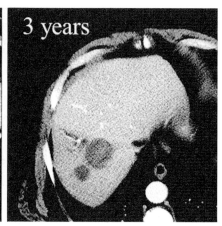

A. Transarterial chemoembolization
B. Transarterial radioembolization
C. Thermal ablation
D. Surgical resection

25   How does CTA compare with a tagged red blood cell (RBC) scan with respect to the detectable rate of active gastrointestinal (GI) bleeding?

A. CTA is more sensitive than tagged RBC scan
B. CTA is equivalent to tagged RBC scan
C. CTA is less sensitive than tagged RBC scan

26 A patient presents for evaluation of severe bilateral calf pain with activity that is relieved by rest. As part of the workup for suspected claudication due to peripheral arterial disease (PAD), an ankle brachial index (ABI) is obtained but measures supraphysiologic at 1.4 (normal 0.9–1.1). The technologist notes "noncompressible arteries due to severe calcification." Which study will best assess the nature and extent of the suspected lower extremity arterial disease?

A. Magnetic resonance angiography (MRA) with gadolinium contrast
B. Duplex ultrasound (US)
C. CTA with iodinated contrast
D. No additional study needed, the ABI is diagnostic

27 In preparation for a fibula free flap harvest from the right lower extremity, a plastic surgeon obtains a lower extremity MRA to evaluate the tibial arteries. Which is the correct interpretation of the right leg 3D volume-rendered MRA images?

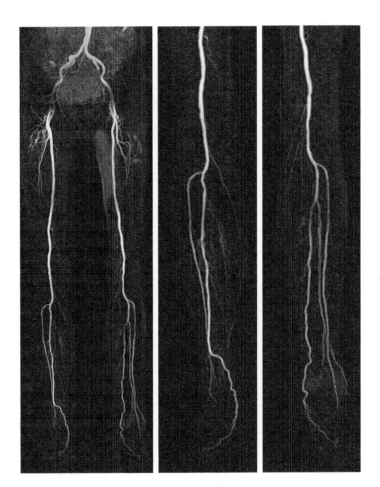

A. Normal tibial branching pattern
B. Dominant right anterior tibial artery, patent posterior tibial artery
C. Dominant right posterior tibial artery, patent peroneal artery
D. Dominant right peroneal artery, patent anterior tibial artery

28   A 43-year-old female chef presents for evaluation of a painful mass in the right forearm. She reports that a doctor once told her she has some sort of malformation. Based on the axial and coronal T1 FS + Gd images, what is the most likely diagnosis?

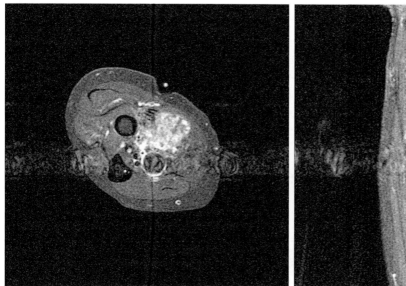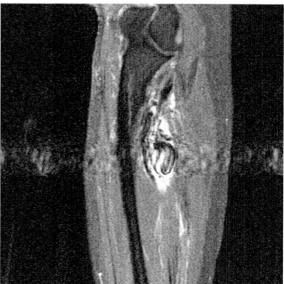

A. Arteriovenous malformation
B. Venous malformation
C. Lymphatic malformation

29   What best explains this spectral Doppler ultrasound image of the left hepatic artery in this patient who is 6 months post cadaveric liver transplant?

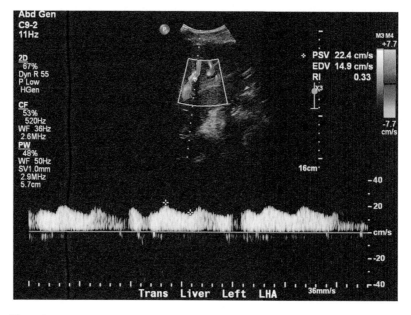

A. Hepatic artery stenosis
B. Transplant rejection
C. Budd-Chiari
D. Portal vein thrombosis

30   Based upon the given velocities, what is the best description for the left internal carotid artery?

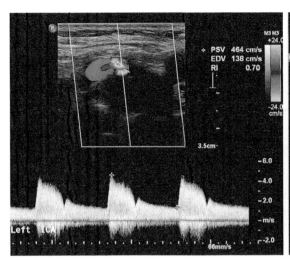 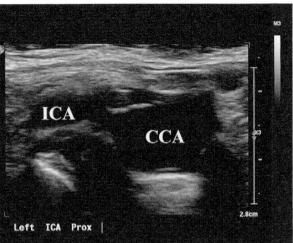

A. <50% stenosis
B. 50% to 69% stenosis
C. >70% stenosis

31   What is the best interpretation of this noninvasive vascular evaluation performed on this patient with suspected lower extremity PAD?

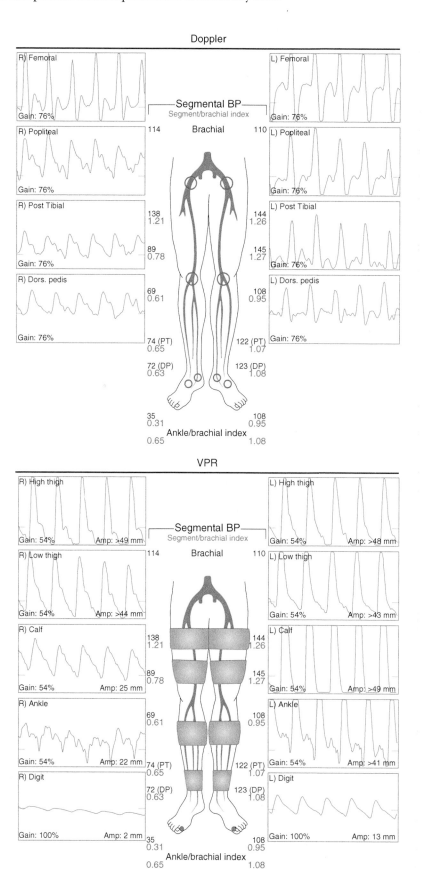

A. Normal bilateral lower extremity arteries
B. Severe right leg PAD, iliac arterial pathology
C. Moderate right leg PAD, SFA pathology
D. Bilateral leg mild PAD, SFA pathology

32 A 65-year-old male with a history of multifocal HCC, cirrhosis, and aortobifemoral bypass graft presents with GI bleeding. Based on the CECT images, what is the most likely diagnosis? Arterial phase on the left; portal venous phase on the right.

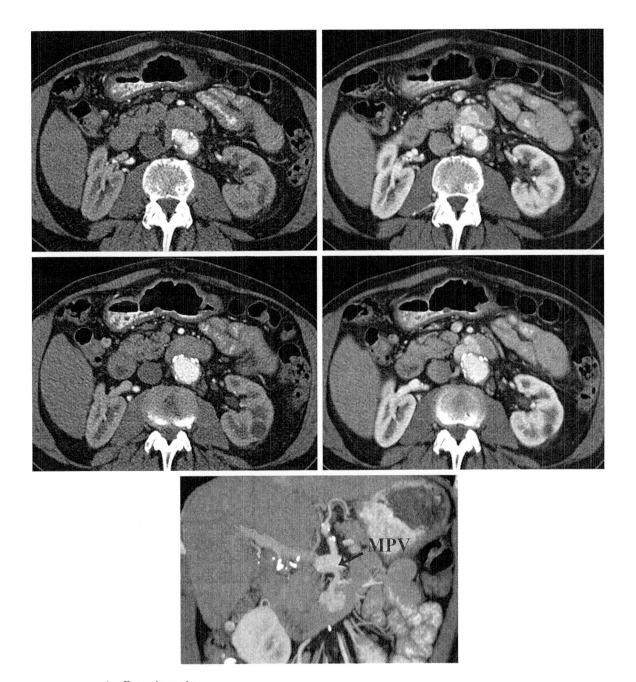

A. Ectopic varices
B. Hypervascular metastasis
C. Aortobifemoral bypass anastomosis aneurysm

33   In what Couinaud segment(s) is the liver lesion denoted by the arrowheads?

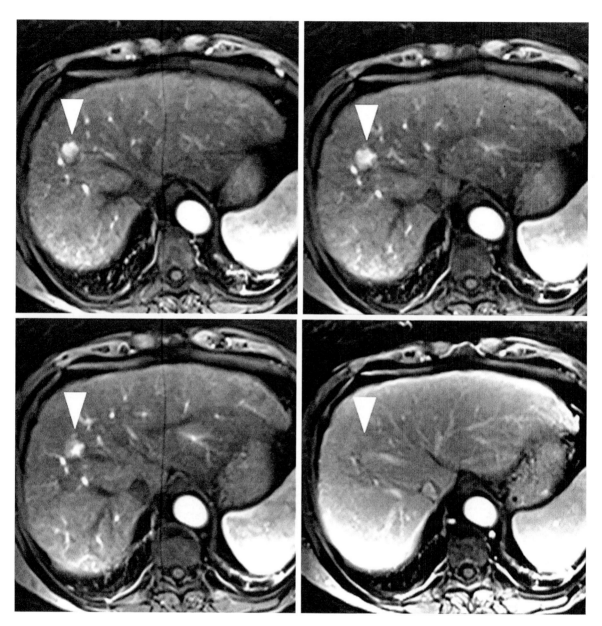

A. I
B. IVb/V
C. VIII
D. IVa/VIII

34   A patient with no history of cancer has a primary tumor which is clearly arising
     from the IVC. What is the most likely pathology?

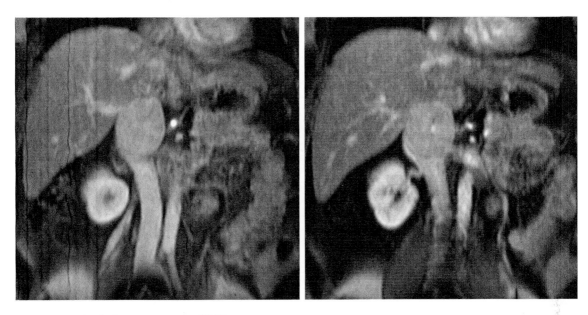

     A. Leiomyosarcoma (LMS)
     B. Angiosarcoma
     C. Angiomyolipoma

35   A patient with a known abdominal aortic dissection presents to establish care. A
     CTA is ordered to establish a new baseline, as no comparison imaging is available.
     Which of the following is true based on these images?

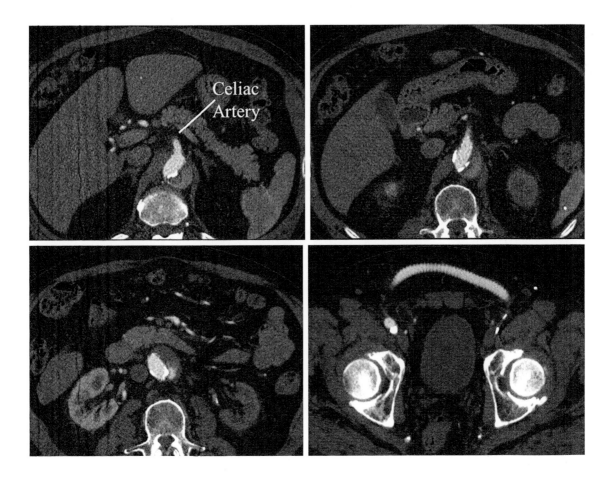

A. The true lumen supplies the celiac artery
B. Urgent intervention is required to save the left kidney
C. An aortobifemoral graft perfuses the legs
D. The false lumen is completely thrombosed

36   In this patient with remote open repair of an infrarenal abdominal aortic aneurysm with interposition graft, which of the following should be considered?

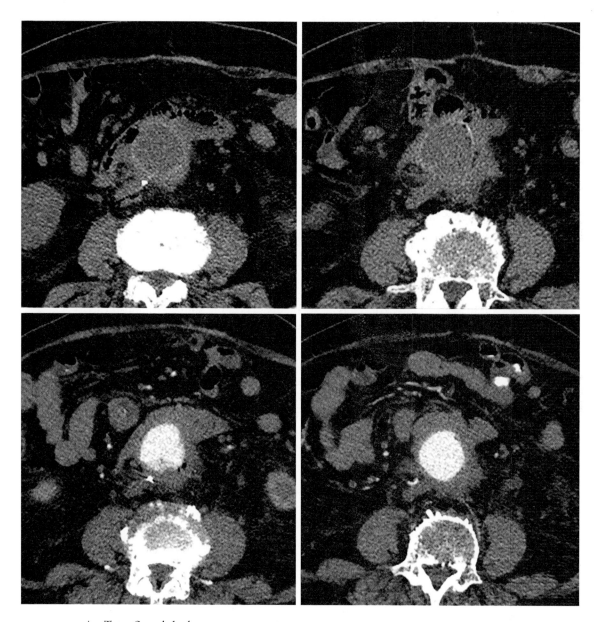

A. Type 2 endoleak
B. Mesenteric fibrosis
C. Expected post-op changes
D. Aortoenteric fistula

37   An 8-year-old boy presents for evaluation of an intermittently painful mass in the suboccipital region. The mass occasionally swells. His parents report that the mass has been present for years and has slowly grown over time. Based on the history and images presented, which is the most likely diagnosis?

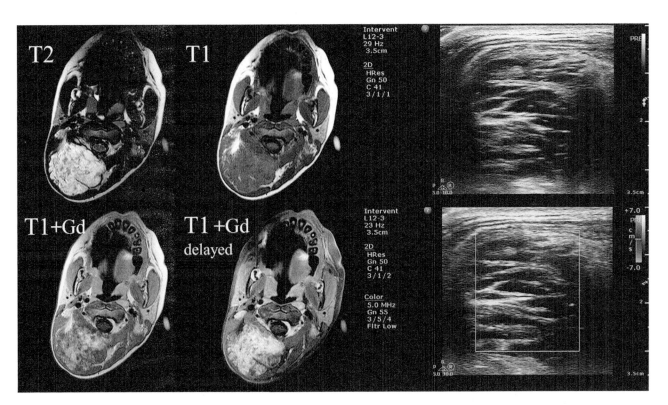

A. Arteriovenous malformation
B. Venous malformation
C. Rhabdomyosarcoma
D. Abscess
E. Hematoma

ANSWERS AND EXPLANATIONS

1   **Answer D.**   As with all contrast-enhanced imaging studies, the interpretation of the images must take into account the timing of intravascular contrast administration. For CTA to evaluate for a suspected PE, optimal contrast opacification of the right heart and pulmonary arterial tree is essential. Notably, the left atrium should not have early dense contrast opacification. Paradoxically, the linear nondependent contrast that has accumulated in the left atrium is denser than the visualized lower lobe pulmonary artery branches. The constellation of findings is consistent with a right to left intracardiac shunt. On the sagittal reformatted image (see Figure 1-1), a clear connection is present between the right and left atria from a patent foramen ovale (PFO). This patient presented with paradoxical emboli and partial right renal infarction as shown in the Hint images. The patient underwent placement of an IVC filter and subsequent PFO closure with a septal occluder device.

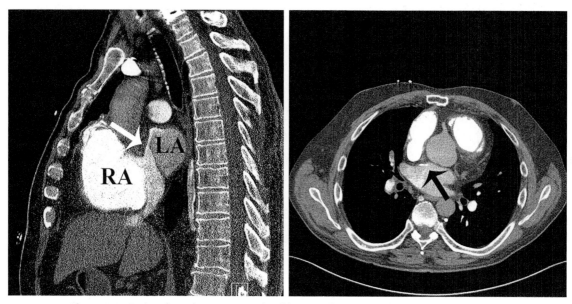

Figure 1-1   Patient from the case example with patent foramen ovale (PFO) (white arrow) producing nondependent contrast (black arrow) layering along the left atrial wall. LA, left atrium; RA, right atrium.

References: Kara K, Sivrioğlu AK, Öztürk E, et al. The role of coronary CT angiography in diagnosis of patent foramen ovale. *Diagn Interv Radiol.* 2016;22(4):341-346.

Saremi F, Channual S, Raney A, et al. Imaging of patent foramen ovale with 64-section multidetector CT. *Radiology.* 2008;249(2):483-492.

2   **Answer A.**   The initial interpretation of the CTA is correct. The right SFA is traumatically transected by the bullet trajectory and is occluded shortly after its origin. Although the profunda femoris artery is patent, it alone is not capable of maintaining the distal pulses. This is especially true in the acute setting, as no arterial collaterals have developed. This lucky patient happens to have the anatomic variant of a persistent sciatic artery (PSA), which occurs in an estimated 0.05% of the population. Normally, the embryologic axial artery regresses to the inferior gluteal artery (coming off of the internal iliac artery) and the SFA becomes the dominant artery to the leg. When this does not occur, the sciatic artery persists as a continuation

from the internal iliac artery, coursing down the posterior buttocks and thigh and ultimately connects up with the popliteal artery. As a result, patients may have hypoplasia or aplasia of the SFA. Unfortunately, its position posteriorly in the gluteal musculature makes it susceptible to repetitive injury leading to aneurysm formation. Those affected can present with a painful gluteal mass or limb ischemia from thrombosis and/or distal embolism.

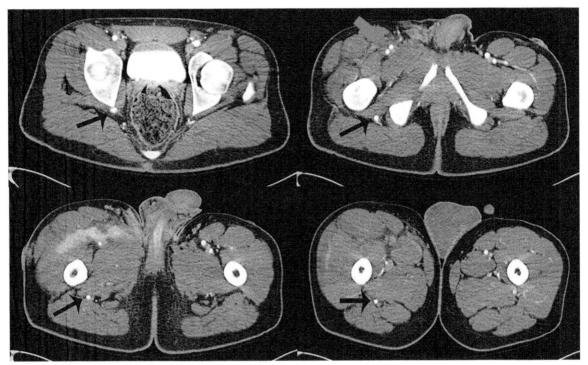

Figure 2-1 Patient from the case example with patent superficial femoral artery (SFA) (red arrow) in the right lower extremity above the site of injury. Note the transversely oriented bullet tract in the soft tissues distally (bottom left image) with only the profunda femoris artery seen. Persistent sciatic artery (PSA) (black arrows) is identified from its origin off the right internal iliac artery coursing through the greater sciatic foramen and then running posteriorly in the thigh.

Reference: Erturk SM, Tatli S. Persistent sciatic artery aneurysm. *J Vasc Interv Radiol.* 2005;16(10):1407-1408.

3   **Answer C.** The abnormality on the CTA images is a tortuous and enlarged artery coursing along the spermatic cord and into the right hemiscrotum. There is no accompanying abnormal vein.

In patients with chronic arterial occlusions (note the infrarenal aortic and iliac artery occlusions), collateral pathways will develop and hypertrophy to continue to supply the organs and/or extremities. A classic example is distal abdominal aortic occlusion, where there is development of enlarged collaterals including the epigastric, intercostal, mesenteric, and lumbar arteries. In this scenario, an uncommon collateral pathway can develop between the gonadal artery (originating from the aorta or renal arteries) and the inferior epigastric artery, as seen in this case. The gonadal artery flows caudally ultimately entering the scrotum and forms a collateral pathway to the inferior epigastric artery with flow back into the common femoral artery and subsequently down the leg. An obvious consideration for an enlarged vessel in the scrotum is a varicocele (choice A); however, this pathology is a group of dilated veins and should not opacify on the arterial phase of imaging. An arteriovenous malformation (choice B) is characterized by enlarged feeding arteries, often a visible nidus, and early opacification of draining veins.

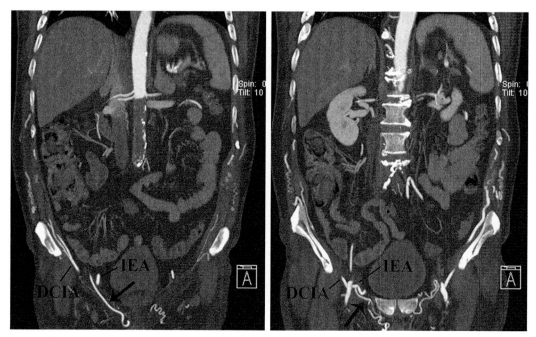

Figure 3-1   Companion case of a patient with a chronic infrarenal aortic occlusion. Note the enlarged deep circumflex iliac artery (DCIA) and inferior epigastric artery (IEA) which provide collateral flow to legs through the abdominal wall. The enlarged and tortuous right gonadal artery (black arrows) is seen crossing the inguinal ligament to enter the scrotum (left image). It then exits the scrotum (right image) and drains into the IEA.

Reference: Hardman RL, Lopera JE, Cardan RA, Trimmer CK, Josephs SC. Common and rare collateral pathways in aortoiliac occlusive disease: a pictorial essay. *AJR Am J Roentgenol.* 2011;197(3):W519-W524.

4   **Answer B.**   There is a central hypodense filling defect in a round structure which is otherwise opacified with iodinated contrast. This appearance is consistent with intravascular clot. The structure is posteriorly located, in the retroperitoneum, making SMV a poor choice. A circumaortic renal vein occurs with the left kidney, and a duplicated IVC would be to the left of the abdominal aorta. Therefore, the finding is most consistent with gonadal vein thrombosis.

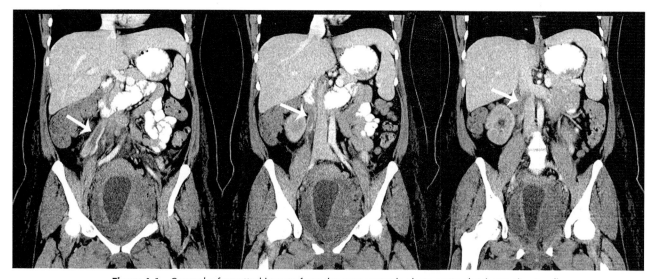

Figure 4-1   Coronal reformatted images from the case example show acute clot (arrows) extending from the right gonadal vein into the inferior vena cava (IVC). The patient could not be anticoagulated, and a suprarenal IVC filter was placed. Gonadal venous thrombosis most commonly occurs in the setting pelvic inflammatory disease, pelvic malignancy, recent childbirth (as with this patient), or surgery.

Reference: Karaosmanoglu D, Karcaaltincaba M, Karcaaltincaba D, Akata D, Ozmen M. MDCT of the ovarian vein: normal anatomy and pathology. *AJR Am J Roentgenol.* 2009;192(1):295-299.

5   **Answer D.** The coronal CECT images demonstrate a filling defect in the SMA at its origin as well as in the more distal SMA branches. This appearance is most consistent with acute mesenteric ischemia due to SMA occlusion. Abdominal pain is the most common presenting symptom. In the acute presentation, patients can have GI bleeding, nausea, and a host of other symptoms, but they are far less common.

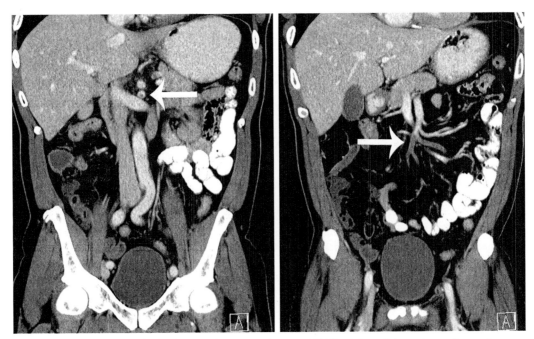

Figure 5-1   Clot in the superior mesentric artery (SMA) origin and downstream (arrows).

References: Clair DG, Beach JM. Mesenteric ischemia. *N Engl J Med.* 2016;374(10):959-968.

Wiesner W, Khurana B, Ji H, Ros PR. CT of acute bowel ischemia. *Radiology.* 2003;226(3):635-650.

6   **Answer A.** A clot associated with an old infarct is present in the left ventricle, serving as the source of the embolic SMA occlusion. Although this is not often seen, it is critical to identify if present. The main etiologies of acute mesenteric ischemia include embolus, in situ thrombosis, dissection, nonocclusive (vasospastic aka NOMI), and venous thrombosis.

References: Clair DG, Beach JM. Mesenteric ischemia. *N Engl J Med.* 2016;374(10):959-968.

Wiesner W, Khurana B, Ji H, Ros PR. CT of acute bowel ischemia. *Radiology.* 2003;226(3):635-650.

7   **Answer C.** The typical structures found in the mid-upper arm neurovascular bundle are the brachial artery, paired brachial veins, and the median nerve. Compression ultrasound is an excellent way to evaluate these structures. When patent, a vein will compress with less pressure than an artery. The artery will appear pulsatile with mild pressure. Spectral Doppler and color flow imaging can be used if there is any doubt. A noncompressible structure could represent a thrombosed vessel or a nerve. With nerves, the hypoechoic fascicles are easily identified with a high-frequency transducer. Scanning more peripheral or proximal is also useful, as vessel branches can be identified, confirming a vascular versus nonvascular structure. PICC placement in the upper arm typically uses the basilic vein, brachial veins, and least likely the cephalic vein. An important variant to be aware of is a high takeoff of the radial artery from the brachial artery. The radial artery will be present in the upper arm

separate from the brachial artery and in a more superficial location. Inexperienced operators can mistake this artery for a vein given its atypical location. Often the variant radial artery will have its associated vein running along with it.

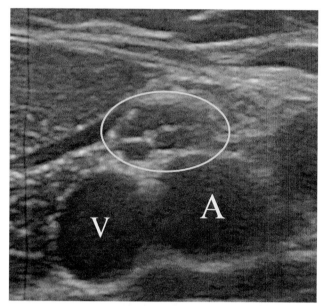

Figure 7-1   Magnified ultrasound image with brachial vein (V) and artery (A). White oval delineating the median nerve comprised of multiple hypoechoic fascicles with intervening hyperechoic connective tissue.

Reference: Chiou HJ, Chou YH, Chiou SY, Liu JB, Chang CY. Peripheral nerve lesions: role of high-resolution US. *Radiographics*. 2003;23(6):e15.

8   **Answer A.**   A popliteal artery is considered aneurysmal once it reaches 1.5x its normal diameter. Given the variance of popliteal artery size in the population, the diameter to define a PAA may range from roughly 7 to 15 mm. Clinically, approximately 45% of PAAs are discovered when the patient is asymptomatic. If there are symptoms, they occur when the aneurysm becomes thrombosed resulting in cessation of blood flow to the distal extremity or if there is distal showering of thromboemboli. In the case example, the left PAA is thrombosed. Peripheral images demonstrate tibial artery occlusions from episodic thromboemboli (see Figure 8-1). Although PAA rupture can occur, it is quite uncommon. PAAs are bilateral 50% to 70% of the time, and 30% to 50% of patients with PAA also have an abdominal aortic aneurysm (choice A). Guidelines are to treat all symptomatic PAA and to treat asymptomatic PAA when the aneurysm is at least 2 cm in diameter.

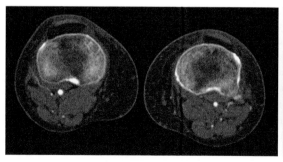 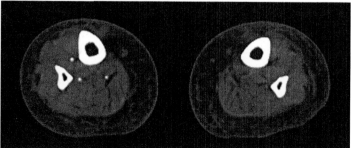

Figure 8-1   Additional images from the case example show reconstitution of the left below-the-knee popliteal artery (left image) with downstream embolic occlusion of all 3 tibial arteries in the left calf (right image).

References: Wolf YG, Kobzantsev Z, Zelmanovich L. Size of normal and aneurysmal popliteal arteries: a duplex ultrasound study. *J Vasc Surg*. 2006;43(3):488-492.

Wright LB, Matchett WJ, Cruz CP, et al. Popliteal artery disease: diagnosis and treatment. *Radiographics*. 2004;24(2):467-479.

9   **Answer C.**   The images demonstrate a normal-appearing below-the-knee popliteal artery. Distally, a central filling defect is noted at the arterial bifurcation with a peripheral ring of iodinated contrast passing beyond. The tibial runoff looks normal further down the leg. The location and appearance of the lesion are most consistent with an acute thromboembolus. With a chronic arterial occlusion, there are often numerous unnamed collateral arteries that have formed over time to compensate for the blockage. The blockage itself will occur at a site of preexisting disease (often atherosclerosis) and, if not completely occlusive, will appear eccentric within the vessel lumen. Venous pathology (choice D) is not evaluated on this purely arterial phase study.

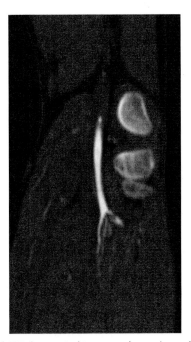

Figure 9-1   Reconstructed CTA (computed tomography angiography) image from the case example showing the thromboembolus draped over popliteal artery bifurcation. Note the otherwise pristine appearance of the arteries in this 25-year-old male with a new diagnosis of atrial fibrillation.

Reference: Fleischmann D, Hallett RL, Rubin GD. CT angiography of peripheral arterial disease. *J Vasc Interv Radiol*. 2006;17(1):3-26.

10   **Answer A.**   The CECT images show enhancing tubular structures in the wall of the gastric cardia and fundus consistent with isolated gastric varices. Additional findings include a normal-appearing liver, lack of esophageal varices, an atrophic distal pancreas, and absence of the splenic vein due to chronic occlusion. In this scenario, a common initial intervention would be endoscopic evaluation and sclerosant or glue injection of the offending gastric varices (choice A). The primary surgical option is a splenectomy, not a gastrectomy. The bleeding in this case is venous, not arterial; therefore, left gastric artery embolization would not be of use. If the bleeding cannot be controlled with endoscopic techniques or recurs, advanced IR techniques are available. Percutaneous transhepatic or transsplenic venous access can be used to recanalize the splenic vein or to sclerose/embolize the varices. Also, a partial splenic arterial embolization can be effective by decreasing the volume of splenic tissue and thereby decreasing splenic venous outflow into the varices.

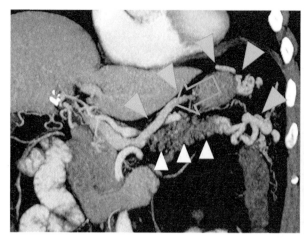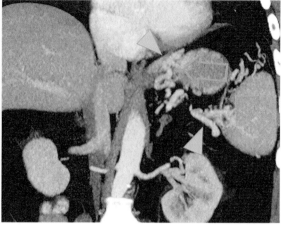

Figure 10-1   Coronal contrast-enhanced computed tomography (CECT) images demonstrating the pathology of chronic splenic vein occlusion with formation of gastric varices. The white arrowheads delineate the expected location of the splenic vein, which is now chronically occluded from prior bouts of pancreatitis. The blue arrows and arrowheads highlight the new venous drainage pathway of the spleen back to the liver through perigastric and submucosal gastric veins. The considerable splenic venous outflow over time causes dilatation of the submucosal gastric veins producing varices. This condition is termed sinistral or left-sided portal hypertension. The importance of this qualifier is that the pathology is both presinusoidal and prehepatic and TIPS would not be of benefit.

References: Kirby JM, Cho KJ, Midia M. Image-guided intervention in management of complications of portal hypertension: more than TIPS for success. *Radiographics*. 2013;33(5):1473-1496.

Kokabi N, Lee E, Echevarria C, Loh C, Kee S. Sinistral portal hypertension: presentation, radiological findings, and treatment options – a case report. *J Radiol Case Rep*. 2010;4(10):14-20.

11   **Answer C.**   This finding can fool even experienced radiologists. The high-attenuation intravenous tubular structure in the left central veins represents a calcified fibrin sheath that formed on a longstanding central venous catheter that is no longer present. The sheath is slightly irregular with varying degrees of calcification. Compare its appearance with the known right-chest central venous catheter. A true catheter (or catheter fragment) has perfectly smooth walls and uniform attenuation. Fibrin sheath formation is common and has some association with underlying venous thrombosis. The sheaths are calcified approximately 50% of the time. Its mere presence without accompanying findings does not warrant any additional treatment. Rarely, the sheaths can become superinfected producing central venous and cardiac vegetations.

References: Krausz DJ, Fisher JS, Rosen G, et al. Retained fibrin sheaths: chest computed tomography findings and clinical associations. *J Thorac Imaging*. 2014;29(2):118-124.

Tang S, Beigel R, Arsanjani R, Larson B, Luthringer D, Siegel R. Infective endovascular fibrin sheath vegetations—a new cause of bacteremia detected by transesophageal echocardiogram. *Am J Med*. 2015;128(9):1029-1038.

12   **Answer C.**   Abdominal pain is one of the most common symptoms that undergoes radiologic evaluation with CT. In this example, it is important to digest the images and work through the findings to pinpoint the diagnosis. The images are obtained in the portal venous phase, with roughly equivalent contrast opacification of the arterial tree, portal venous system, and systemic veins. On the upper left image, all 3 hepatic veins are present and enhancing, indicating patency (excluding choice A). On the upper right image, there is ascites and the proximal SMA courses immediately posterior to the splenic vein as it joins the SMV at the portosplenic confluence. Both the splenic vein and SMA are enhancing. On the bottom left image, which is the most caudal (compare liver and kidneys), a round enhancing structure is seen in the mid abdomen. Note the similar diameter to the SMA at its origin. The SMV should also be present and immediately to the right of the SMA.

Instead, there is a much larger round low-attenuation structure representing the acutely thrombosed SMV. On the more cephalad image, there is partial visualization of a filling defect at the portosplenic confluence, further supporting the diagnosis acute mesenteric ischemia from SMV thrombosis. Extensive bowel wall thickening and ascites are associated findings. The mainstay of treatment is anticoagulation and close observation for complications. Irreversible bowel ischemia, intractable pain, and rapid development of varices can ensue prompting more aggressive surgical and endovascular treatments (beyond the scope of this book, see references). Notably, *Clostridium difficile* colitis shares many similarities to mesenteric venous thrombosis with colonic wall thickening and nodularity, ascites, and pericolonic stranding being the most common imaging features. With SMV thrombosis, if one misses the filling defect, the distribution of bowel wall thickening (large and small bowel) should be a clue that you are not dealing with just a colitis.

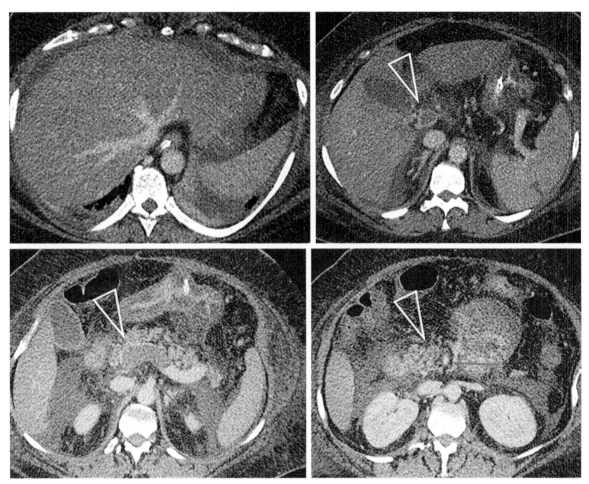

Figure 12-1 Companion case of a 55-year-old female presenting with abdominal pain and fever. Acute thrombus (white arrows) is present in the main portal vein, portosplenic confluence, and superior mesenteric vein (SMV). The superior mesenteric artery (SMA) is identified with red arrows. There are associated ascites and bowel wall thickening.

References: Furukawa A, Kanasaki S, Kono N, et al. CT diagnosis of acute mesenteric ischemia from various causes. *AJR Am J Roentgenol.* 2009;192(2):408-416.

Kim HS, Patra A, Khan J, Arepally A, Streiff MB. Transhepatic catheter-directed thrombectomy and thrombolysis of acute superior mesenteric venous thrombosis. *J Vasc Interv Radiol.* 2005;16(12):1685-1691.

Liu FY, Wang MQ, Fan QS, Duan F, Wang ZJ, Song P. Interventional treatment for symptomatic acute-subacute portal and superior mesenteric vein thrombosis. *World J Gastroenterol.* 2009;15(40):5028-5034.

13   Answer C.   Knowing the characteristic imaging features of liver masses is crucial to making an accurate diagnosis. In this example, 2 MRI images are presented and identified as contrast-enhanced T1 FS. The left image is in the arterial phase (note the intensity of the aorta and heterogeneous perfusion of the spleen), and right image is more delayed (note the homogenous parenchymal enhancement and intensity of the IVC and hepatic veins). There is an arterially enhancing mass in segment 4 of the liver with washout and capsular enhancement on the delayed phase. With the given history of cirrhosis, this is diagnostic for HCC, and a biopsy is not necessary. Additional features that would also support this diagnosis include interval growth, mild to moderate T2 hyperintensity, and diffusion restriction. Intrahepatic cholangiocarcinoma often presents with an irregular mass that demonstrates delayed enhancement and may be accompanied by capsular retraction and peripheral biliary dilatation. Metastases in the liver that are hypervascular most commonly come from neuroendocrine tumors of bowel or pancreas, thyroid carcinoma, renal cell carcinoma, melanoma, or choriocarcinoma. They are most commonly multiple in number and are not associated with an underlying diagnosis of cirrhosis. Hemangioma in the liver classically demonstrates discontinuous peripheral nodular enhancement with centripetal filling over time.

References: Santillan C, Fowler K, Kono Y, Chernyak V. LI-RADS major features: CT, MRI with extracellular agents, and MRI with hepatobiliary agents. *Abdom Radiol (NY)*. 2018;43(1):75-81.

Silva AC, Evans JM, Mccullough AE, Jatoi MA, Vargas HE, Hara AK. MR imaging of hypervascular liver masses: a review of current techniques. *Radiographics*. 2009;29(2):385-402.

14   Answer B.   Many interventionalists perform CECT immediately after thermal ablation of hepatic tumors. This is done to evaluate the ablation zone and margin as well as to look for complications. Heterogeneously attenuating debris, gas, and ill-defined borders are commonly seen at the site of ablation when imaged immediately afterward. There should not be enhancing tissue within the ablation zone, unless there is residual tumor present. As time progresses, a rim of hyperemia characterized by thin peripheral enhancement may develop at the margin of the ablation and last a few months. If the peripheral enhancement enlarges over time or is irregular or nodular, local tumor progression should be considered. Several months after the ablation, the zone shrinks progressively and becomes more well defined and homogenously hypoattenuating. There may be adjacent capsular retraction, dystrophic calcifications, and dilated biliary radicals.

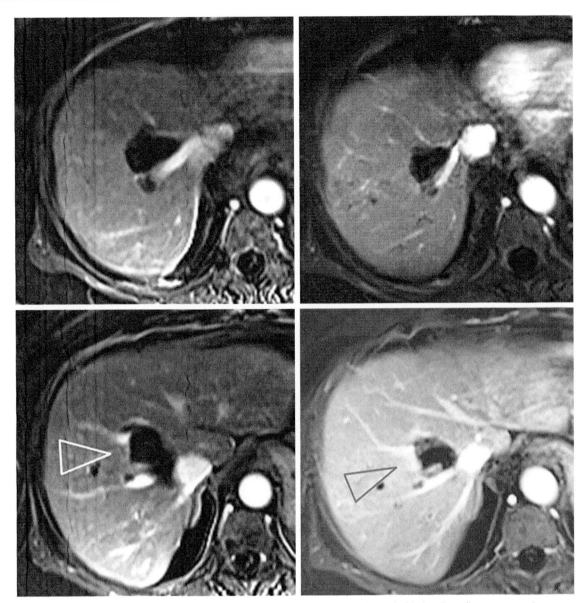

Figure 14-1 Local tumor progression following microwave thermal ablation for solitary metastasis in the liver. Contrast-enhanced T1 FS MRI images at 3 months (left images) show a well-defined ablation zone with thin peripheral enhancement (white arrow). Follow-up study at 9 months shows expected shrinkage of the ablation zone; however, new nodular enhancement (blue arrow) is present at the margin consistent with local tumor progression. This was treated with repeat ablation.

References: Bouda D, Lagadec M, Alba CG, et al. Imaging review of hepatocellular carcinoma after thermal ablation: the good, the bad, and the ugly. *J Magn Reson Imaging*. 2016;44(5):1070-1090.

Wile GE, Leyendecker JR, Krehbiel KA, Dyer RB, Zagoria RJ. CT and MR imaging after imaging-guided thermal ablation of renal neoplasms. *Radiographics*. 2007;27(2):325-339.

15   **Answer A.** Four sequential axial CECT images and a coronal MIP reconstruction demonstrate a communication between the left portal vein and the left hepatic vein. The liver is otherwise normal in appearance. This is an intrahepatic portosystemic shunt. In the absence of trauma or liver disease, the etiology is uncertain but favored to be congenital and due to persistent embryonic venous anastomoses. In children, they can present with a variety of complications including cholestasis, pulmonary hypertension, hepatopulmonary syndrome, and encephalopathy. There is an association with hepatic tumors as well. Occasionally, patients will make it

into adulthood and the shunt will be discovered incidentally, as in the case example. When symptomatic or causing complications, shunt closure via endovascular or surgical means is indicated. In children, even asymptomatic shunts are considered for closure owing to the long-term risk of complications.

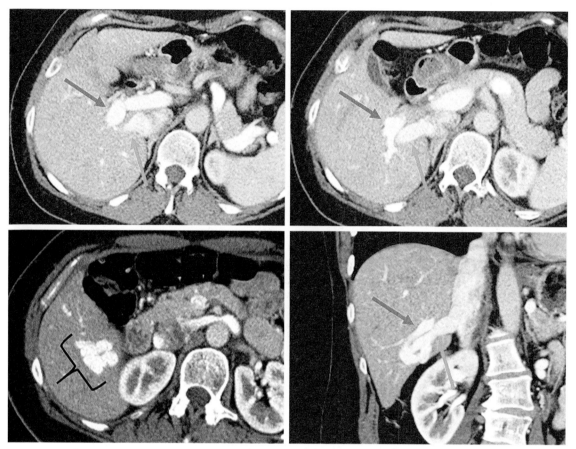

Figure 15-1 Companion case of intrahepatic portosystemic shunt with a connection (bracket) between the right portal vein (red arrows) and the accessory inferior hepatic vein (blue arrows). The connection appears as a tortuous cluster of vessels with dilated feeding and draining veins.

References: Bernard O, Franchi-Abella S, Branchereau S, Pariente D, Gauthier F, Jacquemin E. Congenital portosystemic shunts in children: recognition, evaluation, and management. *Semin Liver Dis.* 2012;32(4):273-287.

Grimaldi C, Monti L, Falappa P, D'Ambrosio G, Manca A, De Ville de Goyet J. Congenital intrahepatic portohepatic shunt managed by interventional radiologic occlusion: a case report and literature review. *J Pediatr Surg.* 2012;47(2):e27-e31.

Remer EM, Motta-Ramirez GA, Henderson JM. Imaging findings in incidental intrahepatic portal venous shunts. *AJR Am J Roentgenol.* 2007;188(2):W162-W167.

16   **Answer D.**   The images show extensive mediastinal hemorrhage with active extravasation anteriorly. The arrows point to a dense linear structure interposed between the descending thoracic aorta and the left pulmonary artery. This structure is a calcified ligamentum arteriosum. Although precontrast images are helpful, they are unnecessary. It is important to recognize this common finding with no clinical implications, as well as the ductus diverticulum, which can masquerade as aortic injury.

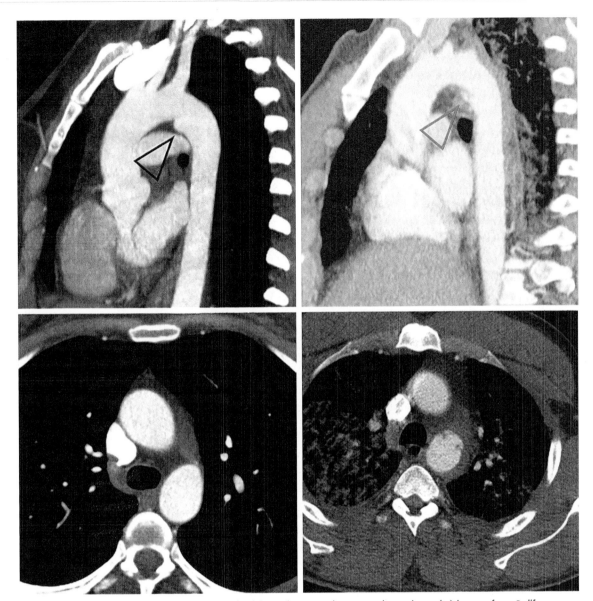

Figure 16-1 Sagittal oblique and axial CTA (computed tomography angiography) images from 2 different patients demonstrating a ductus diverticulum (black arrowhead, left images) and acute traumatic aortic injury (red arrowhead, right images). Both entities are best evaluated in multiple planes given their similarities. The aortic isthmus is the site of up to 90% of visualized traumatic aortic injuries on CT.

References: Batra P, Bigoni B, Manning J, et al. Pitfalls in the diagnosis of thoracic aortic dissection at CT angiography. *Radiographics*. 2000;20(2):309-320.

Patel NR, Dick E, Batrick N, Jenkins M, Kashef E. Pearls and pitfalls in imaging of blunt traumatic thoracic aortic injury: a pictorial review. *Br J Radiol*. 2018:20180130.

Wimpfheimer O, Haramati LB, Haramati N. Calcification of the ligamentum arteriosum in adults: CT features. *J Comput Assist Tomogr*. 1996;20(1):34-37.

17 **Answer A.** There is significant variation in the hepatic arterial blood supply. One of the more common variants is a left hepatic artery arising from the left gastric artery. Angiographically the gastric branches of the artery are proximal, followed by a transversely oriented transition of the artery as it travels into the liver to supply the left lobe segments. This portion of the variant artery is always found in the fissure for the ligamentum venosum, which is otherwise empty of vessels. So with just this single image, one knows confidently there is variant hepatic arterial anatomy present.

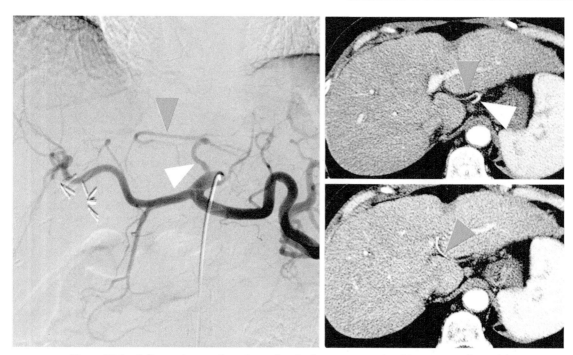

Figure 17-1 Celiac angiogram from the patient in the case example with corresponding axial CTA (computed tomography angiography) images. The celiac artery demonstrates normal branching into the splenic artery, common hepatic artery, and left gastric artery (white arrows). The left gastric artery ascends normally with gastric branches coming off to the patient's left. The artery makes a hairpin turn into a transverse segment that is the replaced left hepatic artery (blue arrows).

Reference: Covey AM, Brody LA, Maluccio MA, Getrajdman GI, Brown KT. Variant hepatic arterial anatomy revisited: digital subtraction angiography performed in 600 patients. *Radiology*. 2002;224(2):542-547.

18   **Answer C.** This is a classic example of Budd-Chiari with characteristic perfusion changes in the liver. To review, Budd-Chiari is hepatic venous outflow obstruction and can be primary (thrombosis or intrinsic venous abnormality) or secondary (extrinsic obstruction or tumor invasion). The hepatic veins and/or IVC may be affected. The clinical presentation may range from mild symptoms to fulminant liver failure, depending on the degree of outflow compromise and hepatic reserve. As the caudate lobe, and sometimes portions of the central right lobe, has separate venous drainage into the IVC, this parenchyma is often spared and will hypertrophy over time. Anticoagulation is the mainstay of early treatment; however, if liver failure progresses, interventions such as hepatic vein recanalization and TIPS may be necessary. In some instances, liver transplant is the only option.

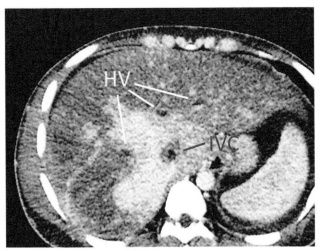

Figure 18-1 A more cephalad contrast-enhanced computed tomography (CECT) image from the case example demonstrates low-attenuation thrombus in the hepatic veins (HVs) and upper segment of the inferior vena cava (IVC). Peripheral hypoenhancement of the parenchyma is present as well.

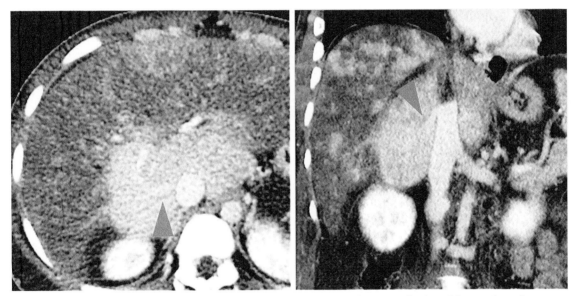

Figure 18-2 Axial and coronal contrast-enhanced computed tomography (CECT) images from the case example with patent hepatic venous branch (orange arrowheads) draining directly to the IVC with associated normal parenchymal enhancement and compensatory hypertrophy on the unaffected liver parenchyma.

Reference: Cura M, Haskal Z, Lopera J. Diagnostic and interventional radiology for Budd-Chiari syndrome. *Radiographics.* 2009;29(3):669-681.

19   **Answer A.**   Many studies have been performed evaluating surveillance ultrasound for TIPS with no consensus as to the frequency and interpretation of the findings. Additionally, some studies were done before the advent of the Viatorr stent graft, which is currently the device of choice. Findings supportive of a TIPS stenosis are elevated peak velocity at a focal point of stenosis (variable thresholds, often >200 cm/s), globally decreased velocity (<40-60 cm/s), and interval changes in velocity and/or direction of portal vein branch flow when compared with a baseline study after TIPS. The direction of flow in the parenchymal portal veins can become hepatofugal after TIPS placement. At follow-up, if the direction changes

to hepatopetal, this can be a sign of dysfunction. Ultimately, as is so often the case in medicine, the clinical picture trumps all. If the duplex study (or patient) shows recurrent ascites (choice A), there is TIPS dysfunction until proven otherwise and portography with intravascular pressure measurements is indicated.

The following case demonstrates the evolution and treatment of TIPS stenosis. A 61-year-old male with recurrent variceal bleeds despite multiple endoscopic band ligation undergoes an uneventful TIPS and variceal coil embolization procedure. The portosystemic gradient drops from 21 to 6 mmHg. Surveillance TIPS ultrasound studies at 6 and 12 months demonstrate a drop in velocity in the TIPS from 128 to 41 cm/s. This was interpreted as concerning for TIPS stenosis. Unfortunately, this was not acted upon and the patient presented with massive hematemesis from variceal rupture in the middle of the night. TIPS venogram (Figure 19-1) shows stenosis at the hepatic venous end of the TIPS with recanalized gastroesophageal varices. This was successfully treated with stent extension into the hepatic vein with adjunctive coil embolization of the recanalized varices.

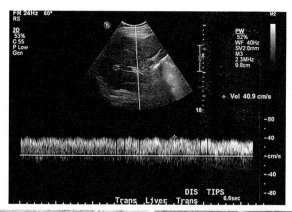

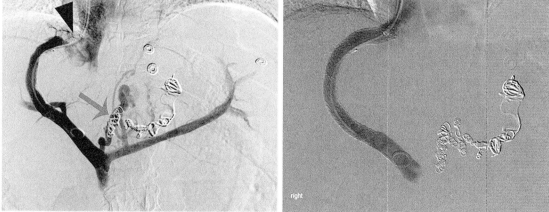

Figure 19-1   TIPS US (transjugular intrahepatic portosystemic shunt ultrasound) study at 12 months with diminished flow in the stent (41 cm/s). TIPS venogram (bottom left) after presentation with variceal rupture shows near-occlusive stenosis at the hepatic vein end of the TIPS (black arrowhead) with retrograde filling of the splenic vein, superior mesenteric vein, and previously coiled variceal complex arising from the left gastric vein (orange arrow). After stent extension across the stenosis with additional coil embolization (bottom right), there is antegrade flow in the TIPS, no residual stenosis, and no filling of the varices.

References: Carr CE, Tuite CM, Soulen MC, et al. Role of ultrasound surveillance of transjugular intrahepatic portosystemic shunts in the covered stent era. *J Vasc Interv Radiol*. 2006;17(8):1297-1305.

Darcy M. Evaluation and management of transjugular intrahepatic portosystemic shunts. *AJR Am J Roentgenol*. 2012;199(4):730-736.

20   **Answer C.**   The images demonstrate a TIPS that has been reduced or constrained. If a TIPS is shunting too much portal venous blood to the systemic veins, it can lead to several problems, the most common of which is encephalopathy. If this is refractory to medical management, a reduction can be performed to alleviate the encephalopathy, with several techniques available. In this case, the reduction technique used 2 additional stents within the preexisting TIPS. A longer self-expanding covered stent is positioned in parallel with a shorter balloon-expandable stent. When the covered stent is deployed, the balloon-expandable stent is trapped between it and the TIPS. The balloon-expandable stent is then deployed. This extrinsically compresses the covered stent narrowing the lumen of the TIPS and reducing its flow.

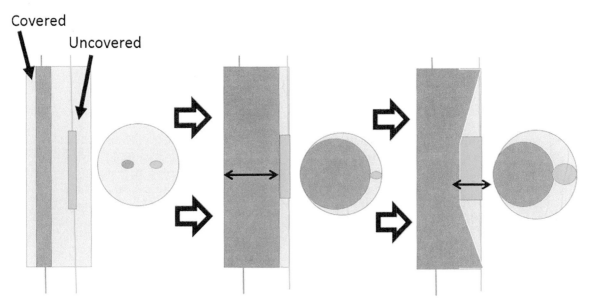

Figure 20-1   Diagrammatic representation of TIPS (transjugular intrahepatic portosystemic shunt) reduction using parallel stent technique. The uncovered balloon-expandable stent can be dilated to various diameters, allowing the operator to customize the degree of TIPS narrowing.

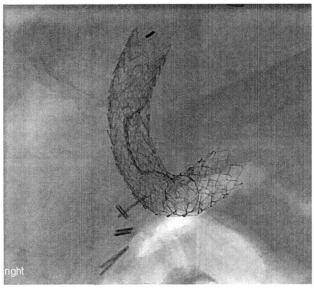

Figure 20-2   Fluoroscopic image of TIPS after reduction using the parallel stent technique.

Reference: Madoff DC, Wallace MJ. Reduced stents and stent-grafts for the management of hepatic encephalopathy after transjugular intrahepatic portosystemic shunt creation. *Semin Intervent Radiol.* 2005;22(4):316-328.

21   Answer C.   Of course physical examiantion is critical in evaluating a patient for vertebroplasty. The best candidate would have point tenderness over the fracture with worsening pain upon axial loading. The osteoporotic patient may certainly have multiple fractures in their lifetime as seen in the case example. With only CT or X-ray, one could get fooled into treating an old quiescent lesion. MRI or even a bone scan will aid in determining which vertebral bodies have acute fractures and thus likely to be symptomatic. In this case, only T11 has increased signal in T2 STIR sequence. There is a minimal amount of retropulsion, but no cord compromise and vertebroplasty is appropriate (choice C). The fractures at T6 and T7 show no bony edema on the MRI and are not likely to be the source of the current symptoms. When it is time for the procedure, ensure you are treating the correct level, as "wrong location" is a surefire way to find legal trouble.

Reference: Baerlocher MO, Saad WE, Dariushnia S, et al. Quality improvement guidelines for percutaneous vertebroplasty. *J Vasc Interv Radiol.* 2014;25(2):165-170.

22   Answer B.   The patient in the case example has undergone aortobifemoral bypass for aortoiliac arterial occlusive disease. There was a previous iliac arterial endovascular intervention with stenting that failed. The curvilinear calcifications surrounding the stent suggest that this is not a venous structure, but rather arterial. With close inspection, the unopacified iliac vein is present as a separate structure adjacent to the psoas muscle. The internal iliac distribution structures are more posteriorly located in the pelvis. The bypass limb parallels the native vessels and can often be delineated by its near-perfect round appearance and absence of atherosclerotic disease. The proximal bypass anastomosis to the aorta can be either end-to-end or end-to-side. In an end-to-side, there can be residual antegrade flow to the native arteries downstream. The distal anastomosis at the inguinal ligament is typically end-to-side which can allow for retrograde filling of the external iliac arteries to potentially supply the internal iliac distribution.

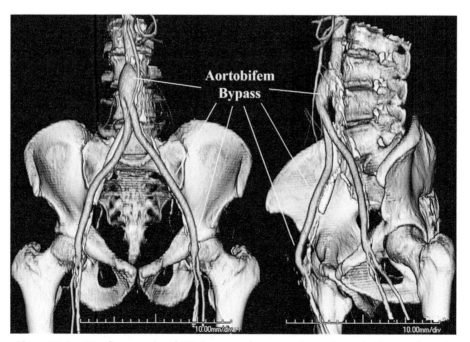

Figure 22-1   3D volume rendered CTA (computed tomography angiography) images from the case example show the proximal and distal end-to-side anastomoses. On the oblique image, the residual diseased infrarenal aorta is patent beyond the anastomosis.

Reference: Dorigo W, Piffaretti G, Benedetto F, et al. A comparison between aortobifemoral bypass and aortoiliac kissing stents in patients with complex aortoiliac obstructive disease. *J Vasc Surg.* 2017;65(1):99-107.

23   **Answer A.**   The pretreatment CECT image demonstrates a hypervascular tumor in the right hepatic dome. On the CT image 4 months later, the lesion is now extremely dense, well beyond what is expected with water soluble iodinated contrast enhancement. The MRI image shows no residual tumoral enhancement. The appearance change on CT is from retained lipiodol. The patient has undergone conventional transarterial chemoembolization (cTACE) with an emulsification of chemotherapy and lipiodol. The lipiodol is an oily iodinated contrast agent which helps create the chemotherapy suspension, provides some degree of arterial embolization, and delineates the distribution and retention of the emulsion in the target tumor through its X-ray attenuation. The retained lipiodol can cause streak artifact on CT, making residual tumor enhancement difficult to see. The lipiodol does not affect the MRI signal, making this a better modality to evaluate for residual disease, recurrent disease, and/or local tumor progression. Of note, transarterial glue (nBCA) embolization could have a similar appearance, as glue is often diluted with lipiodol. However, one would expect a glue cast in the feeding arteries of the tumor, and this option does not make sense as a therapeutic strategy for the pathology.

Reference: Lim HS, Jeong YY, Kang HK, Kim JK, Park JG. Imaging features of hepatocellular carcinoma after transcatheter arterial chemoembolization and radiofrequency ablation. *AJR Am J Roentgenol.* 2006;187(4):W341-W349.

24   **Answer C.**   The CECT images demonstrate the expected changes after thermal ablation. The tumor, a soft tissue attenuation lesion on the pretreatment scan, is replaced by a larger well-circumscribed low-attenuation area on the initial 4 month follow-up study. This represents the zone of ablation. Over time, the zone shrinks in size producing a relative volume loss in that region of the liver. Notice how the smaller cyst appears to move towards the IVC over time. Finally, there is peripheral biliary dilatation, best seen on the 3 year follow-up study, which is an occasionally seen consequence from focal biliary injury after thermal ablation. While radioembolization also produces volume loss, the area affected corresponds to the arterial distribution of the microspheres, whether lobar or sublobar. Lesional necrosis, perilesional edema, biliary injury, and fibrosis can also be seen. Typically the area of lesional necrosis following Y90 is minimally bigger or smaller than the lesion itself, whereas the zone of ablation is often 1 to 2 cm greater (0.5-1 cm circumferential margin) in diameter than the target lesion.

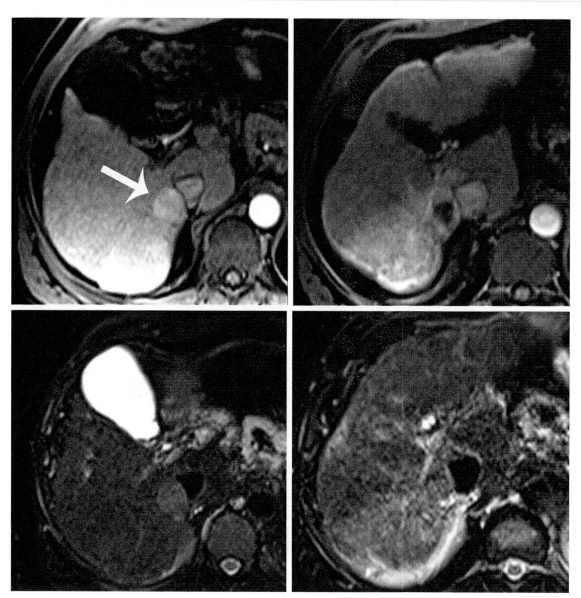

Figure 24-1   Typical findings on CEMRI after segmental radioembolization. Pretreatment images on the left (top, T1FS + Gd; bottom, T2FS) show a 2.5 cm hypervascular tumor (arrow) adjacent to the inferior vena cava (IVC). On the right, images obtained 3 months following treatment (top, T1FS + Gd; bottom, T2FS) show shrinkage of the lesion with no tumoral enhancement. There is geographic hyperenhancement in the posterior right lobe with associated increased T2 signal corresponding the arterial distribution of the microspheres. These changes reflect inflammation and hyperemia from radiation effect. Over time, there will be parenchymal atrophy and often fibrosis in the treatment zone.

References: Bouda D, Lagadec M, Alba CG, et al. Imaging review of hepatocellular carcinoma after thermal ablation: the good, the bad, and the ugly. *J Magn Reson Imaging*. 2016;44(5):1070-1090.

Kallini JR, Miller FH, Gabr A, Salem R, Lewandowski RJ. Hepatic imaging following intra-arterial embolotherapy. *Abdom Radiol (NY)*. 2016;41(4):600-616.

Sainani NI, Gervais DA, Mueller PR, Arellano RS. Imaging after percutaneous radiofrequency ablation of hepatic tumors: part 1, normal findings. *AJR Am J Roentgenol*. 2013;200(1):184-193.

Sainani NI, Gervais DA, Mueller PR, Arellano RS. Imaging after percutaneous radiofrequency ablation of hepatic tumors: part 2, abnormal findings. *AJR Am J Roentgenol*. 2013;200(1):194-204.

25   **Answer C.**   The detectable rate of bleeding for tagged RBC scan is reportedly as low as 0.05 to 0.1 mL/min. The detectable rate of bleeding for CTA is 0.3 to 0.5 mL/min, which is slightly better than catheter angiography (0.5-1.0 mL/min). The use of CTA for the detection of GI bleeding has greatly increased in the past decade. The technique most commonly uses a precontrast phase, followed by intravenous contrast administration with early and delayed phase imaging. No oral contrast should be given. New high-attenuation contrast accumulating in the bowel and increasing on the delayed phase constitutes a positive study. Both upper and lower tract bleeding can be pinpointed, and sometimes the underlying cause (large ulcer, mass, etc,) and source artery can be delineated. The strengths of this noninvasive study include high sensitivity, specificity, accuracy, and positive and negative predictive values.

References: Currie GM, Kiat H, Wheat JM. Scintigraphic evaluation of acute lower gastrointestinal hemorrhage: current status and future directions. *J Clin Gastroenterol*. 2011;45(2):92-99.

García-Blázquez V, Vicente-Bártulos A, Olavarria-Delgado A, et al. Accuracy of CT angiography in the diagnosis of acute gastrointestinal bleeding: systematic review and meta-analysis. *Eur Radiol*. 2013;23(5):1181-1190.

Kennedy DW, Laing CJ, Tseng LH, Rosenblum DI, Tamarkin SW. Detection of active gastrointestinal hemorrhage with CT angiography: a 4(1/2)-year retrospective review. *J Vasc Interv Radiol*. 2010;21(6):848-855.

Martí M, Artigas JM, Garzón G, Alvarez-Sala R, Soto JA. Acute lower intestinal bleeding: feasibility and diagnostic performance of CT angiography. *Radiology*. 2012;262(1):109-116.

26   **Answer A.**   When patients present with a history and examination concerning for PAD, the diagnosis is often first established with a noninvasive arterial examination. At a minimum, this includes Doppler assessment of the pedals arteries and a calculation of the ABI. Like any blood pressure evaluation, the test relies on cuff occlusion of the arteries just above the level of the ankle and Doppler assessment of the return of signal as the cuff is deflated. Extensive arterial wall calcification can diminish the compressibility of the arteries, making the ABI unreliable. If present throughout the arterial tree, which is often the case in diabetics and those with end-stage renal disease, the calcification can be detrimental to other tests. The 3 noninvasive tests often performed to further evaluate lower extremity PAD are an arterial duplex, MRA, and CTA. Arterial duplex can be adversely affected as the calcium prevents acoustic penetration and causes shadowing, precluding accurate evaluation of stenotic and occlusive segments. Though generally an acceptable option, CTA is limited by blooming artifact which can completely obscure arterial pathology in large and especially small arteries. MRA with intravenous gadolinium enhancement is unaffected by arterial wall calcification and provides an excellent assessment in this patient population.

Reference: Pollak AW, Norton PT, Kramer CM. Multimodality imaging of lower extremity peripheral arterial disease: current role and future directions. *Circ Cardiovasc Imaging*. 2012;5(6):797-807.

27   **Answer D.**   This case illustrates an important anatomic variant of the tibial arterial tree. A dominant peroneal artery or peroneal magnus can have a few different appearances. In the most extreme form of dominance, the peroneal artery is the sole tibial artery that continues on below the knee and the anterior and posterior tibial arteries are aplastic or significantly hypoplastic. In this scenario, the dominant peroneal artery at the ankle gives off anterior and medial branches which reconstitute the dorsalis pedis (DP) and posterior tibial (PT) arteries, respectively, into the foot. While only 1 tibial artery is present in the calf, there are palpable DP and PT pulses at the foot! Less severe variants exist, as in this case, where the anterior tibial artery is patent but tapers off in caliber as it enters the foot along the dorsal aspect. The tibioperoneal trunk directly forms the peroneal artery, and there is no visible posterior tibial artery until just above the ankle where the dominant peroneal artery makes a sharp course medially and continues on as the PT into the foot. With peroneal artery dominance, if the vessel is harvested as part of a fibular flap, foot ischemia can develop.

Reference: Lohan DG, Tomasian A, Krishnam M, Jonnala P, Blackwell KE, Finn JP. MR angiography of lower extremities at 3 T: presurgical planning of fibular free flap transfer for facial reconstruction. *AJR Am J Roentgenol.* 2008;190(3):770-776.

28   **Answer A.**   The images presented do not offer much to help characterize the malformation. However, there is an artifact that is key to making the diagnosis off of these 2 images alone. Both the axial and coronal T1 FS + Gd images demonstrate left to right artifact associated with an oval abnormality in the forearm musculature. This is pulsation or motion artifact, which occurs across the entire field of view and vaguely matches the source structure. The artifact manifests as ghosting in the phase-encoded direction.

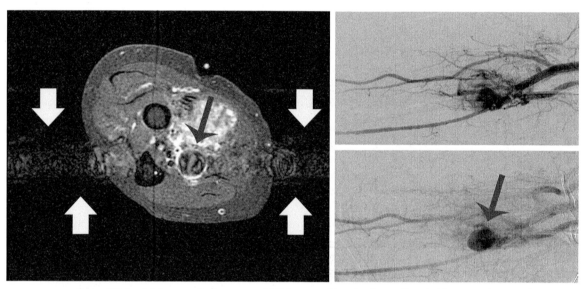

Figure 28-1   Axial magnetic resonance (MR) image with pulsation artifact (white arrows) created by a venous aneurysm (gray arrow) within an arteriovenous malformation. Catheter angiography from the brachial artery (top image, early phase; bottom image, late phase) demonstrates the arteriovenous malformation characterized by numerous tortuous and enlarged feeding arteries, a hypervascular nidus with associated venous aneurysm, and early draining veins. Low-flow anomalies such as venous or lymphatic malformations would not produce motion artifact, as there is no arterial inflow to cause pulsatility.

References: Flors L, Leiva-Salinas C, Maged IM, et al. MR imaging of soft-tissue vascular malformations: diagnosis, classification, and therapy follow-up. *Radiographics.* 2011;31(5):1321-1340.

Morelli JN, Runge VM, Ai F, et al. An image-based approach to understanding the physics of MR artifacts. *Radiographics.* 2011;31(3):849-866.

29   **Answer A.**   The spectral Doppler ultrasound image demonstrates a tardus et parvus waveform in the left hepatic artery. There is prolonged time to peak of the systolic upstroke (tardus), and the peak is blunted and smaller than expected (parvus). This diagnosis is often subjectively made, but some objective guidelines exist. The time to peak is abnormal if >70 ms, and the resistive index (RI) is abnormal if <0.55 (RI is 0.33 in this case). When present, this waveform is consistent with

an upstream arterial stenosis. Typically, this will be at an operative site such as the arterial anastomosis in the posttransplant patient. Catheter angiography confirmed a near-occlusive stenosis of the transplant hepatic artery anastomosis. Following treatment with balloon angioplasty, there was restoration of a normal arterial wave-form on follow-up ultrasound evaluation.

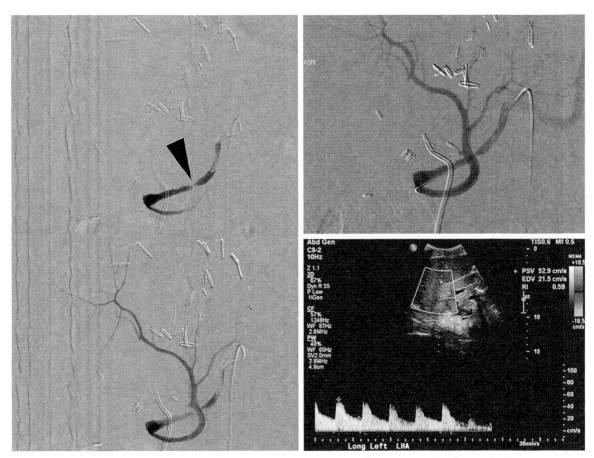

Figure 29-1 Catheter angiography from the case example shows a severe focal stenosis (arrow-head) at the transplant hepatic arterial anastomosis. Following angioplasty (right images), there is minimal residual stenosis, overall improved hepatic arterial flow, and restoration of the normal high-resistance arterial waveform of the hepatic artery.

References: Mcnaughton DA, Abu-Yousef MM. Doppler US of the liver made simple. *Radiographics.* 2011;31(1):161-188.

Saad WE, Davies MG, Sahler L, et al. Hepatic artery stenosis in liver transplant recipients: primary treatment with percutaneous transluminal angioplasty. *J Vasc Interv Radiol.* 2005;16(6):795-805.

30 **Answer C.** A consensus guideline was published in the radiology literature in 2003 regarding interpretation of carotid ultrasound for atherosclerotic narrowing. Per the ABR study guide, knowledge of these criteria is recommended. Of note, not all institutions use these criteria and parameters specific to a vascular laboratory may be used in practice.

TABLE 30-1   Ultrasound Criteria for the Evaluation of Internal Carotid Artery Stenosis

Stenosis	ICA PSV (cm/s)	Visualized Plaque	ICA/CCA PSV Ratio	ICA EDV (cm/s)
None	<125	None	<2	<40
<50%	<125	<50%	<2	<40
50%-69%	125-230	>50%	2-4	40-100
>70%	>230	>50%	>4	>100
Nearly occluded	Abnormal	Yes		
Occluded	No flow	No lumen		

Adapted from Grant EG, Benson CB, Moneta GL, et al. Carotid artery stenosis: gray-scale and doppler US diagnosis–Society of Radiologists in Ultrasound Consensus Conference. *Radiology.* 2003;229(2):340-346.
CCA, common carotid crtery; EDV, end-diastolic velocity; ICA, internal carotid Artery; PSV, peak systolic velocity.

References: Grant EG, Benson CB, Moneta GL, et al. Carotid artery stenosis: gray-scale and Doppler US diagnosis–Society of Radiologists in Ultrasound Consensus Conference. *Radiology.* 2003;229(2):340-346.

Tahmasebpour HR, Buckley AR, Cooperberg PL, Fix CH. Sonographic examination of the carotid arteries. *Radiographics.* 2005;25(6):1561-1575.

31   **Answer C.**   There are several different yet complementary methods commonly used to evaluate the lower extremity arterial system for stenotic and/or occlusive disease. Beginning with the simplest, the ABI is a foundational piece of information. One uses a sphygmomanometer to compress a segment of anatomy while assessing the arterial Doppler signal just downstream. As the cuff is deflated, the arterial signal returns and the systolic pressure is recorded. At the ankle, both the posterior tibial and dorsalis pedis arteries are evaluated and compared with the brachial. The larger of the 2 ankle pressures is traditionally used for the ABI. Although somewhat arbitrary, a value of <0.5 is considered severe disease, 0.5 to 0.7 is moderate disease, 0.71 to 0.9 is mild disease, and 0.91 to 1.1 is normal. This process can be repeated at multiple segments (aka segmental pressures) of the leg as shown here with high thigh, low thigh, and calf. A significant drop in pressure (typically >20 mmHg) across an arterial segment signifies underlying flow-limiting disease.

The Doppler waveform of a specific arterial segment can be evaluated as well. A normal lower extremity arterial waveform has a sharp systolic upstroke, a fall below the baseline on diastole, and a smaller amplitude upstroke before the next beat of systole. If there is an upstream hemodynamically significant stenosis, the waveform will be blunted with a lower amplitude and rounded peak. The normal triphasic signal will become biphasic and, ultimately, monophasic with more significant obstruction.

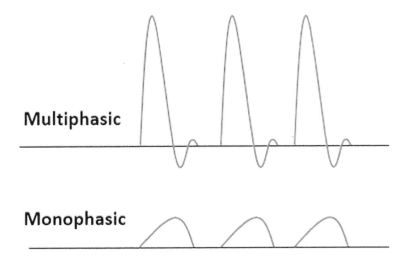

Yet another tool is pulse volume recording (PVR or volume pulse recording VPR). Blood pressure cuffs are positioned at several sites on the leg. The arterial pulse of blood changes the volume of the tissue which can be recorded by the cuffs, resulting in a waveform.

In the case example, the systolic pressure at each level is noted (black number) with corresponding ratio (blue number) to the brachial systolic pressure. In the right lower extremity, the ABI is 0.65 consistent with moderate disease. There is a significant drop in pressure between the upper and lower thigh cuffs from 138 to 89 mmHg. The common femoral Doppler signal is multiphasic, whereas the popliteal and pedal signals are more monophasic. The VPR changes significantly from the high thigh through the calf with loss of amplitude, a more rounded peak, and loss of the normal dicrotic notch. Overall, the information provided by the study is most consistent with pathology present in the right thigh, corresponding to the SFA distribution. The left lower extremity shows essentially normal perfusion for comparison.

Reference: Sibley RC, Reis SP, Macfarlane JJ, Reddick MA, Kalva SP, Sutphin PD. Noninvasive physiologic vascular studies: a guide to diagnosing peripheral arterial disease. *Radiographics*. 2017;37(1):346-357.

32   **Answer A.**   The axial CECT images show an area of lobulated enhancement in the duodenal wall on the portal venous phase suspicious for a vascular abnormality. The phase of imaging suggests a venous source and an outflow vein leading directly to the IVC is present. On the coronal image, the main portal vein is also connected to the abnormal duodenal enhancement. Given the history of cirrhosis and GI bleeding, varices should be considered. Although the majority of varices arising in the setting of portal hypertension occur in the esophagus and stomach, ectopic varices do occur, including duodenal (seen here), small bowel, colonic, and rectal. Other sites include surgical stomas and rarely the gallbladder and pelvic organs. Treatment options mainly include medical management of portal hypertension, endoscopic interventions, and endovascular procedures. Ectopic varices are often overlooked on CTA performed for bleeding given their venous enhancement pattern, atypical location, and lack of bright contrast extravasation. The main causes of variceal formation are generalized portal hypertension (think cirrhosis) and/or

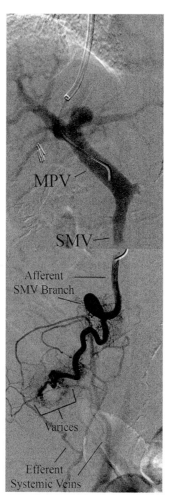

Figure 32-1 Companion case of stomal varices in a patient with cirrhosis, portal hypertension, and an end ileostomy in the right lower quadrant. TIPS (transjugular intrahepatic portosystemic shunt) style access to the portal venous system is obtained with portal venogram show no evidence of obstruction. The portosystemic gradient measures 15 mmHg. Selective catheterization of a superior mesenteric vein (SMV) branch demonstrates reversed flow toward the stoma with circular variceal complex, which was visible on examination. Drainage is back through body wall collaterals to the right common femoral vein (portosystemic shunt physiology). This is subsequently treated with combination of catheter-directed variceal obliteration and placement of a TIPS.

localized portal hypertension (think splenic vein occlusion). Ectopic varices can form with either, and the drainage pathway can be back to the portal venous system (aka portoportal, see question 10) and/or back to the systemic venous system (aka portosystemic shunt) as seen in the case example.

References: Kirby JM, Cho KJ, Midia M. Image-guided intervention in management of complications of portal hypertension: more than TIPS for success. *Radiographics*. 2013;33(5):1473-1496.

Saad WE, Lippert A, Saad NE, Caldwell S. Ectopic varices: anatomical classification, hemodynamic classification, and hemodynamic-based management. *Tech Vasc Interv Radiol*. 2013;16(2):158-175.

33   **Answer D.** Accurately reporting which segment of liver is involved with pathology is critical to surgeons and proceduralists. Anatomically, the liver is frequently described by the Couinaud classification, with 8 segments of relative functional independence. In the case example, the patient is being considered for chemoembolization, and the blood supply to the mass is dictated by its anatomical location.

Given that the tumor is straddling segments IVa and VIII, the arterial supply could be from a branch of the left hepatic artery, right hepatic artery, or both. To further illustrate and evaluate this real world scenario, cone beam CT is performed at the time of the embolization demonstrating the mixed perfusion of the tumor (see Figure 33-1).

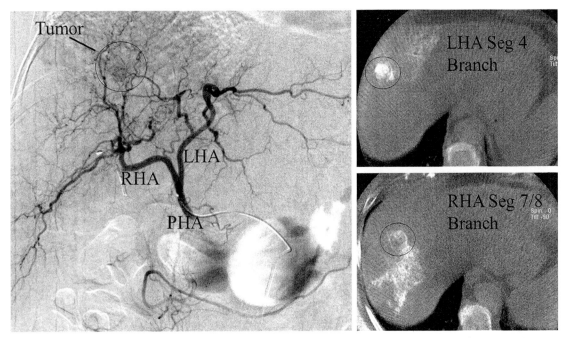

Figure 33-1 Catheter angiography with subsequent cone beam computed tomography (CT) studies from the case example. Cone beam CT performed after contrast is injected into the segment IV artery off the left hepatic, as well as one of the right hepatic artery branches demonstrates that both feed the tumor and will require transarterial treatment for a complete embolization. LHA, left hepatic artery; PHA, proper hepatic artery; RHA, right hepatic artery.

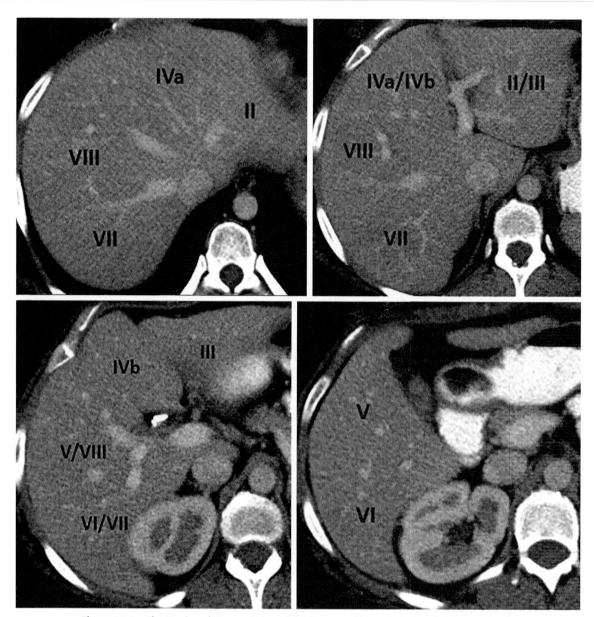

Figure 33-2 The Couinaud segmentation of the liver uses the main left and right portal veins (aka the portal plane) to divide the liver into the superior and inferior segments. Further anterior/ posterior and medial/lateral divisions are made by the right hepatic vein, middle hepatic vein, and falciform ligament. In the superior liver, the right hepatic vein separates segments VII and VIII. The middle hepatic vein separates segments VIII and IVa. An extrapolated line from the falciform ligament separates IVa and II. In the inferior liver, the right lobe segments V and VI are separated by the right hepatic vein. Segments V and IVb are separated by the gallbladder fossa. Segments IVb and III are separated by the falciform ligament. The caudate lobe is segment I.

References: Furuta T, Maeda E, Akai H, et al. Hepatic segments and vasculature: projecting CT anatomy onto angiograms. *Radiographics*. 2009;29(7):e37.

Van Leeuwen MS, Noordzij J, Fernandez MA, Hennipman A, Feldberg MA, Dillon EH. Portal venous and segmental anatomy of the right hemiliver: observations based on three-dimensional spiral CT renderings. *AJR Am J Roentgenol*. 1994;163(6):1395-1404.

34   Answer A.   An LMS is the most common primary tumor of the IVC, accounting for roughly 95% of cases. LMS arising from the vasculature only represents 2% of all LMS and 0.5% of all soft tissue sarcomas. Although malignant, they tend to be slow growing, which lends itself to a delayed diagnosis, at which point it may not be treatable. An LMS of the IVC can metastasize to the lung, liver, and occasionally bone and brain. Tumor growth is intraluminal 5%, extraluminal 62%, and both intra- and extraluminal 33% of the time. When caval tumor pathology is encountered, one must keep in mind the possibility of tumor thrombus, with the kidney, liver, and adrenal gland as potential primary sources. Angiosarcoma can occur in any part of the body, often in the skin, breast, and liver, and is a fairly aggressive tumor with frequent metastases. Angiomyolipoma is a benign lesion most commonly found in the kidney made up of vascular, smooth muscle, and fat components.

References: Gohrbandt AE, Hansen T, Ell C, Heinrich SS, Lang H. Portal vein leiomyosarcoma: a case report and review of the literature. *BMC Surg.* 2016;16(1):60.

Tameo MN, Calligaro KD, Antin L, Dougherty MJ. Primary leiomyosarcoma of the inferior vena cava: reports of infrarenal and suprahepatic caval involvement. *J Vasc Surg.* 2010;51(1):221-224.

35   Answer A.   Evaluating dissections of the abdominal aorta can be challenging. One should report on the true and false lumen relationships, involvement of branch vessels, extent of the dissection, and complications such as end organ ischemia and aneurysmal degeneration. In this example, single-phase imaging in the arterial phase shows the celiac artery is perfused by the true lumen. Features supporting that conclusion include delayed opacification of the false lumen, internally dis- placed intimal calcifications, and acute angle of the false lumen outer wall with the intimal flap (aka beak sign). While the left kidney appears to have no enhancement concerning for ischemia/infarction, the studied is limited by single-phase technique creating a pitfall of imaging diagnosis. Delayed phase images show a patent false lumen with enhancement of the left kidney. At the distal extent of the dissection, the true and false lumens may reconnect with adequate perfusion to the lower extremities. In this patient, a right to left femoral-femoral bypass had been per- formed, as the left external iliac artery was occluded as a result of the dissection.

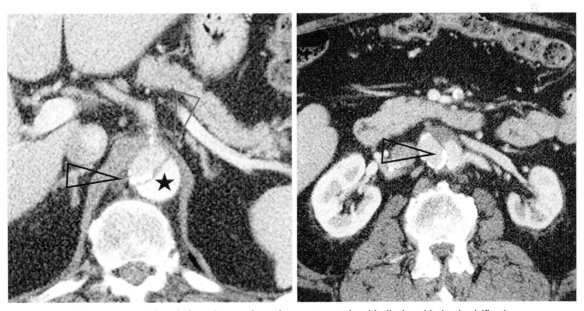

Figure 35-1   Delayed phase images from the case example with displaced intimal calcifications delineating the true lumen (black arrow). False lumen features include delayed enhancement (star) and beak sign (red arrow). Right image shows near-symmetric enhancement of the kidneys.

Reference: Mcmahon MA, Squirrell CA. Multidetector CT of aortic dissection: apictorial review. *Radiographics*. 2010;30(2):445-460.

36   **Answer D.**   In the open aortic aneurysm repair population, aortoenteric fistula has been reported at 0.6% to 2.0% annual incidence. Clinically, it can present as an infectious process with abdominal pain and sepsis or it can present as a hemorrhagic complication. If there is bleeding, a classic scenario is a small self-limited "herald" bleed (representing mucosal erosion) followed by catastrophic intestinal bleeding once the graft is compromised. The bowel affected is nearly always the duodenum. CT findings include perigraft soft tissue edema, fluid, and ectopic gas. Beyond 3 to 4 weeks postoperative, any perigraft gas is abnormal and should clue one in to infection or fistula. Additional suspicious findings are loss of the fat plane between aortic graft and bowel or pseudoaneurysm formation. The pathology can be evaluated with endoscopy as well.

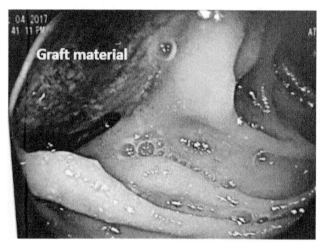

Figure 36-1   Upper endoscopy in the patient from the case example shows exposed graft in the lumen of the duodenum.

A companion case is presented of an even more rare bird (see Figure 36-2). A primary aortoenteric fistula occurs in the absence of prior repair or instrumentation and usually arises in the setting of an aneurysm or other aortic pathology such as a penetrating ulcer.

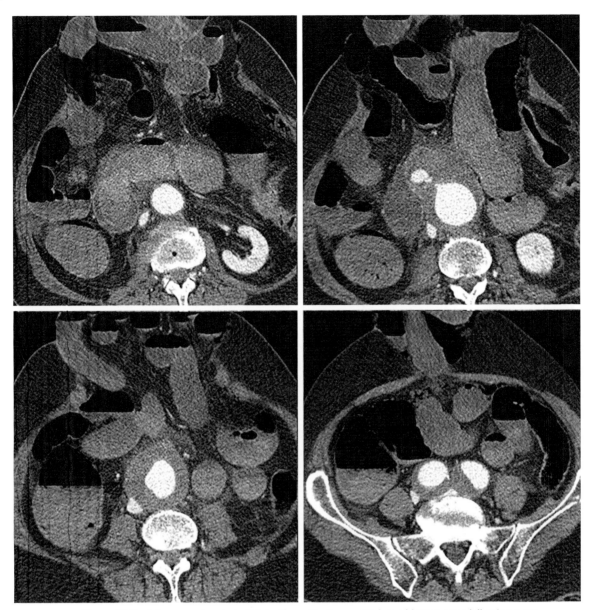

Figure 36-2 Primary aortoenteric fistula. The patient presented as a blunt trauma following a motor vehicle accident. He was profoundly hypotensive and anemic and went straight to the OR (operating room). No internal injuries were discovered; however, a large amount of blood was aspirated from the NG (nasogastric) tube. A computed tomography angiography (CTA) was performed which demonstrated an infrarenal abdominal aortic aneurysm extending into the common iliac arteries. The duodenum was inseparable from the aneurysm sac with a jet of contrast extending from the aortic lumen to the bowel wall. The duodenum and small bowel were distended with acute blood products. The patient was treated with endovascular aortic repair (EVAR) and suppressive antibiotics with planned open reconstruction in the future.

References: Kahlberg A, Rinaldi E, Piffaretti G, et al. Results from the Multicenter Study on Aortoenteric Fistulization After Stent Grafting of the Abdominal Aorta (MAEFISTO). *J Vasc Surg*. 2016;64(2):313-320.e1.

Vu QD, Menias CO, Bhalla S, Peterson C, Wang LL, Balfe DM. Aortoenteric fistulas: CT features and potential mimics. *Radiographics*. 2009;29(1):197-209.

37 **Answer B.** The diagnosis of masses, especially in children, can be challenging as no one wants to miss a malignancy. History, examination, laboratory analysis, and imaging are crucial to noninvasive diagnosis. In the case example, the patient was referred for percutaneous biopsy. The differential diagnosis for this mass is reflected in the answer choices; however, the history and imaging features are classic for a low-flow vascular malformation, specifically a venous malformation, and a biopsy is not indicated.

On the MRI, there is a lobulated mass comprised of cystic spaces with internal septations centered within the posterior cervical musculature that is T2 hyperintense/T1 isointense relative to muscle. There is heterogeneous enhancement that increases over time. Note the lack of flow voids. Ultrasound shows the mass has internal anechoic spaces without demonstrable flow, separated by thin hyperechoic septations. If this were an AVM, we would expect flow voids, neo- and hypervascularity, with early enhancing and enlarged draining veins. Rhabdomyosarcoma is a soft tissue sarcoma that typically presents with rapid growth with MRI features of a soft tissue mass that is often circumscribed but can invade adjacent structures. Intralesional hemorrhage and necrosis can occur. There is typically avid diffuse enhancement of the soft tissue components which are often T2 hyperintense/T1 isointense relative to muscle. Ultrasound can be useful in identifying sarcomas as a soft tissue mass with heterogeneous echogenicity. An abscess or hematoma would have a different clinical presentation and should not demonstrate progressive internal enhancement. With abscess one might expect some perilesional inflammation with peripheral enhancement.

References: Jarrett DY, Ali M, Chaudry G. Imaging of vascular anomalies. *Dermatol Clin.* 2013;31(2):251-266.

Navarro OM. Magnetic resonance imaging of pediatric soft-tissue vascular anomalies. *Pediatr Radiol.* 2016;46(6):891-901.

9

Quality and Safety

1   In preparation for creation of a transjugular intrahepatic portosystemic shunt (TIPS), a wedged carbon dioxide gas (CO_2) hepatoportogram is performed from a right internal jugular vein access. What complication has occurred on the digital subtraction images?

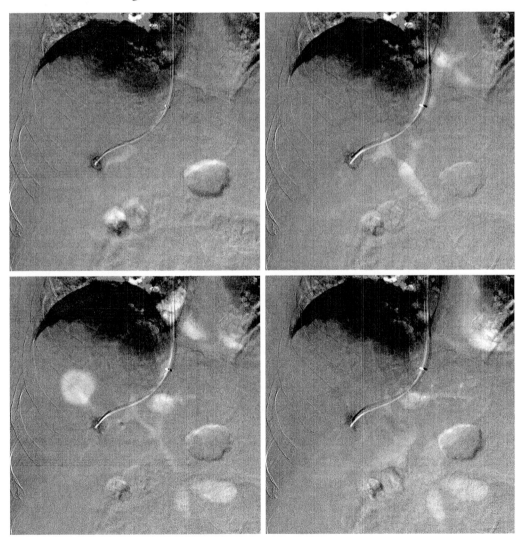

A. Gas embolism to the pulmonary artery
B. Gas laceration of the liver
C. Gas embolism to the hepatic artery
D. Pneumobilia

2   From which catheter position is carbon dioxide gas angiography contraindicated?

A. Left basilic vein
B. Superior mesenteric artery
C. Right subclavian artery
D. Infrarenal abdominal aorta
E. Inferior vena cava (IVC)

3   In which patient population/procedure is a patient most likely to have cardiopulmonary arrest in the interventional radiology (IR) suite?

A. Chronic kidney disease/atrioventricular (AV) graft declot
B. Hepatocellular cancer/chemoembolization
C. Peripheral arterial disease/superficial femoral artery stenting
D. Chronic liver disease/TIPS for ascites

4   A 62-year-old male with chronic biliary obstruction and a capped internal/external biliary drainage catheter calls from home around midnight with new right upper quadrant discomfort and a low-grade fever. Which of the following actions is the best management?

A. Reassurance that this is expected with a biliary drainage catheter
B. Tell the patient to go to the emergency room (ER) for an ultrasound
C. Call in the IR team for emergent biliary drainage catheter exchange
D. Ask the patient to place the catheter to bag drainage and plan for exchange in IR the following day

5   Which of the following falls into the minimum information necessary to review in a preprocedure time-out?

A. Current laboratory values
B. Medication allergies
C. Plan for procedural sedation
D. Correct site for procedure

6   A 40-year-old female is recovering after an uneventful gonadal vein embolization. In the postprocedure area, the nurse becomes concerned, as the patient is now lethargic with the monitor displaying a heart rate of 40 bpm and rhythm that looks like sinus bradycardia. Which medication is the initial treatment?

A. Adenosine 6 mg intravenous (IV)
B. Atropine 0.5 mg IV
C. Amiodarone 300 mg IV
D. Normal saline 500 mL IV bolus

7   During central venous catheter (CVC) placement, a wire is passed into the right atrium. The patient's heart rate immediately changes and is noted to be a narrow complex tachycardia with a rate of 170 bpm. The wire is pulled back out of the heart and the rhythm persists. The patient remains asymptomatic. Which of the following is the best next step?

A. Adenosine 6 mg IV
B. Synchronized cardioversion
C. Vagal maneuvers
D. Amiodarone 300 mg IV

8 How should an uneventful fluoroscopy-guided percutaneous gastrostomy tube placement be classified?

A. Clean
B. Clean-contaminated
C. Contaminated
D. Dirty

9 Which of the following procedures necessitates preprocedure administration of IV antibiotics?

A. IVC filter placement
B. Fistulogram with angioplasty
C. TIPS
D. Venous thrombolysis

10 Which of the following represents best practice for a nontunneled CVC?

A. Routinely exchange nontunneled CVC once per week
B. Administer prophylactic IV antibiotics before CVC insertion
C. Use a CVC with the minimum number of ports or lumens essential for the management of the patient
D. Use topical antibiotics at the insertion site as part of routine dressing change

11 A patient presents for treatment of an acutely thrombosed lower extremity bypass graft. Which of the following histories would be the most concerning before catheter-directed thrombolytic therapy with tissue plasminogen activator (tPA)?

A. Total hip replacement 1 month ago
B. Lower gastrointestinal (GI) bleed 12 months ago
C. TIA (transient ischemic attack) 24 months ago
D. Systolic blood pressure of 196 mmHg

12 Which of the following is true regarding exposure to gadolinium-based contrast agents and the development of nephrogenic systemic fibrosis (NSF)?

A. Patients with chronic kidney disease stage 1 or 2 (estimated glomerular filtration rate [eGFR] 60-119 mL/min/1.73 m^2) require half-dose gadolinium
B. Patients with chronic kidney disease stage 3 (eGFR 30-59 mL/min/1.73 m^2) do not require any special precautions because NSF is exceedingly rare in this population
C. Patients with chronic kidney disease stage 4 or 5 (eGFR <30 mL/min/1.73 m^2) can safely receive gadolinium if there is dialysis within 24 hrs
D. Patients with acute kidney injury are not affected by NSF and require no special precautions

13 Which portion of the capnography graph represents the beginning of inspiration?

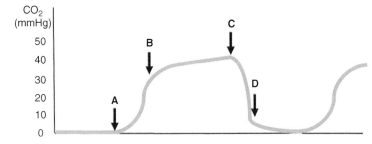

A. A
B. B
C. C
D. D

14   A patient with newly diagnosed colon cancer undergoes uneventful portacath placement. The following morning, the patient calls the office and reports the area around the portacath reservoir and tunneled catheter is red, warm, and tender to touch. He denies having a fever. What is the best initial management?

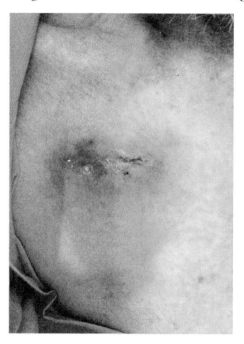

A. Urgent port removal
B. Prescribe 7 to 10 day course of oral antibiotics
C. Ultrasound to evaluate for fluid collection
D. Reassurance and close follow-up

15   Before an interventional procedure using IV moderate sedation, a focused history and physical examination are performed. When assessing the patient's airway, the soft palate and base of the uvula are visualized. Which is the correct modified Mallampati score?

A. Class I
B. Class II
C. Class III
D. Class IV

16   Using Society of Interventional Radiology guidelines, which of the following coagulation parameters would be appropriate for a TIPS procedure?

A. International normalized rate (INR) $\leq$ 1.5; platelets > 50,000/μL
B. INR $\leq$ 2.0; platelets > 100,000/μL
C. INR $\leq$ 2.5; platelets > 150,000/μL
D. INR $\leq$ 3.0; platelets > 200,000/μL

17   A patient needs removal of a nontunneled dialysis catheter. The catheter was uneventfully placed in the right internal jugular vein. How should one position the patient for safe catheter removal?

A. Trendelenburg
B. Reverse Trendelenburg
C. Right lateral decubitus
D. Left lateral decubitus

18 Unfortunately, a patient was not positioned correctly for a nontunneled CVC removal, and to make matters worse, the patient took in a deep breath during the act of removal and an audible sucking noise was heard. Air embolism to the right-sided heart likely occurred. Into which position should the operator now place the patient?

A. Trendelenburg
B. Reverse Trendelenburg
C. Right lateral decubitus
D. Left lateral decubitus

19 A patient is undergoing a complex lower extremity arterial intervention. The nurse suddenly becomes concerned as the blood pressure drops to 75/40, the oxygen saturation is 82%, and the patient is not responsive to stimuli. An additional dose of IV fentanyl is the suspected culprit for the clinical deterioration. What is an appropriate initial dose of naloxone for reversal?

A. 0.01 mg
B. 0.2 mg
C. 10 mg
D. 40 mg

20 Despite opiate reversal with naloxone, a patient remains unarousable during the procedure. The nurse notes that he gave midazolam as well. Which of the following should now be administered?

A. Flumazenil
B. Protamine
C. Dantrolene
D. Disulfiram

21 Which of the following scenarios is acceptable for an adult patient undergoing an IR procedure with moderate sedation?

A. Black coffee 3 hours prior
B. Milk 3 hours prior
C. Orange juice 5 hours prior
D. Cracker 5 hours prior

22 During an adult peripherally inserted central catheter (PICC) placement, the wire will not pass centrally. The technologist suggests performing a venogram to assess vascular patency. A few moments after the contrast venogram, the patient becomes quite uncomfortable. This rapidly progresses to wheezing and frank difficulty with breathing. Which of the following is an appropriate next step?

A. 0.3 mL epinephrine IM (1:1000)
B. 3 mL epinephrine IM (1:10,000)
C. 1 mL epinephrine IV (1:1000)
D. 10 mL epinephrine IV (1:10,000)

23 A patient with shellfish allergy is to undergo an elective outpatient procedure needing iodinated contrast. Which is the appropriate preprocedural regimen?

A. Prednisone 50 mg PO 13, 7, and 1 hour before procedure
B. Diphenhydramine 50 mg PO 1 hour before procedure
C. Procedure is absolutely contraindicated
D. No premedication necessary

24a Immediately before uterine artery embolization for symptomatic fibroids, the interventionalist performs a superior hypogastric nerve block. Under fluoroscopic guidance, a 22 g needle is positioned just caudal to the location of the aortic bifurcation using an anterior approach. Once the needle is in position, 20 mL of 0.5% bupivacaine HCl is injected. The needle is withdrawn. Soon after, the patient becomes unresponsive which evolves into a cardiac arrest. Which is the most likely cause for the arrest?

A. Abdominal aortic injury
B. Iliac venous injury
C. Intravascular injection
D. Vasovagal reaction

24b A diagnosis of local anesthetic systemic toxicity (LAST) from IV bupivacaine is suspected soon after the patient arrests. In addition to advanced cardiac life support (ACLS) protocol, which adjunctive treatment should be considered?

A. Hyperbaric oxygen
B. IV infusion of 20% lipid emulsion
C. Embolization of suspected iliac venous injury
D. Administer subcutaneous lidocaine

ANSWERS AND EXPLANATIONS

1 **Answer B.**   The case images show a catheter from above directed down the right hepatic vein, with small rounded pool of iodinated contrast at the catheter tip (dark gray). As intended, carbon dioxide gas (light gray) crosses the hepatic sinusoids, and retrograde fills the right, left, and main portal veins on the subsequent images. Unfortunately, there is an additional large rounded collection of gas outside of a formed vascular structure consistent with liver laceration and gas extravasation into the perihepatic space (choice B). This occurred when the operator failed to clear the wedged catheter of fluid and then rapidly injected a large bolus of CO_2 gas through the catheter. The gas compresses against the fluid remaining in the wedged end-hole catheter, forming a "gas bullet," so to speak, and it eventually overcomes the pressure needed to expel the fluid in the catheter. In this case, the compressed gas lacerated the liver, rupturing the capsule and causing a large hepatic venous extravasation, which was then treated with coil embolization. By definition, all gas injections from the hepatic vein cause some degree of air embolism to the pulmonary artery (choice A); however, this is expected and tolerated by the patient, as the CO_2 is quickly expelled via gas exchange in the lungs. There is no indication of arterial or biliary filling with gas eliminating choices C and D.

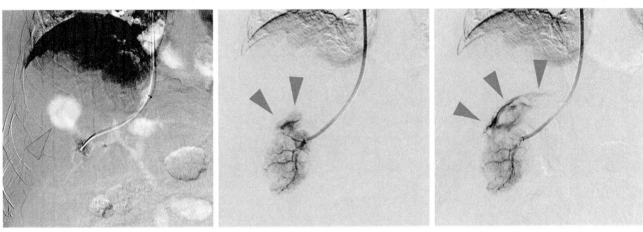

Figure 1-1   Case image on the left with collection of extravasated CO_2 gas (orange arrowhead) arising from near the wedged catheter tip. Subsequent conventional venography (middle and right images) shows enlarging pool of iodinated contrast (blue arrowheads) at the site of hepatic venous injury. The hepatic vein branch was subsequently catheterized and embolized with coils. The transjugular intrahepatic portosystemic shunt (TIPS) was then completed.

Reference: Cho KJ. Carbon dioxide angiography: scientific principles and practice. *Vasc Specialist Int*. 2015;31(3):67-80.

2   Answer C.   Carbon dioxide gas is an extremely useful agent for studying luminal structures such as blood vessels. It can be used in both arteries and veins and has no renal toxicity or allergic potential. However, in certain locations, there is a risk of end organ dysfunction due to gas blockage of a terminal artery. The most susceptible regions are the coronary and cerebral arterial circulation. In animal models, coronary artery injection resulted in arrhythmia and infarction. In the cerebral arteries, injection resulted in neurotoxicity and infarction. Therefore, its use in the thoracic aorta or in branches giving rise to the carotid or vertebral arteries is contraindicated. Use in the mesenteric arteries is acceptable and will not cause any permanent pathology, although temporary flow obstruction typically causes transient abdominal discomfort for the patient.

Reference: Cho KJ. Carbon dioxide angiography: scientific principles and practice. *Vasc Specialist Int.* 2015;31(3):67-80.

3   Answer A.   Although sick patients are frequently encountered in the IR suite, the specialty enjoys low minor and major complication rates, which is in no small part because of the minimally invasive techniques used. However, a busy practice performs many thousands of procedures a year, and it is inevitable that a patient will decompensate. In a study over of 36,000 IR procedures, the most common comorbidity for patients sustaining a cardiopulmonary arrest was chronic kidney disease. The most common procedure type was dialysis access related. With this knowledge, interventionalists should remain vigilant in their periprocedural care of this potentially fragile patient population and take steps to avoid inappropriate risk.

Reference: Rueb GR, Brady WJ, Gilliland CA, et al. Characterizing cardiopulmonary arrest during interventional radiology procedures. *J Vasc Interv Radiol.* 2013;24(12):1774-1778.

4   Answer D.   The patient is presenting with symptoms of cholangitis despite the presence of a biliary drainage catheter. Although the drain cannot be completely assessed over the phone, one should assume that there is some sort of catheter dysfunction causing the patient's symptoms. An internal/external biliary drainage catheter can be capped for bile to drain internally into the bowel, or it can be uncapped to maximize drainage both via the internal route and externally to a bag. At the time of initial placement, discomfort related to the tube is somewhat expected, especially if intercostal. Over time, this should improve. New abdominal pain, jaundice, and/or fever should raise immediate concern for catheter dysfunction and evolving cholangitis. The best first step is to have the patient uncap the tube and attach it to a bag for maximum drainage. As the presumed clogging is typically at the bowel end of the catheter, this maneuver can temporarily drain the bile until a complete fluoroscopic evaluation of the tube can be performed.

Reference: Huang SY, Engstrom BI, Lungren MP, Kim CY. Management of dysfunctional catheters and tubes inserted by interventional radiology. *Semin Intervent Radiol.* 2015;32(2):67-77.

5   Answer D.   A preprocedure time-out is an important tool in minimizing medical error. The Joint Commission Universal Protocol carries a minimum standard of identifying correct procedure, correct patient, and correct site during the time-out. There are of course many other pieces of information which can be reviewed in the time-out (allergies, relevant laboratory test results, etc.); however, these can be tailored to the operative/procedure setting.

Reference: Rafiei P, Walser EM, Duncan JR, et al. Society of interventional radiology IR preprocedure patient safety checklist by the safety and health committee. *J Vasc Interv Radiol.* 2016;27(5):695-699.

6   **Answer B.**   This patient is experiencing symptomatic bradycardia. For patients with asymptomatic bradycardia, close observation is warranted. The symptoms that should trigger therapy beyond observation include hypotension, altered mental status, and signs and/or symptoms of end organ dysfunction such as chest pain. Per ACLS guidelines, atropine 0.5 mg IV is indicated every 3 to 5 minutes with a maximum dose of 3 mg. If the patient does not respond, transcutaneous pacing or vasopressor infusion (dopamine or epinephrine) may be necessary.

Adenosine is the treatment of choice for stable tachycardia. Amiodarone is a complex antiarrhythmic that is most often used for stable tachycardia not responsive to adenosine and as part of the medical treatment for a cardiac arrest. A bolus of normal saline is a good adjunct for many situations such as vagal reactions and hypotension; however, it is not the critical initial treatment for symptomatic bradycardia.

Reference: Hazinski MF. *Handbook of Emergency Cardiovascular Care for Healthcare Providers 2015*; 2015.

7   **Answer C.**   Guidewire-induced tachycardia happens from time to time in the IR suite. Often, the patient will spontaneously revert back to sinus rhythm after the stimulus (guidewire) is removed. If the rhythm persists and the patient is asymptomatic, vagal maneuvers are the best first step in treatment. We use valsalva and unilateral carotid massage. If not successful, obtain a 12-lead electrocardiogram (ECG) and consider adenosine 6 mg IV bolus. For patients with symptomatic tachycardia, synchronized cardioversion is appropriate, or adenosine if the tachycardia is regular and narrow complex.

Reference: Hazinski MF. *Handbook of Emergency Cardiovascular Care for Healthcare Providers 2015*; 2015.

8   **Answer B.**   The commonly used procedure classifications as defined by the National Academy of Sciences/National Research Council are as follows:

Clean: A procedure is regarded as clean, if the GI tract, genitourinary tract, or respiratory tract is not entered; if inflammation is not evident; and if there is no break in aseptic technique. An example of a clean procedure is a routine lower extremity diagnostic arteriogram.

Clean-contaminated: A procedure is regarded as clean-contaminated if the GI tract, genitourinary tract, or respiratory tract is entered; if inflammation is not evident; and if there is no major break in aseptic technique. An example of a clean-contaminated procedure is percutaneous fluoroscopic gastrostomy tube insertion.

Contaminated: A procedure is regarded as contaminated if there is entry into an inflamed or colonized GI or genitourinary tract without frank pus or if a major break in aseptic technique occurs. An example of a contaminated procedure is percutaneous pigtail nephrostomy catheter insertion to treat upper urinary tract obstruction with concomitant nonpurulent infection.

Dirty: A procedure is regarded as dirty if it involves entering an infected purulent site such as an abscess, a clinically infected biliary or genitourinary site, or a perforated viscus. An example of a dirty procedure is percutaneous drainage of an abscess from a colonic anastomosis breakdown.

Reference: Chan D, Downing D, Keough CE, et al. Joint practice guideline for sterile technique during vascular and interventional radiology procedures: from the society of interventional radiology, association of perioperative registered nurses, and association for radiologic and imaging nursing, for the Society of Interventional Radiology [corrected] Standards of Practice Committee, and Endorsed by the Cardiovascular Interventional Radiological Society of Europe and the Canadian Interventional Radiology Association. *J Vasc Interv Radiol*. 2012;23(12):1603-1612.

9   **Answer C.**   The use of prophylactic antibiotics for procedures in IR suffers from a lack of high-quality randomized data. Some of the recommendations are extrapolated from the surgical literature. Others are expert consensus. In an effort to create a uniform practice pattern, guidelines have been published by the Society of Interventional Radiology. In general, clean procedures that do not violate colonized or infected tracts do not require preprocedural antibiotics (CVC insertion, arterial and venous interventions). The notable exception here would be a procedure with an implanted device such as a stent graft. Patients undergoing procedures that may violate colonized or infected tracts are recommended to receive preprocedural antibiotics (TIPS, percutaneous biliary or nephrostomy catheter insertion). In addition, for embolization procedures whereby the intent of the procedure is to create ischemia/infarction (uterine artery embolization, transarterial chemoembolization, and partial splenic embolization), preprocedure antibiotics are typically administered.

Reference: Venkatesan AM, Kundu S, Sacks D, et al. Practice guidelines for adult antibiotic prophylaxis during vascular and interventional radiology procedures. Written by the Standards of Practice Committee for the Society of Interventional Radiology and Endorsed by the Cardiovascular Interventional Radiological Society of Europe and Canadian Interventional Radiology Association [corrected]. *J Vasc Interv Radiol.* 2010;21(11):1611-1630.

10   **Answer C.**   There exists an extensive Centers for Disease Control guideline regarding the prevention of intravascular catheter-related infections. Operators should be familiar with the guideline, especially IR physicians, given the volume of CVC insertion that occurs in most practices. Catheters should not be routinely exchanged to prevent infection; prophylactic IV antibiotics should not be administered before CVC insertion; and a topical antibiotic should not be placed on the dressing, as it can promote fungal infections and/or antimicrobial resistance. These recommendations, including the correct answer, are classified as Category IB—strongly recommended for implementation and supported by some experimental, clinical, or epidemiologic studies and a strong theoretical rationale—or an accepted practice (e.g., aseptic technique) supported by limited evidence.

Reference: Miller DL, O'Grady NP. Guidelines for the prevention of intravascular catheter-related infections: recommendations relevant to interventional radiology for venous catheter placement and maintenance. *J Vasc Interv Radiol.* 2012;23(8):997-1007.

11   **Answer D.**   Intravascular catheter-directed thrombolytic therapy carries a small but real risk of major and minor hemorrhage. Depending on the source, the listed contraindications may vary; however, there are many universally agreed upon contraindications that practitioners should assess for before performing this treatment. In the case example, the patient should get reliable blood pressure control (we prefer an IV agent) before starting the tPA infusion, such that the goal blood pressure can be maintained throughout the treatment window without significant lability. All contraindications should be considered in the context of the patient and clinical setting. The care of patients should be individualized, and violating a contraindication may be appropriate.

TABLE 11-1   Frequently Cited Absolute and Relative Contraindications for Catheter-Directed Thrombolytic Therapy

Contraindications to Catheter-Directed Thrombolysis
Absolute
• Active bleeding
• Intracranial hemorrhage
• Disseminated intravascular coagulation
• Contraindication to anticoagulation
Relative
• Cerebrovascular event within the past 2 mo
• Craniospinal surgery or trauma within the past 3 mo
• Intracranial tumor, vascular malformation, or aneurysm
• Major surgery or trauma within the past 10 d
• Uncontrolled hypertension (>180/>110 mmHg)
• Major gastrointestinal bleeding within the past 10 d
• Age > 80 yr
• Pregnancy
• Preexisting coagulopathy or severe thrombocytopenia

References: Adams HP, Brott TG, Furlan AJ, et al. Guidelines for thrombolytic therapy for acute stroke: a supplement to the guidelines for the management of patients with acute ischemic stroke. A statement for healthcare professionals from a Special Writing Group of the Stroke Council, American Heart Association. *Circulation*. 1996;94(5):1167-1174.

Patel NH, Krishnamurthy VN, Kim S, et al. Quality improvement guidelines for percutaneous management of acute lower-extremity ischemia. *J Vasc Interv Radiol*. 2013;24(1):3-15.

Vedantham S, Sista AK, Klein SJ, et al. Quality improvement guidelines for the treatment of lower-extremity deep vein thrombosis with use of endovascular thrombus removal. *J Vasc Interv Radiol*. 2014;25(9):1317-1325.

12   **Answer B.**   Gadolinium-based contrast agents are classified into groups I, II, and III. Group I agents have the greatest number of NSF cases reported. Group II agents have few if any reported cases. Group III agents have few if any cases reported, but data are limited. Patients with chronic kidney disease (CKD) stage 1 or 2 have no increased risk for NSF. NSF is exceedingly rare in patients with CKD stage 3, and therefore no special precautions are required. Regarding gadolinium use in patients with CKD stage 4 and 5, group I agents are contraindicated, and if gadolinium is to be used, it should be a group II agent. Use of gadolinium in this scenario requires a risk-to-benefit evaluation with the patient and referring physician. Patients with acute kidney injury are at risk for the development of NSF and should essentially be treated as CKD stage 4 or 5, as true kidney function is difficult to determine in this setting.

References: ACR. *Manual on Contrast Media, Version 10.3*; 2018. Available Online.

Beckett KR, Moriarity AK, Langer JM. Safe use of contrast media: what the radiologist needs to know. *Radiographics*. 2015;35(6):1738-1750.

13   **Answer C.**   In 2010, the American Society of Anesthesiologists updated the recommendations for procedural sedation, essentially making capnography monitoring a requirement. Many physician groups have adopted this policy; therefore, some working knowledge of capnography is important. Built into or attached to the nasal cannula, nonrebreather, or advanced airway is a channel which communicates to a sensor determining the expired CO_2 level. As expiration begins (point A), the level of exhaled CO_2 increases (point B), typically plateaus, and then descends at the end of expiration/beginning of inhalation (point C). End-tidal CO_2 (etCO_2) is measured at the peak of the expiratory plateau (point C). A normal etCO_2 is 35 to 45 mmHg.

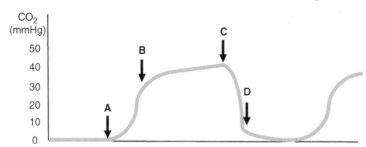

If the patient is bradypnic, as can occur with oversedation, they will retain CO_2 with resultant elevation of etCO_2 levels. Data suggest that changes in CO_2 capnography precede a drop in oxygen saturation levels by 30 to 90 seconds. Meta-analysis has shown that cases of respiratory depression were >17x more likely to be detected if CO_2 capnography was used.

References: Baerlocher MO, Nikolic B, Silberzweig JE, et al. Society of Interventional Radiology position statement on recent change to the ASA's moderate sedation standards: capnography. *J Vasc Interv Radiol*. 2013;24(7):939-940.

Waugh JB, Epps CA, Khodneva YA. Capnography enhances surveillance of respiratory events during procedural sedation: a meta-analysis. *J Clin Anesth*. 2011;23(3):189-196.

14   **Answer D.**   When placing a portacath for prolonged central venous access, it is important to be familiar with the expected postprocedure appearance and possible complications. While a red, warm, and tender portacath site may raise concern for port pocket infection, the important detail in this case is the appearance of these symptoms in under 24 hours. It is virtually impossible (without gross negligent contamination) for a clean or even a minorly contaminated insertion to result in a symptomatic pocket infection in this time period. Patients may mount a sterile inflammatory response in the first 24 to 48 hours after placement, which mimics infection early on, but gradually goes away over a few days. Additional differential considerations are hematoma formation in the pocket or contact dermatitis from

the cleaning solutions, dressings, or surgical drapes. Contact type allergic reactions can often be discerned by their geographic distribution which corresponds to the area of contact with the offending agent. Portacaths have a relatively low infection rate documented from 0.15 to 0.43 per 1000 catheter days. If truly infected, clinical presentation can range from nearly asymptomatic to devastating septicemia.

Reference: Bamba R, Lorenz JM, Lale AJ, Funaki BS, Zangan SM. Clinical predictors of port infections within the first 30 days of placement. *J Vasc Interv Radiol.* 2014;25(3):419-423.

15 **Answer C.** When considering a sedation plan for patients undergoing procedures in IR, it is important to consider the airway in the initial assessment. Although uncommon, during procedures using IV moderate or deep sedation, the airway can become compromised necessitating urgent or emergent endotracheal intubation. The modified Mallampati score is a visual physical examination assessment that can help identify a patient with an airway that may be challenging for endotracheal intubation.

Class I: Soft palate, fauces, uvula, pillars

Class II: Soft palate, fauces, uvula

Class III: Soft palate, base of uvula

Class IV: Soft palate not visualized

Patients with Class IV airways can be challenging to perform direct laryngoscopy with endotracheal intubation, and the operator may consider anesthesia provider consultation or altering the sedation plan before the procedure. Additional airway factors the operator should consider before procedures using IV sedation include the mouth opening capability, thyromental distance, neck size/obesity, and neck range of motion.

References: Johnson S. Sedation and analgesia in the performance of interventional procedures. *Semin Intervent Radiol.* 2010;27(4):368-373.

Lee A, Fan LT, Gin T, Karmakar MK, Ngan Kee WD. A systematic review (meta-analysis) of the accuracy of the Mallampati tests to predict the difficult airway. *Anesth Analg.* 2006;102(6):1867-1878.

Martin ML, Lennox PH. Sedation and analgesia in the interventional radiology department. *J Vasc Interv Radiol.* 2003;14(9 Pt 1):1119-1128.

16 **Answer A.** Management of coagulation parameters to minimize the bleeding risk of a procedure can be challenging, as there is a wide range of procedural complexity and of patient bleeding propensity. To assist with decision-making, the Society of Interventional Radiology publishes guidelines for coagulation parameters and groups procedures into one of three categories. TIPS, being one of the more invasive IR procedures, falls into category III, which carries the strictest recommendation of INR $\leq$ 1.5 and platelets > 50,000 (choice A). Category III procedures carry a significant risk of bleeding, which is difficult to detect or control.

References: Patel IJ, Davidson JC, Nikolic B, et al. Consensus guidelines for periprocedural management of coagulation status and hemostasis risk in percutaneous image-guided interventions. *J Vasc Interv Radiol.* 2012;23(6):727-736.

Patel IJ, Davidson JC, Nikolic B, et al. Addendum of newer anticoagulants to the SIR consensus guideline. *J Vasc Interv Radiol.* 2013;24(5):641-645.

17 **Answer A.** A nontunneled CVC is fairly straightforward to remove, but one must keep in mind some potential risks. The most devastating complication is air embolism to the heart, which can result in cardiopulmonary failure, or systemic embolism in the setting of a right to left shunt. To minimize this risk, it is standard practice to have the patient in Trendelenburg position (head down) for removal of the catheter. The removal should also be performed with Valsalva or during expiration. After hemostasis is achieved, placement of an impermeable dressing over the access site is recommended.

References: Thielen JB, Nyquist J. Subclavian catheter removal. Nursing implications to prevent air emboli. *J Intraven Nurs.* 1991;14(2):114-118.

Vesely TM. Air embolism during insertion of central venous catheters. *J Vasc Interv Radiol.* 2001;12(11):1291-1295.

18   **Answer D.**   Of course, the best way to deal with this problem is to avoid it in the first place. Trendelenburg position along with Valsalva or expiration increases intrathoracic and central venous pressure. These maneuvers during CVC removal from the neck or chest prevent atmospheric air from entering through the skin into the access vein. If air embolism does occur, the immediate goal is to trap the air in the right-sided heart to prevent further migration into the pulmonary arterial system. To achieve this goal, the patient is positioned left lateral decubitus (choice D), which puts the right atrium in a nondependent orientation (see Figure 18-1). Depending on the size of the embolus and the clinical effect, further management includes 100% oxygen administration and ICU monitoring. If the embolism occurs intraprocedurally, catheter aspiration of intravascular air may be possible.

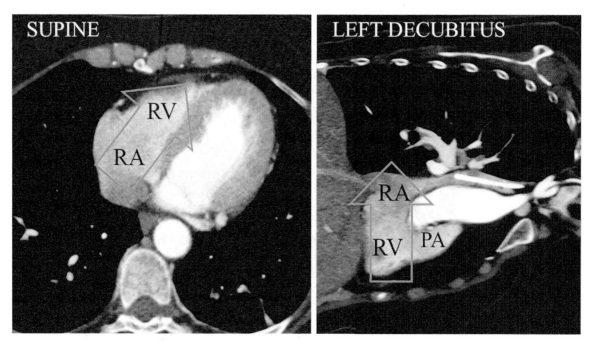

Figure 18-1   Movement of intravascular air (blue arrows) in the right-sided heart in the supine and left lateral decubitus position with computer tomography (CT) correlation. In the left lateral decubitus position, the right atrium becomes nondependent. PA, pulmonary artery; RA, right atrium; RV, right ventricle.

References: McCarthy CJ, Behravesh S, Naidu SG, Oklu R. Air embolism: practical tips for prevention and treatment. *J Clin Med.* 2016;5(11):93.

Shaikh N, Ummunisa F. Acute management of vascular air embolism. *J Emerg Trauma Shock.* 2009;2(3):180-185.

19   **Answer B.**   The initial dose for opiate reversal using naloxone is 0.1 to 0.3 mg IV. The maximum recommended total dose is 10 mg. The onset of action is within 2 minutes, and repeated dosing is often necessary if longer acting opiates remain in the system. A continuous infusion can be used for prolonged reversal. Opiate reversal should only be used when absolutely necessary, as side effects include immediate cessation of analgesia, hypertension, nausea, and vomiting.

References: Arepally A, Oechsle D, Kirkwood S, Savader SJ. Safety of conscious sedation in interventional radiology. *Cardiovasc Intervent Radiol*. 2001;24(3):185-190.

Olsen JW, Barger RL, Doshi SK. Moderate sedation: what radiologists need to know. *AJR Am J Roentgenol*. 2013;201(5):941-946.

20   **Answer A.**   The reversal agent for benzodiazepines such as midazolam is flumazenil. The recommended dose is 0.2 mg IV, with repeated dosing often necessary. A total of 1 mg can be given. The onset of action is within minutes. Protamine reverses heparin. Dantrolene is a treatment for malignant hyperthermia. Disulfiram is an alcohol abuse deterrent.

References: Arepally A, Oechsle D, Kirkwood S, Savader SJ. Safety of conscious sedation in interventional radiology. *Cardiovasc Intervent Radiol*. 2001;24(3):185-190.

Olsen JW, Barger RL, Doshi SK. Moderate sedation: what radiologists need to know. *AJR Am J Roentgenol*. 2013;201(5):941-946.

21   **Answer A.**   The NPO status of children and adults is an important piece of information to obtain before administering procedural sedation. For adults, the recommended fasting period for clear liquids is 2 hours. Solids and nonclear liquids should be avoided for a minimum of 6 hours.

References: Johnson S. Sedation and analgesia in the performance of interventional procedures. *Semin Intervent Radiol*. 2010;27(4):368-373.

Olsen JW, Barger RL, Doshi SK. Moderate sedation: what radiologists need to know. *AJR Am J Roentgenol*. 2013;201(5):941-946.

22   **Answer A.**   The patient is having a severe reaction to iodinated contrast. There is bronchospasm (wheezing) with respiratory compromise. Prompt administration of epinephrine is appropriate. The dilution for IM is 1:1000 and IV is 1:10,000. The initial dose is 0.1 to 0.3 mg, which equates to 0.1 to 0.3 mL epinephrine IM (1:1000) or 1 to 3 mL epinephrine IV (1:10,000). Up to 1 mg can be given. Epinephrine should be used for moderate to severe bronchospasm, laryngeal edema, and anaphylactoid/anaphylaxis reactions. Mild bronchospasm is treated with beta-agonist inhalation therapy. Urticaria (hives) is managed with antihistamines such as diphenhydramine, which can be given PO, IM, or IV.

References: Beckett KR, Moriarity AK, Langer JM. Safe use of contrast media: what the radiologist needs to know. *Radiographics*. 2015;35(6):1738-1750.

Boyd B, Zamora CA, Castillo M. Managing adverse reactions to contrast agents. *Magn Reson Imaging Clin N Am*. 2017;25(4):737-742.

23   **Answer D.**   A patient with a history of shellfish allergy can safely receive iodinated contrast. The cross-reaction has been fully debunked, but for some reason, this myth persists in clinical practice. Patients with unrelated allergies (food, medication, other) to contrast media do have a 2- to 3-fold increased risk of subsequent allergic-like reactions to contrast media. This increased risk, however, should not prompt routine use of a premedication protocol nor deter physicians from ordering radiologic examinations requiring contrast media.

References: Beckett KR, Moriarity AK, Langer JM. Safe use of contrast media: what the radiologist needs to know. *Radiographics*. 2015;35(6):1738-1750.

Boyd B, Zamora CA, Castillo M. Managing adverse reactions to contrast agents. *Magn Reson Imaging Clin N Am*. 2017;25(4):737-742.

24a **Answer C.**   Nerve blocks and neurolysis can be performed with different types of guidance including anatomic landmarks, fluoroscopy, ultrasound, and CT. In the case example, the exact location of the needle tip is not known. The needle is advanced under fluoroscopic guidance using bony and vascular landmarks into the anatomic location of the superior hypogastric nerve plexus. There are arterial and venous structures in close proximity. If the operator does not do due diligence and ensure extravascular positioning of the needle with contrast injection and lack of blood return, inadvertent intravascular injection of medications and neurolytic agents can occur, sometimes with disastrous consequences. This question illustrates an example of bupivacaine toxicity from inadvertent IV injection. LAST may present initially with neurological symptoms such as tinnitus, lightheadedness, circumoral numbness, and drowsiness. With severe toxicity, seizures, coma, hypotension, dysrhythmias, and cardiopulmonary arrest can occur.

References: Bourne E, Wright C, Royse C. A review of local anesthetic cardiotoxicity and treatment with lipid emulsion. *Local Reg Anesth*. 2010;3:11-19.

Sekimoto K, Tobe M, Saito S. Local anesthetic toxicity: acute and chronic management. *Acute Med Surg*. 2017;4(2):152-160.

24b **Answer B.**   When witnessed cardiac arrest occurs at the time of a procedure, ACLS protocol should begin immediately. In the case example, a diagnosis of LAST is suspected given the temporal association of the nerve block to the cardiac arrest. Treatment of LAST begins with early recognition and cessation of further injection of the offending anesthetic. Airway problems can occur, and management with intubation may be necessary. If seizures occur, benzodiazepines should be given as first-line. In the case example, the patient has cardiac arrest. The ACLS protocol is initiated. Lipid emulsion therapy should be strongly considered as soon as possible. Some groups recommend initiating 20% lipid emulsion (given as bolus followed by continuous infusion) treatment at the first sign of LAST. The exact mechanism of IV lipid therapy is unclear but is thought to affect both pharmacokinetic and pharmacodynamic effects.

References: Bourne E, Wright C, Royse C. A review of local anesthetic cardiotoxicity and treatment with lipid emulsion. *Local Reg Anesth*. 2010;3:11-19.

Sekimoto K, Tobe M, Saito S. Local anesthetic toxicity: acute and chronic management. *Acute Med Surg*. 2017;4(2):152-160.

10 Physics

1   During a complex splenic artery aneurysm embolization, fluoroscopy time exceeds 60 minutes with an estimated skin dose of 4 Gy. A second aneurysm remains that will require a second embolization procedure. What is the most accurate description of potential radiation toxicity for this patient?

   A. Skin erythema may occur; deterministic effect
   B. Deep ulceration may occur; stochastic effect
   C. No cancer risk below threshold of 6 Gy; stochastic effect
   D. No increased risk of skin damage for second procedure in 1 week; deterministic effect

2   Which of the following regarding skin radiation exposure is true?

   A. If there is radiation damage to the skin, it will appear within 1 week
   B. It is ideal to keep the X-ray beam in the same orientation to minimize the area of skin exposed
   C. The majority of skin complications are seen on the anterior chest from coronary intervention
   D. Radiation injury is unexpected below 2 Gy

3   During a busy first 3 months of IR training, a fellow accrues 1000 mrem of total effective dose equivalent (TEDE). Assuming a similar workload for the remainder of the year, which statement is most accurate?

   A. The fellow will exceed the annual limit TEDE for radiation workers
   B. The fellow will not exceed the annual limit TEDE for radiation workers
   C. There is no annual limit TEDE for radiation workers

4   What is the annual maximum radiation dose to the lens of the eye?

   A. 15 mrem
   B. 150 mrem
   C. 15 rem
   D. 150 rem

5   What is the fetal dose limit during pregnancy?

A. 0.5 mrem
B. 5 mrem
C. 50 mrem
D. 500 mrem

6   An IR attending reveals that she is 4 months pregnant and is concerned about accurately measuring radiation exposure to her fetus. Which is correct regarding radiation dosimeter position for measuring fetal exposure?

A. Radiation dosimeter is worn underneath lead apron at the waist level
B. Radiation dosimeter is worn outside of lead apron at the level of uterine fundus, based on physical examination
C. There is no specific recommendation for radiation dosimeter position and measuring fetal exposure

7   What is a typical lead equivalent thickness for shielding aprons?

A. 0.05 mm
B. 0.5 mm
C. 5 mm
D. 50 mm

8   During a lengthy fluoroscopic-guided procedure, an ALARA-conscious attending tells a pregnant medical student to step back during a digital subtraction angiogram. The attending receives 50 mGy at a distance of 1 foot from the source. At a distance of 5 feet, how much radiation will the medical student receive?

A. 46 mGy
B. 25 mGy
C. 2 mGy
D. 0.5 mGy

9   In preparation for a routine, uncomplicated, internal-external biliary drainage catheter exchange, the technologist asks what fluoroscopic pulse rate would be acceptable for the procedure. Keeping in line with minimizing radiation exposure while maintaining image quality, which pulse rate is appropriate?

A. 60 pulses/s
B. 30 pulses/s
C. 7.5 pulses/s
D. 0.5 pulse/s

10   Which position will produce the most scatter radiation exposure to the operator during a fluoroscopic-guided procedure?

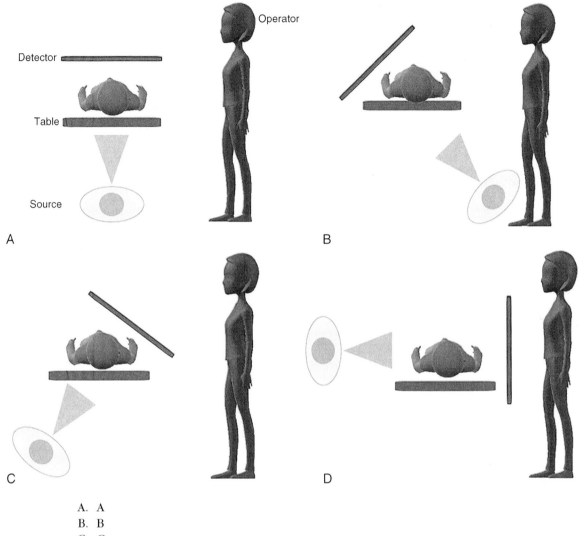

A. A
B. B
C. C
D. D

11   During a TIPS procedure, the technologist narrows the hard collimators to exclude much of the abdomen. Which of the following will occur as a result of this action?

A. Reduced image quality
B. Increased skin radiation dose to the patient
C. Reduced scatter radiation exposure to the operator
D. Magnifies image 2x

12   Which of the following is the most optimal relationship of source to patient to detector?

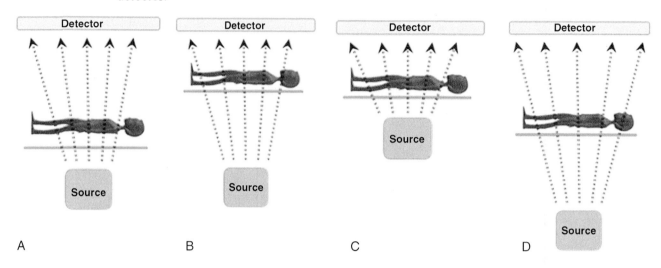

A   B   C   D

A. A
B. B
C. C
D. D

13   Which of the following is true regarding geometric and electronic magnification?

A. Neither affects dose
B. Geometric magnification increases dose, electronic magnification does not
C. Electronic magnification increases dose, geometric does not
D. Both increase dose

14   The following 3 images are obtained without moving the metallic clamp placed on the patient's skin. What effect has occurred to explain the clamp position relative to the femoral head?

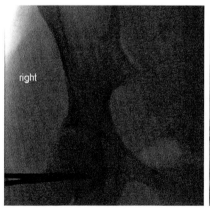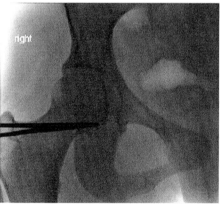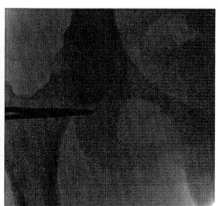

A. Parallax
B. Motion artifact
C. Detector lag
D. Pincushion distortion

15   What explains the difference in appearance of the right lower thorax (circle) in this patient undergoing a transvenous liver biopsy?

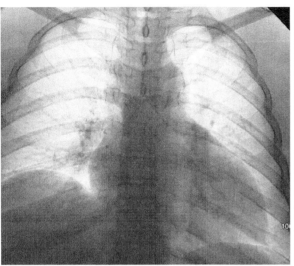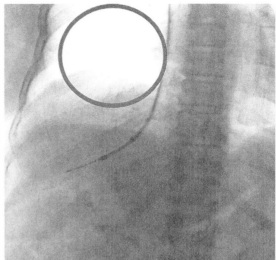

   A. Automatic brightness control
   B. Faulty anode
   C. Cracked detector
   D. Vignetting

16   In preparation for US-guided placement of a percutaneous nephrostomy catheter, the operator selects the curved transducer (right) rather than the hockey-stick transducer (left). What characteristic does the curved transducer have to be beneficial in this situation?

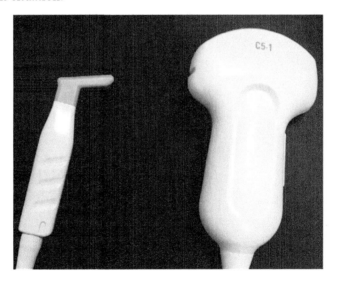

   A. Lower frequency
   B. Higher pulse repetition
   C. Higher resolution

17   What type of decay does Yttrium-90 undergo?

    A. Alpha

    B. Gamma

    C. Omega

    D. Beta

18   A patient with colon cancer metastatic to the liver is treated with bilobar yttrium-90 radioembolization. Regarding immediate postprocedure precautions, which of the following is true?

    A. Patient is a radiation hazard to others; maintain 1 meter separation for 5 half-lives

    B. Patient is a radiation hazard to children (<18 y) only, maintain 1 meter separation for 5 half-lives

    C. Patient is not a radiation hazard to others; resume normal interactions

19   What is the half-life of yttrium-90?

    A. 64 minutes

    B. 64 hours

    C. 64 days

    D. 64 years

ANSWERS AND EXPLANATIONS

1   **Answer A.**   It is vital for radiologists, and in particular, interventional radiologists, to understand the effects of radiation exposure on patients and others. The 2 types of biologic radiation effects are stochastic and deterministic. Stochastic effects have several key features: they occur by chance; there is no threshold for effect; the probability of occurrence is related to the cumulative exposure; the severity of the effect is independent of the dose. Deterministic effects have several key differences: they do not occur by chance; there is a threshold for effect; the severity of the effect increases with the dose. Operators should be familiar with basic thresholds for deterministic effects on different tissues (as discussed in additional questions).

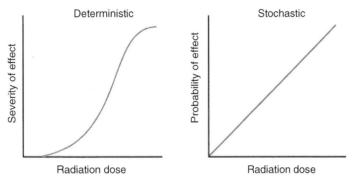

Figure 1-1   Graphic comparison of deterministic versus stochastic radiation effects.

Reference: Mahesh M. Fluoroscopy: patient radiation exposure issues. *Radiographics*. 2001;21(4):1033-1045.

2   **Answer D.**   One of the hallmarks of deterministic effects from radiation is a threshold dose. If a high dose is reached, damage to the skin is naturally of concern. The skin at the X-ray beam entry point receives the highest dose compared with other organs, as the photons attenuate as they travel through the body (roughly half of the available photons are attenuated for every 45 mm tissue). The most commonly accepted threshold for skin effect is 2 Gy. Regarding time of onset for skin change, the earliest it can be seen is within hours as a transient histaminelike response. With higher doses, reaching above 6 Gy, additional effects can be seen, including epilation, desquamation, and even dermal necrosis if exposure is high enough. It is important to make note of higher skin exposures, as the changes can appear weeks or months after exposure.

TABLE 2-1   Radiation Dose and Skin injury

Single-Dose Skin Effects		
Effect	Gy	Onset
Early erythema	2	hours
Temporary epilation	3	~3 wk
Main erythema	6	~10 d
Permanent epilation	7	~3 wk
Dry desquamation	10	~4 wk
Moist desquamation	15	~4 wk
Dermal necrosis	18	>10 wk

Since the beam enters the skin from below in a typical fluoroscopic examination, the supine patient will see effects on the posterior skin (not on the anterior chest as in choice C). One method to combat high exposure to the skin is to periodically reorient the X-ray beam, dividing the dose among a larger area of skin (see Figure 2-1).

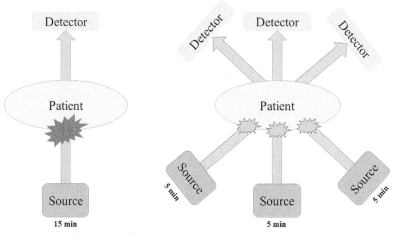

Figure 2-1   Skin radiation dose is greater with unchanged X-ray beam orientation (left) compared with using different obliques throughout the examination (right).

References: Mahesh M. Fluoroscopy: patient radiation exposure issues. *Radiographics.* 2001;21(4):1033-1045.

Wagner LK, Eifel PJ, Geise RA. Potential biological effects following high X-ray dose interventional procedures. *J Vasc Interv Radiol.* 1994;5(1):71-84.

3   **Answer B.**   Assuming a uniform workload, a little math tells us that the fellow will accumulate 4000 mrem (4 rem) TEDE over their year of training. The NRC (Nuclear Regulatory Commission) occupational annual dose limits for adults are as follows:

Whichever is more limiting of (1) TEDE of 5 rem or (2) the sum of deep dose equivalent plus committed dose equivalent to any organ (except the lens of the eye) totaling 50 rem.

Reference: *NRC Regulations Title 10, Code of Federal Regulations. Part 20 - Standards for Protection Against Radiation*; 2018 (updated annually).

4   **Answer C.**   NRC occupational annual dose limits for adults:

Whichever is more limiting of (1) TEDE of 5 rems or (2) the sum of deep dose equivalent plus committed dose equivalent to any organ (except the lens of the eye) totaling 50 rems.

Itemized annual limits:

Lens of the eye: 15 rems (150 mSv)

Shallow dose equivalent to the skin of whole body or extremity: 50 rems

Leaded glasses and gloves are available for protection.

Reference: *NRC Regulations Title 10, Code of Federal Regulations. Part 20 - Standards for Protection Against Radiation*; 2018 (updated annually).

5   **Answer D.**   According to the NRC, the dose equivalent to a fetus shall not exceed 500 mrem (0.5 rem) for the entire pregnancy. Pregnancy lead aprons do exist, with double the lead protection in the fetal area.

Reference: *NRC Regulations Title 10, Code of Federal Regulations. Part 20 - Standards for Protection Against Radiation*; 2018 (updated annually).

6   **Answer A.**   Standard practice is for pregnant women to wear 2 radiation dosimeters: one is worn outside the lead to estimate the maternal dose, while the second dosimeter is worn inside the lead at waist level to estimate fetal dose.

Reference: Chandra V, Dorsey C, Reed AB, Shaw P, Banghart D, Zhou W. Monitoring of fetal radiation exposure during pregnancy. *J Vasc Surg*. 2013;58(3):710-714.

7   **Answer B.**   The most common lead equivalent thickness is 0.5 mm, though some slightly lighter options exist. A 1.0 mm equivalent is often used in pregnancy. A 0.5 mm lead equivalent reduces photon transmission to 3.2% at 100 kVp and 0.36% at 70 kVp.

Reference: Brateman L. Radiation safety considerations for diagnostic radiology personnel. *Radiographics*. 1999;19(4):1037-1055.

8   **Answer C.**   Radiation dose decreases via the inverse square law: $1/\text{Distance}^2$. At twice the distance, the dose is divided by 4. At 5 times the distance, the dose is divided by 25.

Reference: Parry RA, Glaze SA, Archer BR. The AAPM/RSNA physics tutorial for residents. Typical patient radiation doses in diagnostic radiology. *Radiographics*. 1999;19(5):1289-1302.

9   **Answer C.**   Many fluoroscopic units have the ability to pulse the X-ray beam rather than producing a continuous exposure. A rate of 10 pulses/s is a common baseline setting in IR. When performing work that requires precise catheter and wire manipulation, we use 10 and occasionally 15 pulses/s. For routine catheter exchanges, central venous access, and other basic IR procedures, we use 4 to 7.5 pulses/s. Interestingly, the radiation exposure decrease does not decrease in 1:1 fashion with the pulse decrease. In order to limit degradation of image quality due to noise, the manufacturer will often increase the milliamperage with the lower pulsed setting. Therefore dropping from 30 pulses/s to only 15 pulses/s will result in only 25% to 28% dose reduction rather than the expected 50%.

Reference: Mahesh M. Fluoroscopy: patient radiation exposure issues. *Radiographics*. 2001;21(4):1033-1045.

10   **Answer B.**   Scatter radiation to the operator is an important concept for not only the operator to understand, but for anyone in the interventional suite in close proximity to the patient such as the nurse, technologist, assistant, or anesthesiologist. The amount of scatter radiation varies with several X-ray tube parameters including the source to image distance (SID), source to object distance (SOD), and object to image distance (OID). In addition, the obliquity of the tube with respect to the patient has a significant impact on scatter production. When working in a steep oblique or lateral position, more radiation is needed to penetrate the patient to produce a quality image (increased relative tissue thickness). As scatter is highest from patient tissues that are closest to the X-ray source, the scenario depicted in B will result in the highest scatter radiation exposure to the operator.

Reference: Meisinger QC, Stahl CM, Andre MP, Kinney TB, Newton IG. Radiation protection for the fluoroscopy operator and staff. *AJR Am J Roentgenol*. 2016;207(4):745-754.

11   **Answer C.**   To review, hard collimators are the shutters that shape the X-ray beam produced prior to it passing through the patient. If the beam is optimized to evaluate only a small region of interest, this will result in improved image quality and decreased radiation dose and scatter. It will not affect the magnification.

Reference: Schueler BA. The AAPM/RSNA physics tutorial for residents: general overview of fluoroscopic imaging. *Radiographics*. 2000;20(4):1115-1126.

12   **Answer B.**   Source to patient distance should be maximized, given the inverse square law of radiation. Additionally, the detector/image intensifier should be kept as close to the patient as possible, maximizing the photons intercepted, thusly decreasing the dose needed for good imaging.

References: Mahesh M. Fluoroscopy: patient radiation exposure issues. *Radiographics*. 2001;21(4):1033-1045.

Parry RA, Glaze SA, Archer BR. The AAPM/RSNA physics tutorial for residents. Typical patient radiation doses in diagnostic radiology. *Radiographics*. 1999;19(5):1289-1302.

13   **Answer D.**   Geometric magnification occurs when moving the object closer to the source, with a constant source to image distance. If one has a flashlight fixed in position shining on a wall, the closer your hand to the flashlight, the larger the shadow on the wall.

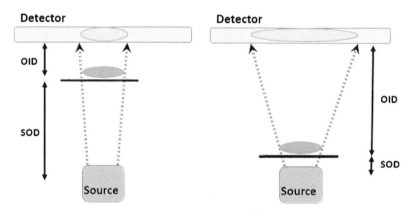

Figure 13-1   Geometric magnification. OID, object to image distance; SOD, source to object distance.

In this scenario, as the patient is closer to the source, the inverse square law dictates that the dose is going to be increased. With electronic magnification, changing the patient position is not necessary. However, the smaller field of view with electronic magnification requires an increased dose to combat noise. Dose increases of 1.4-2.0× per magnification level have been reported with conventional image intensifiers. This effect is significantly decreased with flat-panel detectors, but most manufacturers still increase the dose somewhat to reduce the perception of noise.

Reference: Nickoloff EL. AAPM/RSNA physics tutorial for residents: physics of flat-panel fluoroscopy systems: Survey of modern fluoroscopy imaging: flat-panel detectors versus image intensifiers and more. *Radiographics*. 2011;31(2):591-602.

14   **Answer A.**   Parallax in an illusion of image formation that occurs when assessing the relative position of 2 objects when viewed along different lines of sight. In the case example, if the source and detector are lined up exactly with the femoral head and the clamp, the true relationship is observed on the image. If the source is too caudal, the clamp will project inferior to the femoral head. If the source is too cranial, the clamp will project superior to its true relationship with the femoral head. The greater the distance between the 2 objects of interest, the greater the effect of parallax can be.

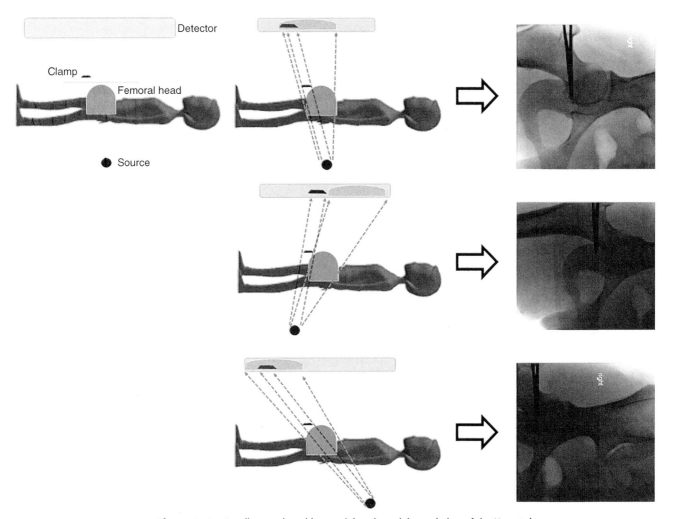

Figure 14-1   Parallax produced by cranial and caudal angulation of the X-ray tube.

References: Buckle CE, Udawatta V, Straus CM. Now you see it, now you don't: visual illusions in radiology. *Radiographics*. 2013;33(7):2087-2102.

Walz-Flannigan A, Magnuson D, Erickson D, Schueler B. Artifacts in digital radiography. *AJR Am J Roentgenol*. 2012;198(1):156–161.

Wang J, Blackburn TJ. The AAPM/RSNA physics tutorial for residents: X-ray image intensifiers for fluoroscopy. *Radiographics*. 2000;20(5):1471-1477.

15 **Answer A.** Naturally, there is intra- and interpatient variability regarding thickness/density and therefore the photon requirements for a good picture. The fluoroscopic system has a feedback mechanism called automatic brightness control (ABC) as a means to maintain the appropriate amount of photons passing through an area of study. The mechanism will adjust the mA or kVP as needed. This can produce specific problem areas, notably at the interface of regions of different density, eg, thorax and abdomen. If the detector is sensing not enough photons getting through the abdomen (as in the case example), it will significantly increase the tube output and result in a burned-out appearance of the lower density lung field. To combat this, one must center upon the area of interest and/or use hard and soft collimators. Pincushion distortion and vignetting are additional artifacts seen with fluoroscopy. Because of the internal geometry of the image intensifier, the periphery of the image may differ from the center. Distortion of truly straight lines to look curved on the periphery is referred to as pincushion distortion; vignetting refers to the fact that the center of the image may be brighter than the periphery.

References: Geise RA. Fluoroscopy: recording of fluoroscopic images and automatic exposure control. *Radiographics*. 2001;21(1):227-236.

Nickoloff EL. AAPM/RSNA physics tutorial for residents: physics of flat-panel fluoroscopy systems: Survey of modern fluoroscopy imaging: flat-panel detectors versus image intensifiers and more. *Radiographics*. 2011;31(2):591-602.

16 **Answer A.** Ultrasound pulses are attenuated by friction, scatter, and conversion to heat as they travel in tissue. Attenuation is proportional to the distance traveled and affected by the frequency of the US wave. The higher the frequency, the greater the attenuation. In order to examine deeper structures in the body such as the kidney, a lower frequency will be necessary to overcome these attenuating factors. The curved transducer in the case example performs with a frequency range of 1 to 5 MHz, whereas the small hockey-stick transducer utilizes a range of 7 to 15 MHz for fine-tuned examination of more superficial structures.

Reference: Hangiandreou NJ. AAPM/RSNA physics tutorial for residents. Topics in US: B-mode US: basic concepts and new technology. *Radiographics*. 2003;23(4):1019-1033.

17 **Answer D.** Selective internal radiation therapy (SIRT) has become increasingly popular in the last 10 years for the treatment of primary and secondary malignancies in the liver. Also known as radioembolization, SIRT involves the intra-arterial administration of millions of microscopic spheres coated or impregnated with Y-90. The administration can be performed superselectively, treating only a segment or subsegment of the liver, or done on a lobar or whole liver basis. The delivered particles are contained by the treated zone of the liver with typically only a small percentage shunted through and deposited in the lungs. There are 2 types of beta decay: beta minus and beta plus. Beta minus (B−) decay involves the conversion of a neutron into a proton, an electron, and an antineutrino. Yttrium-90 undergoes B− decay to zirconium-90. The decay energy is 2.28 MeV, with 0.1% of the energy decay via 1.7 MeV photons.

Beta plus (B+) decay involves the conversion of a neutron into a proton, a positron, and a neutrino. Alpha decay (as seen with the formerly used Thorotrast contrast agent) involves the emission of an alpha particle (2 protons, 2 neutrons) from the nucleus. The decay results in a different atom with mass number reduced by 4 and atomic number reduced by 2. Gamma decay is a spontaneous dissipation of gamma rays (high-energy photons) from relatively unstable atomic nuclei. There is no change to the atomic mass or number, as the energy carries no charge or mass. Omega decay does not exist.

Reference: Salem R, Thurston KG, Carr BI, Goin JE, Geschwind JF. Yttrium-90 microspheres: radiation therapy for unresectable liver cancer. *J Vasc Interv Radiol*. 2002;13(9 Pt 2):S223-S229.

18   **Answer C.**   A unique feature of yttrium-90 SIRT is its precision, as the beta radiation only travels a few millimeters (average 2.5 mm, max 11 mm) in tissue. Additional photons are produced through bremsstrahlung interactions, and this is of interest when handling the dose as well as considering radiation exposure to others around the patient after delivery. Research has indicated that the risk to people near patients treated with Y-90 is very low, and no specific proximity restrictions are necessary. Currently, there are 2 available microspheres, glass and resin. With resin microspheres, the Y-90 is bound to the particle surface, and a trace amount may be free and released into the body. Because of this, the manufacturer recommends (1) handwashing after using the toilet and (2) cleaning up any spills of body fluids and disposing of them in the toilet.

References: Kim YC, Kim YH, Uhm SH, et al. Radiation safety issues in y-90 microsphere selective hepatic radioembolization therapy: possible radiation exposure from the patients. *Nucl Med Mol Imaging*. 2010;44(4):252-260.

Salem R, Thurston KG, Carr BI, Goin JE, Geschwind JF. Yttrium-90 microspheres: radiation therapy for unresectable liver cancer. *J Vasc Interv Radiol*. 2002;13(9 Pt 2):S223-S229.

19   **Answer B.**   In interventional radiology, there are few radioactive isotopes that an operator can come into contact with during routine work. Certainly, yttrium-90 SIRT has been widely adopted, and some basic knowledge is imperative for users to obtain. The half-life is roughly 64.2 hours. This equates to about 97% of the energy being released in the first 2 weeks, and 99% released by 4 weeks. The relatively long half-life is most important to remember, as an inadvertent spill of particles containing Y-90 can result in a prolonged quarantine of that area. Technetium-99m, commonly used during the mapping component of SIRT as well as red blood cell scanning, has a half-life of 6 hours.

Reference: Salem R, Thurston KG, Carr BI, Goin JE, Geschwind JF. Yttrium-90 microspheres: radiation therapy for unresectable liver cancer. *J Vasc Interv Radiol*. 2002;13(9 Pt 2):S223-S229.

INDEX

Note: Page numbers followed by "f" indicate figures, "t" indicate tables and "b" indicate boxes.